Colorectal Surgery Consultation

Sang W. Lee • Scott R. Steele
Daniel L. Feingold
Howard M. Ross • David E. Rivadeneira
Editors

Colorectal Surgery Consultation

Tips and Tricks for the Management of Operative Challenges

Springer

Editors
Sang W. Lee
Keck School of Medicine
of University of Southern California
Los Angeles, CA
USA

Scott R. Steele
Cleveland Clinic
Cleveland, OH
USA

Daniel L. Feingold
Columbia University
New York, NY
USA

Howard M. Ross
Lewis Katz School of Medicine
Temple University
Philadelphia, PA
USA

David E. Rivadeneira
Hofstra-Northwell School of Medicine
Woodbury, NY
USA

ISBN 978-3-030-11180-9 ISBN 978-3-030-11181-6 (eBook)
https://doi.org/10.1007/978-3-030-11181-6

This Springer imprint is published by the registered company Springer Nature Switzerland AG
The registered company address is: Gewerbestrasse 11, 6330 Cham, Switzerland

Preface

The art of surgery takes a lifetime to master and develops only through repetition and deliberate practice. Despite long years of surgical training, it is challenging for surgeons to individually acquire operative experiences and pattern recognition that results from years of high-volume clinical practice. Expectedly, significant operative learning and judgment occurs during our first several years of practice. Some of us may be fortunate enough to start our careers in a group practice with senior partners that can impart their knowledge and experience when we encounter difficult operative situations. Many of us may not be so fortunate and find ourselves in a situation in which we rely only on our training and limited experience. With this book, we wanted to gather together operative tips and techniques that are not commonly addressed during our training. We wanted to create a compilation of techniques and tips that might be useful in dealing with unusual, difficult, or unexpected operative situations that may arise during our practice.

At times, we are called by our colleagues to help with unexpected intraoperative problems. These situations have specific challenges as we lack significant knowledge of the patient's history or even what occurred before we walked into the operating room. The need to make expeditious assessment of the patient and act is complicated by the technical complexities and medicolegal ramifications.

This book brings together operative tips and tricks we have learned from our many years of practices in high-volume, specialized, academic centers over the years. For this reason, all the chapters were either personally guided and reviewed or written by one of the editors. It is not surprising that in the process of working on this book, we the editors have learned a lot from each other's experiences. Although the book is by no means all encompassing, we tried to cover a wide variety of situations encountered during endoscopy, anorectal surgery, and open and laparoscopic abdominal surgeries. We also do not pretend that the techniques described are the only way to approach a similar situation, or conversely, that the described approach guarantees success. Yet we hope to provide a few ideas, tip, and tricks to approach these challenging and, at times, demanding circumstances. We designed the text to be simple and succinct and provide salient key points and practical techniques that may make the difference in patient outcomes. We tried to provide as many illustrations and photos as possible to accompany the text and guide operations. We are truly grateful for everyone involved for their time and contributions. We hope our textbook will stimulate further discussions and lead to better patient outcomes.

Los Angeles, CA, USA	Sang W. Lee, MD, FACS, FASCRS
Cleveland, OH, USA	Scott R. Steele, MD, MBA, FACS, FASCRS
New York, NY, USA	Daniel L. Feingold, MD, FACS, FASCRS
Philadelphia, PA, USA	Howard M. Ross, MD, FACS, FASCRS
Woodbury, NY, USA	David E. Rivadeneira, MD, MBA, FACS, FASCRS

Acknowledgments

Thank you to my fellow editors and Marianna, Michele, Piper, and Flynn.

Scott R. Steele, MD

Success is not final, failure is not fatal: it is the courage to continue that counts.

–Winston Churchill

My gratitude to my fellow editors Howard, Danny, and Scott for all of their guidance and hard work and in addition Sang for the leadership and vision for this project. Forever grateful to my family Anabela, Sophia, and Gabriella for their love and support.

David E. Rivadeneira, MD, MBA, FACS, FASCRS

One of the greatest joys of my career has been the friendships I have made with other surgeons. The relationships forged in training and on efforts such as this textbook have enriched my life. The editors and authors of this book have supported me while tackling difficult clinical challenges and caused me to belly laugh too many times to count. I encourage all trainees to take extra effort to get to know your peers (and to read this excellent textbook). Thank you to my family who continue to make every day special.

To Stacy, Fin, Leo, and Emily...all my love.

Howard M. Ross, MD, FACS, FASCRS

To my fellow editors, it has been a joy and an honor collaborating with you over the years. To my wife, Tonja, and Judah, Ethan, Noa, and Lily, for your unwavering understanding, love, and support. And to my parents who supported and inspired me from the very beginning.

Daniel L. Feingold, MD, FACS, FASCRS

I would like to acknowledge and thank my colleagues and friends for volunteering their time and expertise. I extend special thanks to Yuko Tonohira for providing beautiful illustrations. To my editors, David, Howard, Scott, and Danny, thank you for your hard work, dedication, and friendship. Finally to my family, Crystal, Eric, and Ryan, thank you for the unwavering support and love and for making everything worthwhile.

Sang W. Lee, MD, FACS, FASCRS

Contents

Contributors

Titilayo Adegboyega, MD, MPH Huntington Hospital-Northwell Health, Department of Colorectal Surgery, Huntington, NY, USA

Alison Althans, BA University Hospitals Cleveland Medical Center, Cleveland, OH, USA

Anuradha R. Bhama, MD Department of Colorectal Surgery, Cleveland Clinic, Cleveland, OH, USA

Richard Cohen, MD, FRCS University College London Hospitals, NHS Foundation Trusts, Department of Surgery and Interventional Sciences, London, UK

Daniel L. Feingold Division of Colorectal Surgery, Department of Surgery, Columbia University, New York, NY, USA

Daniel Fish, MS, MD Department of Colorectal Surgery, Cleveland Clinic, Cleveland, OH, USA

Garrett Friedman, MD Mike O'Callaghan Federal Medical Center, Department of Colon and Rectal Surgery, Las Vegas, NV, USA

Daniel P. Geisler, MD, FACS, FASCRS NewYork-Presbyterian/Columbia, Department of Colorectal Surgery, New York, NY, USA

Andrew Godwin, MD Northwell Health-Lenox Hill Hospital, New York, NY, USA

Laura Greco, MD Department of Surgery, Temple University Hospital, Philadelphia, PA, USA

Meredith Gunder, MD Department of Surgery, Temple University Hospital, Lewis Katz School of Medicine at Temple University, Philadelphia, PA, USA

Christine Hsieh, MD Keck School of Medicine – University of Southern California, Los Angeles, CA, USA

Mehraneh D. Jafari, MD UC Irvine Health, Department of Surgery, Division of Colorectal Surgery, Orange, CA, USA

Deborah S. Keller, MS, MD Department of Surgery, NewYork-Presbyterian, Columbia University Medical Center, New York, NY, USA

J. Mark Kiely, MD Division of Colorectal Surgery, Department of Surgery, Columbia University, New York, NY, USA

Ravi P. Kiran, MS, FACS, FASCRS Division of Colorectal Surgery, Department of Surgery, Columbia University, New York, NY, USA

David A. Kleiman, MD Lahey Hospital and Medical Center, Department of Colon and Rectal Surgery, Burlington, MA, USA

Sarah Koller, MD Department of Surgery, Lewis Katz School of Medicine at Temple University and the Temple University Health System, Philadelphia, PA, USA

Sang W. Lee, MD, FACS, FASCRS Department of Surgery – Colon and Rectal Surgery, Keck School of Medicine of University of Southern California, Los Angeles, CA, USA

Steven A. Lee-Kong, MD, FACS, FASCRS Division of Colorectal Surgery, Department of Surgery, Columbia University, New York, NY, USA

Jason Lei, MD Virtua Medical Center, Department of Colon and Rectal Surgery, Vorhees, NJ, USA

Nivedh V. Paluvoi, MD University of Miami, Department of Surgery, Division of Colorectal Surgery, Pasadena, CA, USA

Matthew M. Philp, MD, FACS, FASCRS Division of Colon and Rectal Surgery, Temple University School of Medicine, Philadelphia, PA, USA

David E. Rivadeneira, MD, MBA, FACS, FASCRS Surgical Strategic Initiatives, Northwell Health, New Hyde Park, NY, USA

Surgical Services and Colorectal Surgery, Huntington Hospital, Huntington, NY, USA

Hofstra University-Northwell School of Medicine, Hempstead, NY, USA

Howard M. Ross, MD, FACS, FASCRS Division of Colon and Rectal Surgery, Lewis Katz School of Medicine at Temple University and the Temple University Health System, Philadelphia, PA, USA

Andrew T. Schlussel, DO, FACS Madigan Army Medical Center, Department of Surgery, Tacoma, WA, USA

Shirley Shih, MD Northwell Health, Department of Colorectal Surgery, Woodbury, NY, USA

Scott R. Steele, MD, FACS, FASCRS Case Western Reserve University School of Medicine, Cleveland, OH, USA

Department of Colorectal Surgery, Cleveland Clinic, Cleveland, OH, USA

Emily Steinhagen, MD University Hospitals Case Medical Center, Department of Surgery, Cleveland, OH, USA

Part I

Introduction

How to Avoid Getting into Difficult Operative Situations

1

Sang W. Lee

Clinical Scenario

A 67-year-old male who underwent sigmoidectomy with high ligation of his inferior mesenteric artery (IMA) for sigmoid cancer presents 3 years later with a second primary colon cancer located in the mid-descending colon.

Key Points

1. As surgeons, we occasionally encounter difficult operative situations.
   (a) Avoidable situations often result from inadequate preparation. Try to gather as much of the relevant information as possible, and optimize the situation. Anticipate and plan ahead for potential operative difficulties.
   (b) Unavoidable or unexpected situations can occur despite appropriate preparation. Chapter 2 will review strategies dealing with unanticipated intraoperative difficulties.
2. Review relevant medical records and operative reports. Try to obtain and review as much of the relevant medical and surgical information as possible.
   (a) Which parts of the colon were resected? What mesenteric vessels were taken previously? In patients who underwent high ligation of the IMA for colon cancer, the left side of the colon proximal to the anastomosis is perfused only by the marginal vessels. In the event of a subsequent tumor in the left side of the colon, the blood flow to the colon requires that the resection includes the previous anastomosis and the margin should be distal to the previous anastomosis (Figs. 1.1 and 1.2).
   (b) Was the splenic flexure mobilized previously?
   (c) How much of the small intestine remain?
   (d) Is the ileocecal valve still present?
   (e) What was the extent of adhesions during the last surgery? Although a history of multiple previous surgeries is not a contraindication to performing laparoscopy, early proactive conversion should be made in appropriate situations.
   (f) Review all relevant radiologic reports and images.
   (g) Review pathology reports. Make note of the length of the specimen and number of lymph nodes retrieved.
3. Consider performing additional preoperative studies.
   (a) For malignancies, obtain pathologic slides and have them reviewed at your home institution for a second opinion.

S. W. Lee (✉)
Department of Surgery – Colon and Rectal Surgery, Keck School of Medicine of University of Southern California, Los Angeles, CA, USA

S. W. Lee et al. (eds.), *Colorectal Surgery Consultation*,
https://doi.org/10.1007/978-3-030-11181-6_1

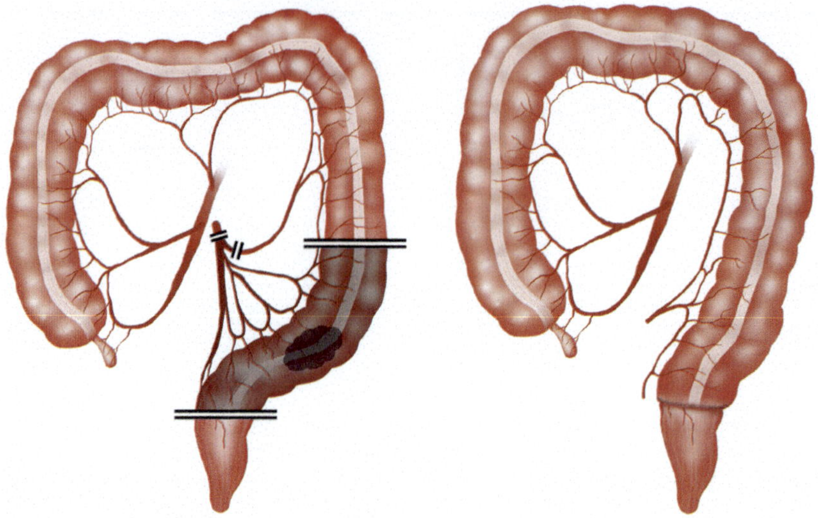

Fig. 1.1 In patients who underwent high ligation of IMA for colon cancer, the left side of the colon proximal to the anastomosis is perfused only by marginal vessels

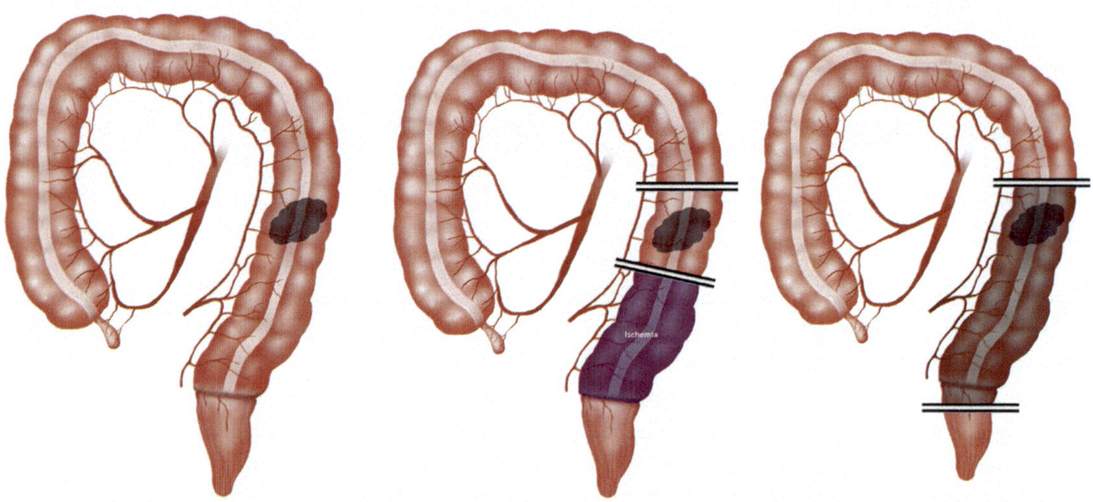

Fig. 1.2 In case of recurrent tumor in the left side of the colon, the distal resection margin has to include the previous anastomosis and be distal to the previous anastomosis

(b) Sigmoidoscopy should be performed for all patients who present with a presumed left-sided colonic lesion to rule out actually having rectal cancer. Rectal cancer needs to be properly staged for possible neoadjuvant therapy prior to operation.

(c) Tattoo should be placed for localizing smaller lesions or pathologies not visible by radiologic studies.

(d) CT of the abdomen or MR of the pelvis if recent radiologic studies are not available.

(e) In cases of Hartmann reversal, routinely obtain a Hypaque, Gastrografin, or barium study performed through the rectum and, if needed, via the colostomy. Assessment of the rectal stump length and quality and the colon length proximal to the stoma will allow better planning for the reversal surgery. Flexible sigmoidoscopy can also be helpful in this situation.

(f) Examination under anesthesia in the OR prior to definitive surgery can often provide additional findings.

4. When in doubt, prep the bowel and mark the patient for a stoma.
   (a) Routine bowel preparation is somewhat controversial as related to preventing surgical site infections.
   (b) Prepped bowel allows for intraoperative colonoscopic localization of the tumor and primary repair of the colon in case of injury.
   (c) In high-risk situations, it is important to anticipate the need for diversion. Alerting the patient of this possibility should be a routine part of the preoperative process.
   (d) Having the patient marked in multiple sites can be helpful in reoperative surgery.
5. Anticipate the need for assistance from other specialties.
   (a) For reoperative pelvic surgeries, placement of stents may be helpful in identifying the ureters.
   (b) Urology, gynecology, or neurosurgery consultation prior to surgery may be indicated in certain situations.
6. Optimize patient's condition in elective settings.
   (a) Medical clearance.
   (b) Optimization of nutrition.
   (c) Reversal of anticoagulation, antiplatelet agents.
   (d) Hold immunosuppressive medications, if possible.
   (e) Appropriate timing for elective surgery needs to be individualized for patients with history of recent MI or stroke.
7. Timing of reoperative surgery (Fig. 1.3).
   (a) During the immediate perioperative period, the decision to reoperate should be made as quickly as possible so that it is done, ideally, within 7–10 days postoperatively.
   (b) If the 7–10-day reoperative window is missed, it is preferable to defer the reoperation for at least 3–6 months, if possible. If the situation is urgent or emergent, re-exploration needs to be performed without delay.
8. Consider alternative plans such as medical management and less risky and less extensive surgery, especially in high-risk patients.

Operative Assessment

1. What is the best surgical approach based on previous history?
2. Can it be done laparoscopically? Although a history of multiple previous surgeries is not a contraindication to performing laparoscopy, early proactive conversion should be made in appropriate situations.
3. Determine the extent of the pathology and come up with road map.
4. Do what is best and safe for the patient.

Operative Checklist

1. Have additional equipment available in the operating room.
   (a) Head lights or lighted pelvic retractors, if available.
   (b) Flexible sigmoidoscopy can be helpful in localizing the pathology and assessing perfusion to the tissues.
   (c) Additional imaging such as indocyanine green (ICG) perfusion system may be helpful in assessing tissue perfusion.
2. Mark for possible stoma site.
3. Additional specialty consultants available for possible OR help.
   (a) Urology consult for preoperative ureteral stent placement.
4. Exposure.
   (a) Early proactive conversion to hand-assisted or laparotomy.
   (b) Consider epidural catheter placement for extensive laparotomy cases.
5. Positioning.
   (a) Consider placing all difficult cases in lithotomy position or split leg position.
      (i) Provides exposure to anus, rectum, and pelvis

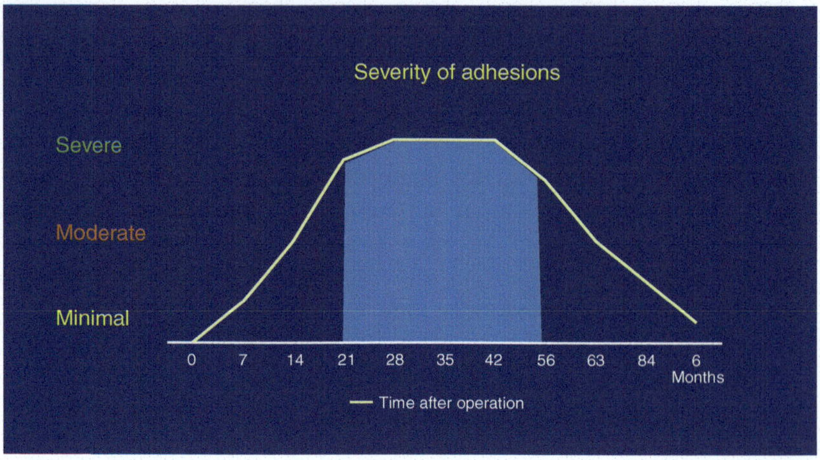

Fig. 1.3 If the 7–10-day reoperative window is missed, it is preferable to defer the reoperation for at least 3–6 months, if possible. If the situation is urgent or emergent, re-exploration needs to be performed without delay

(ii) Allows endoscopic evaluation of the colon and the rectum
(iii) Allows transanal stapled anastomosis
(iv) Allows placement of ureteral stents

Operative Techniques

Intraoperative considerations and strategies will be discussed in Chap. 2.

Technical Pearls (Tips and Tricks)

1. Anticipate and plan ahead for potential operative difficulties—plan for the unexpected.
2. Anticipate the need for assistance from other specialties.
3. Mark for a stoma.
4. Consider placing ureteral stents in reoperative pelvic surgery.
5. Have experienced help available.
6. Schedule difficult cases early in the day, and limit the number of cases scheduled on the same day.
7. Prior to committing to the operation, confirm the operative plan.
8. Have checkpoints throughout the operation, and know when and how to back out safely.

Special Postoperative Care

1. Possible telemetry and ICU care should be planned.
2. Appropriate postoperative care will be based on the operative findings and procedures performed.

Suggested Reading

1. Bailey HR, Isaacson TC. The intraoperative consult. In: Steele SR, Maykel JA, Champagne BJ, Orangio GR, editors. Complexities in colorectal surgery. New York: Springer Publ; 2014. p. 463–76.

Principles in Approaching Difficult Operative Situations

2

Deborah S. Keller and Scott R. Steele

Clinical Scenario

You are called in by the urology team during a robotic prostatectomy for a "small tear" in the anterior rectal wall. On the monitor, you see the pelvis filled with dark venous blood. With suctioning, the rectum appears significantly injured and the bleeding continues. The senior urologist tells you to try to fix it robotically and that "this guy will not accept a bag."

Key Points

1. The initial assessment is critical. The surgeon must verify through their own examination what the real purpose of the consultation is and should determine the clinical status of the patient in order to decide on the best next steps in any given situation.
   (a) Use a controlled, stepwise approach, just like starting with the ABCs in trauma. At the initial assessment, look at the whole patient: airway, breathing, circulation, disability, and exposure. How is your exposure?
   (b) Take the time to assess the urgency of the situation prior to making your first move.
   (c) Do not commit to an operation by performing an irreversible maneuver such as ligating a major vessel or performing a bowel resection without first assessing resectability and surveying the abdomen.
2. Ensure you have adequate exposure.
   (a) In laparoscopic or robotic cases that require better visualization or exposure, take the time to insert additional trocars, as needed, or convert the minimally invasive surgical platform to an open procedure, if needed.
   (b) In open cases, extend the existing operative incision as needed, insert an abdominal wall retractor, as deemed appropriate, and pack away the small bowel and other structures to obtain the ideal view of the region of interest.
   (c) Ask for the retractors and equipment that you are comfortable using.
   (d) Pay attention to positioning, using gravity to have the omentum, bowel, and viscera fall away from your field of intended view.
   (e) Ensure that you feel comfortable with the exposure. If the requesting surgeon is robotic or laparoscopic and you feel the

D. S. Keller
Department of Surgery, New York-Presbyterian, Columbia University Medical Center, New York, NY, USA

S. R. Steele (✉)
Case Western Reserve University School of Medicine, Cleveland, OH, USA

Department of Colorectal Surgery, Cleveland Clinic, Cleveland, OH, USA

S. W. Lee et al. (eds.), *Colorectal Surgery Consultation*,
https://doi.org/10.1007/978-3-030-11181-6_2

need to open to do what needs to be done, *do it*!

3. Damage control procedures may be required to temporize the situation.
   (a) Pack the abdomen to stop bleeding.
   (b) Oversew enterotomies and staple off unsalvageable portion of the bowel to control feculent spillage and stop ongoing contamination.
   (c) Decompress fluid-filled, edematous, or obstructed bowel to facilitate dissection via a controlled enterotomy or colotomy in a segment of bowel that will, ideally, be resected (Fig. 2.1).
   (d) Transfer to the intensive care unit, and resuscitate the patient before definitive surgery is attempted.
   (e) Communicate with the critical care team the plan to optimize and return to the operating suite for definitive surgery, so all team members are aligned.
4. Use your experience and sound judgment to do what is best for the patient.
   (a) Keeping in mind the enemy of good is better, know when to bail out of the elective operation and move the patient to damage control or a resuscitation phase.
   (b) Ask for additional help, if available, for insight into management and technique. In certain situations even students or trainees can provide invaluable retraction.

Operative Assessment

1 What is the stability of the patient?
   (a) In your initial assessment, talk to the consulting surgeon as well as the anesthesiologist about the patient's fitness for exploration and surgical procedures.
   (b) Take notice of the vital signs and if blood products or vasopressor medications are hanging or were given.
   (c) Determine if the operating room is still the best place for the patient or if damage control measures should be undertaken and the patient transferred to intensive care for resuscitation, warming, etc.

2 Determine the location and extent of the injury.
   (a) Understanding the mechanism of the injury can help determine if this is a tissue or vascular injury and can guide management.

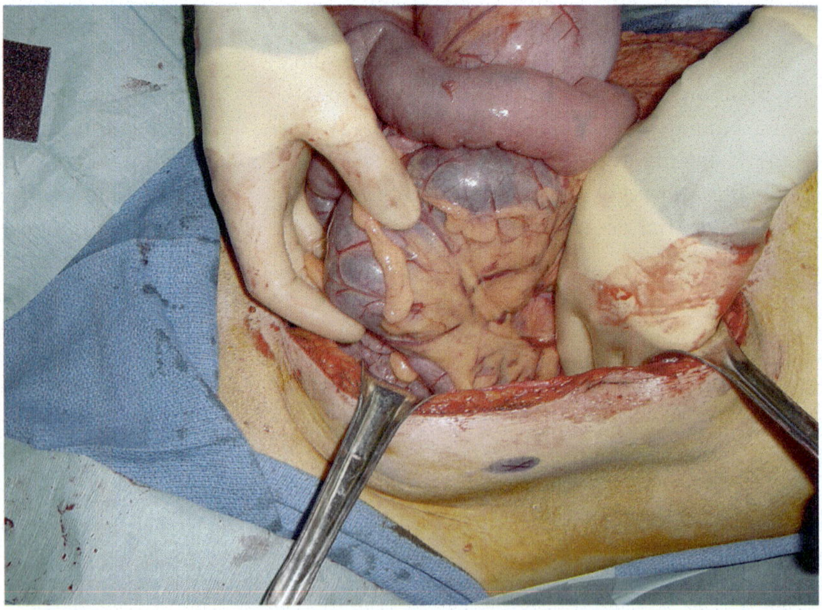

Fig. 2.1 Dilated bowel

(b) During a prostatectomy, the rectum is most commonly injured when developing the extraperitoneal plane between the prostate and rectum or when retracting the seminal vesicles anteriorly and incising Denonvilliers fascia to develop the plane between the prostate and the rectum for the anterior dissection.

3 Is the robotic approach the best approach?
   (a) Use the approach you are most comfortable with and can work most efficiently regardless of the current robotic setup.
   (b) If there is a need for better visualization, better retraction, direct pressure, or tactile sense, convert from a robotic approach to a laparoscopic, hand-assisted, or open approach, as needed.

4 Always do what's best for the patient.
   (a) While it may be reported that the patient does not want an ostomy, use your best surgical judgment, and perform the procedures necessary for the best patient outcome. A stoma can generally be reversed, but major complications may be permanent.
   (b) The risk of needing a diverting stoma may have been covered in the informed consent, but if it was not explicitly listed under the possible procedures, the consent often covers any procedure deemed necessary by the surgical team abating any medicolegal fears of performing a stoma. In this situation, it may be helpful to talk with the waiting family to update them and review your recommendation for fecal diversion at that time.
   (c) Document accordingly. Make sure to make note of who called you into the case, time in and out for your procedure, and discussions had with family members.

Operative Checklist

1. Additional helpful equipment.
   (a) Long pelvic instrument tray
   (b) Long continuous sutures
   (c) Pelvic retractors, such as a St. Marks or a Sweetheart (lighted retractors, if available), if making a lower midline or Pfannenstiel incision
   (d) Bookwalter retractor if making a midline laparotomy incision
   (e) Rigid proctoscope
   (f) Headlight
2. Exposure.
   (a) Consider making a low midline, full midline, or Pfannenstiel incision, as needed, to assess and manage the complication.
   (b) Put in additional ports, as needed, to help retract omentum, small bowel, or other organs (e.g., large uterus). Simply adding a 5 mm port can help tremendously.
3. Positioning.
   (a) Reverse Trendelenburg allows gravity to help move the small bowel out of the pelvis and can lower the hydrostatic pressure in the presacral veins.

Operative Techniques

1. Control the bleeding.
   Pack the pelvis with laparotomy pads. If needed, maintain the packs to let anesthesia catch up. In an unstable patient, this may be your first and last operative maneuver that day. In a stable patient, cycles of packing combined with irrigation and suctioning the irrigant will help clear the blood and clots from the field, localize the site of the injury, and highlight ongoing bleeding. With these initial maneuvers, you can determine if the bleeding is coming from the rectum itself or torn presacral veins (Fig. 2.2).
2. Assess the damage to the rectum.
   If the area and extent of the rectal injury are not immediately apparent after packing and controlling the bleeding in the pelvis, perform a rigid proctoscopy for an intraluminal view. The insufflation can help delineate the injury.
3. Repair the rectum or divert.
   For injuries to less than 50% of the rectal wall circumference, consider a primary repair.

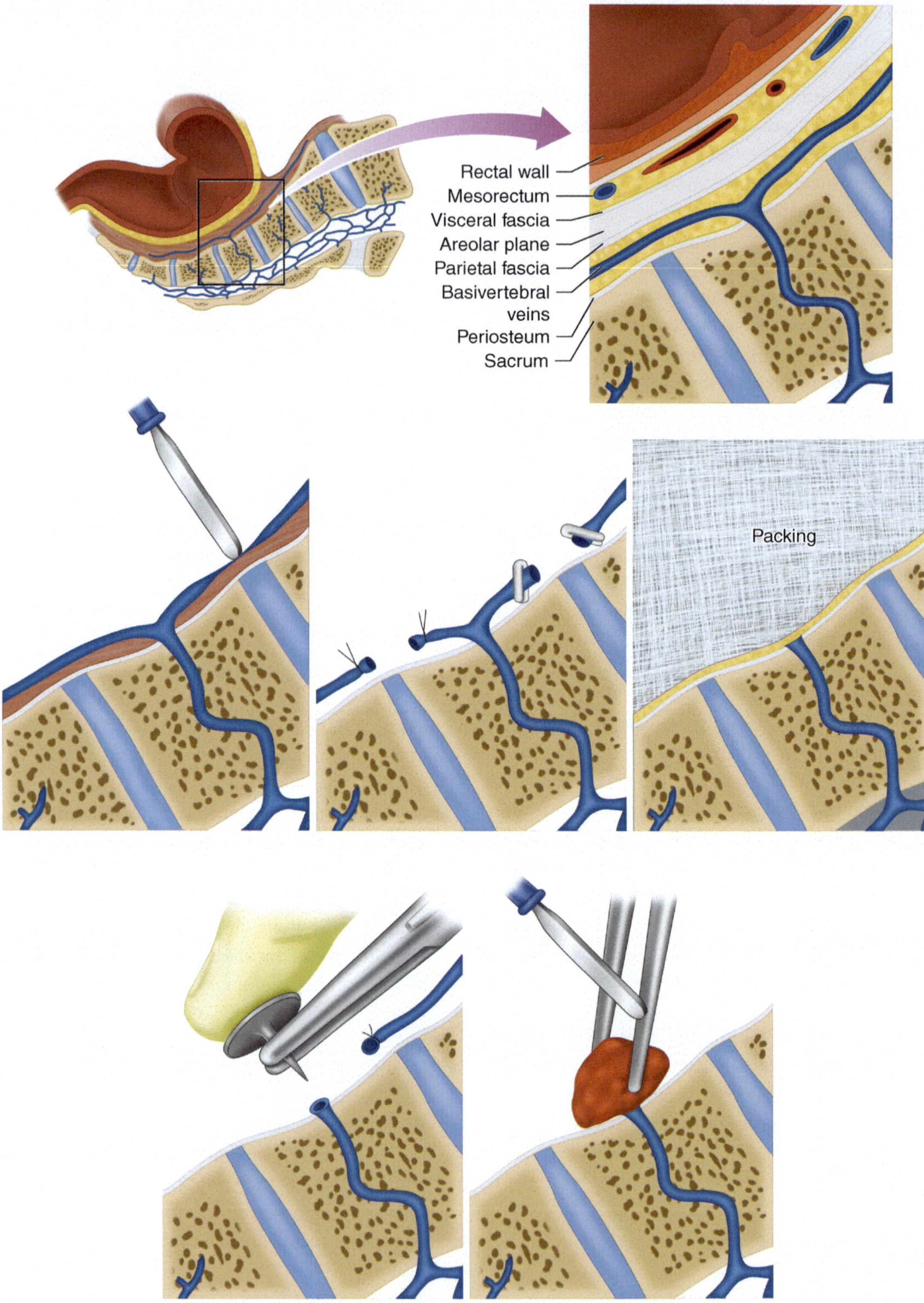

Fig. 2.2 Pelvic bleeding

Sharply freshen the edges of the injury, and place sutures in the edges to direct a transverse closure. This can be performed in one or two layers. For more extensive injuries, first determine if the patient's hemodynamic state and degree of bleeding/contamination are conducive to an anastomosis. If so, staple off the proximal and distal ends of the rectum, releasing the attachments up to the splenic flexure as needed for adequate length for a tension free anastomosis. The anastomosis can be fashioned using the anvil in the proximal limb and pairing it to an intraluminal stapler introduced into the rectum, in standard fashion. Consider proximal diversion if creating an anastomosis. If it is not the ideal situation to perform a repair or anastomosis, staple off the rectum distal to the injury, and divert the proximal limb as an end colostomy. Plan to return to the OR and restore continuity under better conditions.

Technical Pearls (Tips and Tricks)

1. If the patient is hemodynamically stable and it is appropriate in your surgical judgment to maintain a minimally invasive approach, it may aid your initial assessment—the pneumoperitoneum may help tamponade bleeding, and the camera may afford better visualization than what would be possible through an open approach.
2. In cases where there has been significant bleeding and gross contamination, defer more complex techniques such as resection and primary anastomosis for a second procedure in a more controlled setting to reduce the risk of further complications.
3. In certain situations, consider performing a repair or anastomosis with a proximal diverting loop ileostomy. This will make the subsequent stoma reversal procedure easier.
4. Don't forget about a scope when needed to air leak test, assess viability of the bowel, or search for other pathology. A colonoscope can provide additional information than just what the initial situation was assumed to be.

Special Postoperative Care

1. If there is significant contamination, 24 hours of IV antibiotics should be considered.
2. While it is not our preference to leave drains in the pelvis routinely, if the rectum is repaired below the mid-rectum level or there is any concern for a urinary leak, leave a closed suction drain in the dependent portion behind the rectum.

Suggested Reading

1. Bailey HR, Isaacson TC. The intraoperative consult. In: Steele SR, Maykel JA, Champagne BJ, Orangio GR, editors. Complexities in colorectal surgery. New York: Springer Publ; 2014. p. 463–76.

Part II

How to Deal with Commonly Encountered Intra-operative Findings/Complications

Extensive Intra-abdominal Adhesions

3

Jason Lei and David E. Rivadeneira

Clinical Scenario

A 48-year-old female with a history of ulcerative colitis and several extensive open operations, which include a three-stage restorative proctocolectomy, is scheduled for a hysterectomy for a bleeding myomatous uterus. The gynecologist would like for you to be there because of possible adhesions.

Key Points

1. The formation of adhesions is multifactorial.
   (a) The extent and frequency of prior surgical procedures is of paramount importance. Review of previous operative reports is important as they may indicate the level of difficulty you should expect. Mention of the extent of adhesions and difficulty of the procedure is important.
   (b) Make note of prior resections and anastomoses, prior ostomies, and repair of enterotomies as these may be areas of increased adhesion formation.
   (c) Prior history of pelvic radiation may indicate significant adhesions of the small bowel in the pelvis, and the option of intestinal bypass may be more prudent than extensive dissection or resection.
   (d) Patients with keloid scars on the abdomen will often present with significant intra-abdominal adhesions.
2. Careful, cautious, and meticulous dissection.
   (a) Sharp dissection with either Metzenbaum scissors or scalpel should be the preferred method of adhesiolysis. It is important to avoid the use of energy such as monopolar electrocauterization or ultrasonic or bipolar devices as they can cause thermal injury that may not be immediately apparent but can lead to devastating delayed perforations.
   (b) When dealing with dense, thick adhesions, it is better to leave a piece of peritoneum, muscle, or fascia on the bowel rather then attempt dissection and risk perforation (Fig. 3.1).
   (c) Hydrodissection can facilitate the visualization of anatomical planes. The convenient and easy method of infiltrating the

J. Lei
Virtua Medical Center, Department of Colon and Rectal Surgery, Vorhees, NJ, USA

D. E. Rivadeneira (✉)
Surgical Strategic Initiatives, Northwell Health, New Hyde Park, NY, USA

Surgical Services and Colorectal Surgery, Huntington Hospital, Huntington, NY, USA

Hofstra University-Northwell School of Medicine, Hempstead, NY, USA
e-mail: DRivadeneira@northwell.edu

S. W. Lee et al. (eds.), *Colorectal Surgery Consultation*,
https://doi.org/10.1007/978-3-030-11181-6_3

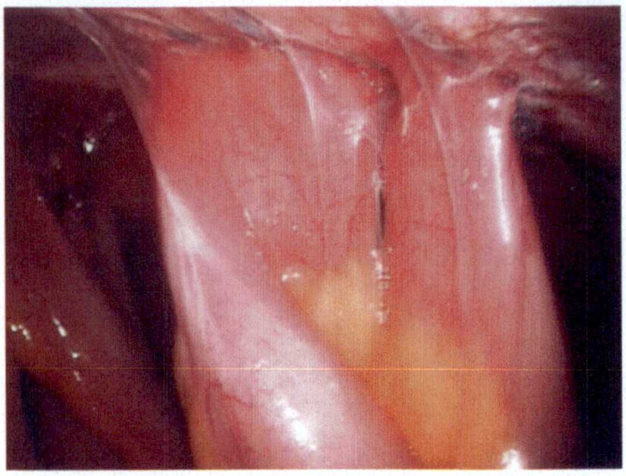

Fig. 3.1 Adhesions

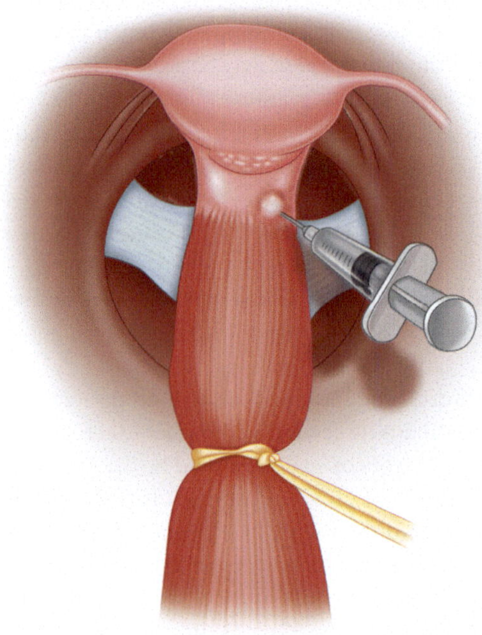

Fig. 3.2 Injection of saline with syringe, hydrodissection of planes allows for improved tissue plane visualization

tissue between adherent loops of the bowel with sterile saline can help separate the tissues, thereby creating a plane of safe dissection. This can be performed in an open procedure with a piston or bulb syringe (Fig. 3.2) and in laparoscopic or robotic procedures with a powered suction/irrigation device.

Operative Assessment

1. Should I perform the case open or laparoscopically?
   (a) In this case scenario, the patient has undergone several extensive open procedures, and the surgeon must decide which approach should be performed. This is often up to the comfort level and experience of the surgeon. Our practice is to start most of our cases laparoscopically with a 5 mm zero degree laparoscope through a left subcostal approach (Palmer's point). It is important to initially access the abdomen away from any prior midline incisions.
   (b) "Extensive" and "difficult" are subjective terms. If the case can be done safely with a minimally invasive approach, then that would be the preferred method. However, in the authors' experience, a minimally invasive approach is often not possible with extensive adhesions, particularly when inter-loop small bowel adhesions are present. It is often better to convert early than subject the patient to longer anesthesia time and risk inadvertent injuries.
   (c) Careful, meticulous dissection is imperative. Hemostasis must be maintained for proper visualization. Areas of serosal injury to the bowel should be immediately repaired to avoid progression to full-thickness perforation and contamination.

Operative Checklist

1. Additional equipment.
   (a) Extra long instruments will be useful for pelvic dissection.
   (b) Powered irrigator for laparoscopic saline injection or large syringe and needle for open.
   (c) Lighted pelvic retractors.
   (d) Adhesion barrier placement at the end of the case can reduce further adhesion formation.

Operative Technique

1. Enter the abdomen carefully: the initial entry into the abdomen without any inadvertent injury to other organs, particularly loops of small intestine, is of paramount importance. In a laparoscopic approach, the left subcostal (Palmer's point) is often a safer area. Stay away from previous midline incisions. If the open approach is used, then entry must be done cautiously and sharply with a scalpel or Metzenbaum scissors. If possible, initiate the laparotomy in an area of the midline that does not have any prior incisions.
2. The use of hydrodissection can facilitate the visualization of anatomical planes. The convenient and easy method of infiltrating the tissue between an adherent loop of bowel with sterile saline can help the tissue balloon out, thus creating and displaying the correct plane of dissection. This can be performed in an open procedure with a piston or bulb syringe and in laparoscopic or robotic procedures with a powered suction/irrigation device and may provide a better separation of planes.
3. When dealing with extensive abdominal adhesions, it is often best to start in area that has less adhesions and deliberately head to the more challenging, more adherent areas. When dealing with adhesions, it's best "to start with the easy, and then the difficult becomes easy."
4. If you encounter bowel that is extremely adherent to the abdominal wall and at high risk of enterotomy; then, it is acceptable to leave the anatomical plane and excise the area of the peritoneum or fascia leaving residual peritoneum or fascia stuck to the bowel wall. In these scenarios, it is better to denude the abdominal wall and avoid a bowel injury.
5. Sharp dissection is preferred as the avoidance of electrocautery is encouraged.
6. Immediate repair of enterotomies or areas of deserosalization should be done as to avoid spillage and contamination.

Technical Pearls (Tips and Tricks)

1. Timing. Re-operative surgery and adhesions go hand in hand. Remember that adhesions are easier to deal with either immediately or soon after surgery (up to 7 days) or wait a significant amount of time. The most difficult time to reoperate is between 7 and 30 days due to the active inflammation and friability of bowel walls make them more susceptible to injury.
2. Gain entry into the abdomen away from previous incisions. This can be accomplished laparoscopically usually through a left subcostal approach in Palmer's point. The author prefers entry through this area with a 5 mm laparoscope. Often a loop or several loops of small bowel are adherent to a previous midline incision, and entry via this method will avoid inadvertent injury. If performing an open approach, then gain access by starting at a "virgin" area cephalad to the prior midline incision.
3. In general, cautery should be avoided in favor of sharp dissection in scalpel or scissors.
4. Use cross-sectional imaging: there may be adhesion free areas in the abdomen that may not be noticed on physical examination.
5. Tag any areas of potential injury so they can be reassessed and repaired as needed.
6. Use hydrodissection: both in laparoscopic and open approaches, the use of hydrodissection is useful to separate bowel wall from other structures.
7. A scalpel can be extremely useful when you have dense adhesions. Kelly claps may be placed onto the edges of the fascia as this will allow it to be distracted from underlying bowel. Then, a deliberate layer-by-layer dissection with a scalpel is performed.

Special Postoperative Care

1. Although there are no special postoperative needs/care required for these cases, a nasogastric tube may be needed preemptively as many patients with extensive lysis of adhesions will have a protracted ileus.

2. The surgeon should have a high index of suspicion for possible inadvertent bowel injury as this can lead to peritonitis and formation of enterocutaneous fistulas. This is particularly evident if the patient develops tachycardia, fevers, or unexpected drainage from the incisions.

Suggested Reading

1. ten Broek R, et al. Epidemiology and prevention of postsurgical adhesions revisited. Ann Surg. 2016;263(1):12–9.

Intraoperative Injury to Small or Large Bowel

4

Laura Greco and Howard M. Ross

Clinical Scenario

Mrs. P understood she had an endoscopically unresectable carpet lesion of her cecum and that at 40 years of age, leaving the polyp in presented an unacceptably high risk of developing cancer. Mrs. P also was quite hesitant to have surgery because she did not want a large scar and had four prior laparoscopic procedures for advanced endometriosis. Mrs. P spent a significant amount of time in the gym and came to your practice because you are a recognized expert in minimally invasive approaches to colon and rectal diseases. During laparoscopic ileocolectomy, as you try to free the small bowel from the pelvis, you notice a few drops of succus exiting from an injury in a fixed small bowel loop.

Key Points

1. Intraoperative bowel injury occurs in roughly 0.2% of laparoscopic cases. Of these injuries, the majority affects the small bowel (55–58%). Most of these injuries are caused by electrocautery or other type of thermal injury.
2. The majority of cases complicated by an unplanned bowel injury will require conversion to an open approach. Options for addressing these injuries include primary repair or resection of the injured bowel.
3. Prevent laparoscopic penetrating bowel injury by directly visualizing ports and instruments during insertion.
4. Prevent inadvertent crush injury to bowel by making sure that the instrument is not grabbing onto the bowel during withdrawal.
5. Intraoperative recognition of a bowel injury is critical!
6. If an injury cannot be evaluated completely, conversion to open midline incision and direct examination must occur.
7. Recognition and then safe repair of an intraoperative bowel injury is far more important than completing an operation in a minimally invasive fashion.

L. Greco
Department of Surgery, Temple University Hospital, Philadelphia, PA, USA

H. M. Ross (✉)
Division of Colon and Rectal Surgery, Lewis Katz School of Medicine at Temple University and the Temple University Health System, Philadelphia, PA, USA
e-mail: Howard.Ross@tuhs.temple.edu

S. W. Lee et al. (eds.), *Colorectal Surgery Consultation*,
https://doi.org/10.1007/978-3-030-11181-6_4

Operative Assessment

1. Complete identification of the injury is mandatory.
2. If complete visualization can be performed, laparoscopic repair and or resection can be considered (Fig. 4.1).
3. A tension-free repair or resection demands soft healthy bowel.
4. If conversion to a midline laparotomy is required to adequately address the injury, then it must be performed.

Operative Checklist

1. Additional helpful equipment:
   (a) Excellent surgical assistance
   (b) Appropriate lighting, including possible headlight
   (c) All retractors in room so exposure is maximized
   (d) If laparoscopic suturing is to be performed, appropriate needle holders and suture

Operative Techniques

1. Transverse primary closure.
   (a) Injuries to the small bowel that result in violation of the lumen of the small bowel that are less than 50% of the bowel wall circumference can be sutured closed transversely to prevent future stricture at the site of repair.
   (b) Injuries of the colon without significant destruction of the colon wall (<50% of the circumference) can be closed primarily either with suture closure or through stapling. In a patient who has not undergone bowel preparation preoperatively, the decision whether or not to repair a colon perforation laparoscopically or through laparotomy may be determined by the amount of fecal spillage. If there is significant fecal contamination, laparotomy with copious irrigation is indicated. If there is minimal spillage, laparoscopic repair may be prudent. In either case, primary repair is still an acceptable choice without need for colostomy or resection if

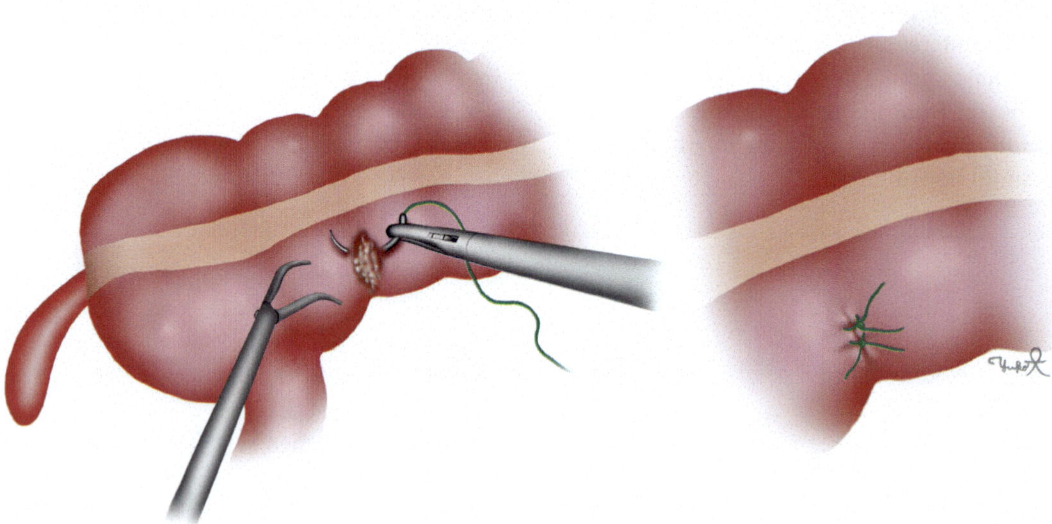

Fig. 4.1 Colon repair

the size of the defect and health of the colon permit this.
   (c) Several studies have shown no difference in the rate of leak with single compared to double layer anastomosis. Whether to close the defect in single or double layer fashion is up to the individual surgeons' discretion.
2. When to resect and anastomose.
   (a) Small Bowel. Decisions regarding small bowel injury are usually dictated by the extent of the injury to the wall of the small bowel in relation to the circumference of the lumen. If the injury is over 50% of the wall, in most cases, it would be appropriate to resect and anastomose that portion of bowel.
   (b) Colon. Similar to the small bowel, whether to directly repair or resect a segment of colon can be determined by the extent of injury to the wall in relation to the circumference of the lumen. For injuries greater than 50%, resection and anastomosis are indicated. If the injury is proximal to the middle colic artery, the surgeon may consider performing a right hemicolectomy with an ileocolonic anastomosis. For injuries distal to the middle colic artery, a colo-colonic anastomosis is indicated.
   (c) Resection and anastomosis are also indicated in cases where the injured small or large bowel is too inflamed or if there is questionable viability of the bowel that would lead to increased risk of delayed anastomotic leak.
3. Enterotomy in inflamed tissue.
   (a) In the case of an enterotomy in inflamed small bowel, freshening the edges and performing a primary repair are usually not appropriate. These situations typically require conversion, mobilization of the diseased segment, and resection and anastomosis. If the bowel is unable to be resected due to inflammation restricting the ability to mobilize the bowel, another option is to patch the defect and leave drains.
   (b) Patch options include making an omental patch by suturing a tongue of omentum over the defect or securing a serosal patch if there is no omentum that can reach the defect. In these rare situations, it is prudent to drain the area and bowel rest the patient until you are confident the injury is not leaking.
   (c) If an enterotomy is made distally in the small bowel or in the colon and is unable to be repaired to healthy tissue and without tension, another management option is to bring up an ostomy to divert the flow of stool from the defect.
4. Serosal injury.
   (a) Serosal abrasion occurs in up to 0.6% of cases. In animal models, it has been shown that serosal injuries to the small bowel do not perforate at normal physiologic pressures, but are associated with increased formation of peritoneal adhesions. It is recommended that serosal injuries be repaired at the time they are recognized. This can be treated with imbricating the healthy serosa of the small bowel together by placing interrupted sutures transversely through the seromuscular layer over the area of injury (Lembert sutures).
5. Delayed bowel injury.
   (a) Unrecognized Bowel Injury. Unrecognized bowel injury after laparoscopic surgery carries a high morbidity and mortality and can present in the postoperative period with abdominal pain, peritonitis, ileus, leukocytosis, and sepsis. In one large case series, up to 69% of small bowel injuries made during laparoscopy were not recognized at the index surgery, and of those 80% were ultimately treated with laparotomy.

(b) Delayed Thermal Injury. Delayed thermal injury describes the process whereby the bowel wall is exposed to heat which, over time, breaks down the bowel potentially resulting in a delayed perforation. In this situation, patients usually become symptomatic 4–11 days after the index surgery. Pathologic examination of the effected bowel may show necrotic amorphous tissue without polymorphonuclear infiltrate.

Technical Pearls (Tips and Tricks)

1. The best bowel injury is one not made…be careful with adhesiolysis and thermal devices.
2. If you need to convert to laparotomy, do so. The cost of not evaluating an injury is enormous.
3. Whether performing repair or resection, the bowel must be healthy and tension-free. Take the extra time to do it right. A single area of concern can be marked with a suture and exteriorized through a specimen extraction site. This allows for inspection and repair directly while still maintaining the benefits of a laparoscopic operation. This can also be performed with an ENDOLOOP (Ethicon, Cincinnati, OH) laparoscopically.
4. A leak test can be performed by milking contents across a concerning area and look for effluent leaking or air.
5. Betadine-saline mixture can be instilled through an injury or an ostomy to look for other sites of leakage.

Special Postoperative Care

1. Understand that a missed enterotomy can occur. A high index of suspicion must be maintained.

Suggested Reading

1. Binenbaum SJ, Goldfarb MA. Inadvertent enterotomy in minimally invasive abdominal surgery. JSLS J Soc Laparoendosc Surg. 2006;10(3):336–40.
2. Binnebösel M, Klink CD, Grommes J, et al. Langenbeck's Arch Surg. 2011;396:133. https://doi.org/10.1007/s00423-010-0672-8.
3. Bishoff JT, et al. Laparoscopic bowel injury; clinical incidence and presentation. J Urol. 1999;161(3):887–90. ISSN 0022-5347. https://doi.org/10.1016/S0022-5347(01)61797-X.
4. Chen C. The art of bowel anastomosis. Scand J Surg. 2012;101:238–40.
5. Goulder F. Bowel anastomoses: the theory, the practice and the evidence base. World J Gastrointest Surg. 2012;4(9):208–13. https://doi.org/10.4240/wjgs.v4.i9.208.
6. Kar S, et al. Single layered versus double layered intestinal anastomosis: a randomized controlled trial. J Clin Diagn Res. 2017;11(6):PC01–4. https://doi.org/10.7860/JCDR/2017/24817.9983. Epub 2017 Jun 1.
7. Reich H. Laparoscopic bowel injury. Surg Laparosc Endosc. 1992;2(1):74–8.
8. Stahl R. Laparoscopic anastomotic techniques. SAGES.org. Copyright 2018.
9. Tsai MC, Candy G, Costello MA, Grieve AD, Brand M. Do iatrogenic serosal injuries result in small bowel perforation in a rabbit model? S Afr J Surg. 2017;55(2):18–22.
10. van der Voort M, Heijnsdijk EAM, Gouma DJ. Bowel injury as a complication of laparoscopy. Br J Surg. 2004;91:1253–8. https://doi.org/10.1002/bjs.4716.

Injury to the Rectum During Pelvic Surgery

5

Daniel L. Feingold and Mehraneh D. Jafari

Clinical Scenario

While using a scalpel to transect the vaginal cuff during a hysterectomy, the gynecologist pass-points and creates a full-thickness proctotomy in the anterior wall of the mid-rectum. You are asked to provide intraoperative consultation to address the injury.

Key Points

1. Recognizing and repairing an injury to the rectum during the index procedure is paramount to reducing the morbidity of this kind of injury.
2. While it is tempting to simply repair a rectal injury, some rectal injuries will require proctectomy and/or fecal diversion.

D. L. Feingold (✉)
Division of Colorectal Surgery, Department of Surgery, Columbia University, New York, NY, USA
e-mail: df347@cumc.columbia.edu

M. D. Jafari
UC Irvine Health, Department of Surgery, Division of Colorectal Surgery, Orange, CA, USA

Operative Assessment

1. Obtain a patient-specific history.
   (a) It is important to consider whether the patient has had prior pelvic radiotherapy or has undergone prior colorectal surgery or colonoscopy as this information can influence the plan.
      (i) What was the mechanism of the injury?
         A. Injuries created sharply can often be repaired primarily, while injuries created with an energy device may need to be debrided to healthy tissue prior to closure. Bipolar energy devices can have a larger footprint compared with monopolar technology and can have a degree of crush injury, as well.
      (ii) How distal is the injury?
         A. As these injuries are almost always created transabdominally and lay along the anterior plane, the preferred approach for repair will most commonly be transabdominal. Rarely, it may be easier to approach the injury transanally.
      (iii) What are the details of the injury?
         A. While full-thickness injuries require repair, more superficial

S. W. Lee et al. (eds.), *Colorectal Surgery Consultation*,
https://doi.org/10.1007/978-3-030-11181-6_5

injuries may not. Given the difficulty in accurately appreciating the actual depth of a partial-thickness injury as well as the inability to predict which injuries may declare themselves as full-thickness over time, it is recommended to repair all recognized rectal injuries. A flexible sigmoidoscopy or other technique should be used to assess the injury prior to repair.

Operative Checklist

1. Additional resources and equipment
   (a) Pelvic tray including long instruments, lighted pelvic retractors, and EEA sizers
   (b) Depending on the circumstances (obesity, bleeding, prior radiation, degree of contamination, etc.), it is helpful to have an experienced assistant join you for the repair.
   (c) A flexible sigmoidoscope or other means to evaluate the injury and the integrity of the repair.

Operative Technique

1. As the rectal injury likely changes the surgical wound classification of the case, consider giving additional antibiotics appropriate for a colorectal resection, and thoroughly irrigate the field to address the contamination encountered.
2. Typically begin by utilizing the surgical platform that is already underway (robotic, laparoscopic, open). The specifics of the injury and the requirements of the repair may necessitate a change in the operative approach.
3. The capacious rectum usually permits tension-free closure along the plane of the injury whether this is transverse, longitudinal, or oblique. Details like single versus double layer repairs and running versus interrupted closures are up to the preference of the surgeon. Large, irregular injuries that result in significant loss of the anterior rectal wall or that are otherwise not amenable to primary closure and complex injuries involving pathology (cancer, endometriosis, poor quality of tissues, etc.) will require proctectomy. Injury to the mesorectum is rare but may necessitate proctectomy, as well.
4. While some surgeons prefer to leave a drain in this situation, pelvic drains are not usually required given the timeliness of the repair.
5. The majority of these rectal injuries are repaired primarily and are left unprotected. The decision whether or not to divert is a judgment call that should take into consideration whether or not a bowel preparation was taken, the degree of stool burden in the colon, the quality of the tissues involved in the repair, the clinical status of the patient on the table, and whether or not the patient has been irradiated. Appreciate that the surgeon who created the injury and consulted you will often want to avoid stoma creation in this setting. As the consultant responsible for addressing the rectum, consider the treatment options and make the best decision for the patient. Options for diversion include creating a stoma proximal to the rectal repair/anastomosis or, if the pelvis is particularly hostile, dividing the rectum and exteriorizing an end colostomy. A later section in this chapter describes stoma creation in patients not preoperatively marked.

Technical Pearls (Tips and Tricks)

1. Assess the patient when consulted, but usually allow for completion of the primary procedure (like hysterectomy or prostatectomy) before definitively addressing the rectal injury. This approach prevents completing the index procedure from manipulating the rectal repair but may need to be modified in situations where there is ongoing contamination from the open rectum.
2. In cases of hysterectomy, leaving the stay sutures on the vaginal cuff closure long can help manipulate the field. Similarly, leaving the rectal repair sutures long while completing the repair helps with exposure.

3. In cases requiring dissection of the anterior peritoneal reflection, it may be helpful to have an assistant manipulate the vagina and/or rectum digitally or with the EEA sizers. Care should be taken when introducing a sizer into an already injured rectum; a smaller sizer usually works better than a larger sizer. Using a sizer to manipulate the rectum can also help with exposure for the repair by moving the injury cephalad in the pelvis.
4. Evaluate the integrity of the repair with a leak test, and confirm you did not "back wall" the rectum during the repair and that the lumen of the rectum is still patent.
5. If time and circumstances permit, mobilize an omental pedicle to place over the repair. In cases where there is a nearby suture line (like a fresh vaginal cuff), using the omentum as an interposition may prevent fistula formation (Fig. 5.1).

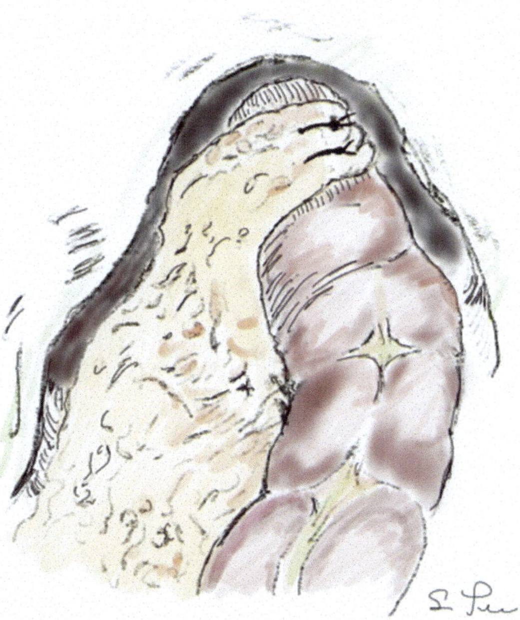

Fig. 5.1 An omental pedicle interposed between the vaginal cuff and the rectal repair

Special Postoperative Care

1. Nothing per anus given the location of the injury.
2. Consider continuing antibiotics for 24 hours or longer depending on the degree of contamination encountered and the specifics of the patient.
3. Full disclosure to the patient including operative details and risk of leak, infection, potential functional issues, etc.

Suggested Reading

1. Jo EJ, Lee Y, Kim T, et al. Management and outcome of rectal injury during gynecologic laparoscopic surgery. J Minim Invasive Gynecol. 2013;20:166–71.

6 Appendectomy Pathology Report Returns Adenocarcinoma, Carcinoid, or Appendiceal Mucinous Neoplasm

Daniel L. Feingold and Steven A. Lee-Kong

Clinical Scenario

A few days after performing laparoscopic appendectomy for apparent appendicitis, the pathology report reveals adenocarcinoma, carcinoid, or a mucinous neoplasm.

Key Points

1. Appendiceal adenocarcinoma is rare and can be difficult to diagnose prior to or even during appendectomy. In the post-appendectomy situation, evaluation involves typical colon cancer staging with CT scans of the chest, abdomen, and pelvis and a CEA level. While the benefit of right colectomy in the setting of margin negative appendiceal adenocarcinoma remains controversial, the majority of patients undergo right colectomy according to oncologic principles with removal of the lymph node basin.
2. The management of appendiceal carcinoid, a rare, usually indolent neuroendocrine tumor, is controversial. Factors related to developing locally recurrent or metastatic disease include size ≥2 cm, location at the base of the appendix, Ki-67 index >2% (higher-grade tumors), lymphovascular or mesoappendix invasion, and positive surgical margins. Published management recommendations are consensus based, and treatment should be individualized to each patient. Patients with a poor prognostic factor are typically recommended to undergo right colectomy. In addition to usual CT staging, preoperative evaluation may include chromogranin A levels and somatostatin receptor imaging. Carcinoid syndrome is extremely rare from an appendiceal primary and indicates metastatic disease; 24-hour urine 5-HIAA levels may be useful in this setting. Goblet cell tumors and composite carcinoid-adenocarcinomas are more aggressive neoplasms and are treated with right colectomy.
3. Appendiceal mucinous neoplasms can be difficult to diagnose and classify. Current classification includes low-grade mucinous neoplasm (LAMN), high-grade mucinous neoplasm (HAMN), and neoplasms with signet ring cells. In the setting of LAMN with no peritoneal surface disease and negative margins, observation with CT scans at 1 year is indicated. In the setting of HAMN or signet ring cell pathology, right colectomy and exploration is recommended despite a typically low positive lymph node yield with these histologies. The surgeon should maintain a high index of suspicion for peritoneal

D. L. Feingold (✉) · S. A. Lee-Kong
Division of Colorectal Surgery, Department of Surgery, Columbia University, New York, NY, USA
e-mail: df347@cumc.columbia.edu

S. W. Lee et al. (eds.), *Colorectal Surgery Consultation*,
https://doi.org/10.1007/978-3-030-11181-6_6

metastasis in the setting of a perforated appendix and/or high-grade or signet ring cell tumors, and referral for consideration of cytoreductive surgery and HIPEC should be made. Preoperative MRI may be helpful prior to surgery to better determine the extent of the peritoneal disease.

4. Patients found to have appendiceal neoplasia should be evaluated by a multidisciplinary tumor board to optimize treatment.

Operative Assessment

1. Oftentimes in this situation, the preoperative cross-sectional imaging does not suggest an occult neoplasm, nor do the operative findings suggest the presence of a tumor. While it is good practice for the surgeon to examine the gross appendix specimen once it is exteriorized, an underlying neoplasm may not be appreciated.

Technical Pearls (Tips and Tricks)

1. Patients who require colonoscopy to complete their evaluation typically wait an interval of a few weeks due to the fresh cecal staple line.
2. Patients who, after staging and appropriate counselling, require right colectomy typically undergo resection after an interval of a few weeks taking into consideration the recent operative findings and course and the degree of anticipated postoperative inflammatory adhesions that might be present.
3. In the setting of interval colectomy for appendiceal adenocarcinoma or a mucinous neoplasm, in addition to routine intraoperative assessment, a careful survey of the peritoneal surfaces and ovaries is required to evaluate for metastatic disease as these histologies may have a propensity to metastasize in this distribution.
4. If peritoneal disease is found in the setting of interval colectomy, referral to a HIPEC center for evaluation and treatment is warranted. In this setting it is recommended, if possible, to place midline ports to allow for port site excision during subsequent cytoreductive surgery.

Special Postoperative Care

1. These patients are usually under the impression they "just" had an appendectomy for appendicitis and require disclosure and a plan for staging and medical oncology consultation.

Suggested Reading

1. Elias H, Galata C, Warschkow R, et al. Survival after resection of appendiceal carcinoma by hemicolectomy and less radical than hemicolectomy: a population-based propensity score matched analysis. Color Dis. 2017;19:895–906.
2. Groth SS, Virnig BA, Al-Refaie WB, et al. Appendiceal carcinoid tumors: predictors of lymph node metastasis and the impact of right hemicolectomy on survival. J Surg Oncol. 2011;103:39–45.
3. Pape U, Niederle B, Costa F, et al. ENETS consensus guidelines for neuroendocrine neoplasms of the appendix. Neuroendocrinology. 2016;103:144–52.
4. Shaib WL, Assi R, Shamseddine A, et al. Appendiceal mucinous neoplasms: diagnosis and management. Oncologist. 2017;22:1107–16.

Unexpected Findings: Normal Appendix During Appendectomy

7

Daniel L. Feingold and Steven A. Lee-Kong

Clinical Scenario

A 36-year-old woman presents with right-sided abdominal pain for 2 days, an elevated white blood cell count, and a CT scan with what appears to be a somewhat dilated appendix but upon laparoscopy is found to have a normal appearing appendix.

Key Points

1. Appreciating that the appendix is normal and does not grossly appear to explain the patient's clinical presentation facilitates an alternative accurate diagnosis.
2. Consider the patient's unique presentation, and survey the abdomen and pelvis for other potential etiologies for their presentation.

D. L. Feingold (✉) · S. A. Lee-Kong
Division of Colorectal Surgery,
Department of Surgery, Columbia University,
New York, NY, USA
e-mail: df347@cumc.columbia.edu

Operative Assessment

1. Evaluate the appendix as the intended target of the operation and recognize that the gross operative findings do not support a diagnosis of suppurative appendicitis.
2. Position the patient in Trendelenburg, and evaluate the uterus, tubes, ovaries, pelvic colon, and internal inguinal rings looking for any pathology.
3. Position the patient in slight reverse Trendelenburg, and run the small bowel from the ileal fat pad (ligament of Treves) to the ligament of Treitz looking for ileitis or other small bowel inflammation, etc. Take care to evaluate the anti-mesenteric wall looking for a Meckel's diverticulum, the ascending colon, and cecum.
4. Inspect the stomach and duodenum for peptic ulcer disease, the gallbladder, and liver.

Technical Pearls (Tips and Tricks)

1. Re-review the CT imaging in the operating room looking for an alternative explanation for the patient's presentation.
2. The standard laparoscopic appendectomy port setup can usually be used to survey the abdomen and search for another explanation for the patient's presentation.

S. W. Lee et al. (eds.), *Colorectal Surgery Consultation*,
https://doi.org/10.1007/978-3-030-11181-6_7

3. Use laparoscopic bowel graspers to run the bowel by keeping the laparoscope stationary and moving the small bowel in a hand-over-hand fashion across the field of view. This expedites running the bowel by maintaining the orientation of the field and is less disorienting.
4. In most situations, when a grossly normal appendix is found with or without a different intraoperative diagnosis to explain the patient's presentation, it makes sense to proceed with appendectomy to prevent the patient from re-presenting in the future with actual appendicitis. An exception to this rule of thumb is the presence of cecal inflammation (typhlitis, Crohn's disease, etc.).
5. Removing an otherwise "normal appendix" is supported as well by the fact that a proportion of patients presenting clinically with appendicitis but with a normal appearing appendix found laparoscopically may have "endoluminal appendicitis" with evidence of inflammation only evident histologically.

Special Postoperative Care

1. Usual post-appendectomy care.
2. Patients with unexpected operative findings require disclosure.
3. If no alternative diagnosis is found upon exploration, consider obtaining a urine analysis and culture, if not done preoperatively, and a CT urogram looking for nephrolithiasis and other pathology.

Suggested Reading

1. Jaunoo SS, Hale AL, Masters JP, Jaunoo SR. An international survey of opinion regarding investigation of possible appendicitis and laparoscopic management of a macroscopically normal appendix. Ann R Coll Surg Engl. 2012;94:476–80.
2. Phillips AW, Jones AE, Sargen K. Should the macroscopically normal appendix be removed during laparoscopy for acute right iliac fossa pain when no other explanatory pathology is found? Surg Laparosc Endosc Percutan Tech. 2009;19:392–6.

During Sigmoid Resection for Diverticulitis, the Patient Is Found to Have Diffuse Diverticulosis

8

Daniel L. Feingold and Steven A. Lee-Kong

Clinical Scenario

During sigmoidectomy for diverticulitis, the colon is resected and delivered off the field. You excise the colonic linear staple line in order to place a purse-string suture to secure the circular stapler's anvil and find diverticula lining the descending colon that you were going to use for the colorectal anastomosis.

Key Points

1. As per convention, the extent of resection in this setting should include the entire sigmoid colon with margins of healthy colon and rectum. The purpose of the resection is not to remove all proximal diverticula.
2. Care should be taken to avoid incorporating diverticula into the mechanism of the circular stapler as false diverticula are comprised of only mucosa, submucosa, and serosa and stapling across a diverticulum can result in anastomotic leak.
3. The distal transection point should be the most proximal healthy rectum.

Technical Pearls (Tips and Tricks)

1. The goal is to exclude diverticula from where the head of the stapler and the body of the anvil come together when the stapler mechanism is married.
2. Once the linear staple line is removed and prior to placing the purse string suture, incise any diverticulum along the cut edge of the colon so that the purse string will pull in a circumference of full-thickness colon wall.
3. Secure the anvil with a purse string, and if a diverticulum lays on the edge of the circumference of the anvil, use a "u" stitch around the shaft of the anvil to pull the diverticulum in toward the shaft of the anvil (Fig. 8.1). This maneuver can be repeated, as needed, to pull in other diverticula causing the diverticula to be included in the proximal donut. After firing the device, check the donuts to confirm the anticipated tissue was in fact pulled in (this can be verified by looking for the "u" stitch suture that was placed). Using colonoscopy to leak test will also confirm that no diverticula were incorporated in the anastomosis.
4. When using "u" stitches as described above, avoid pulling in too much colon and making

D. L. Feingold (✉) · S. A. Lee-Kong
Division of Colorectal Surgery, Department of Surgery, Columbia University, New York, NY, USA
e-mail: df347@cumc.columbia.edu

S. W. Lee et al. (eds.), *Colorectal Surgery Consultation*,
https://doi.org/10.1007/978-3-030-11181-6_8

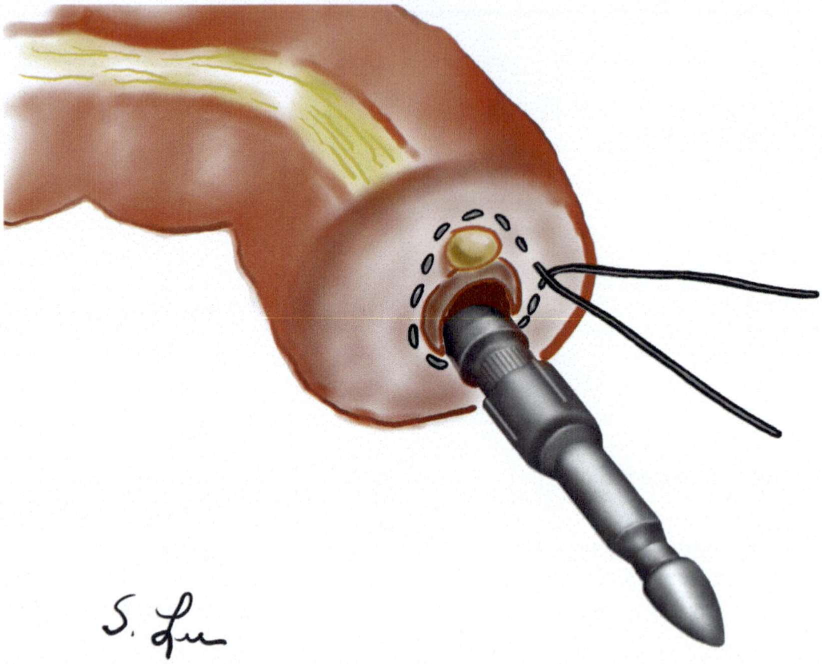

Fig. 8.1 Use a "u" stitch to pull in a diverticulum and exclude it from the anastomosis

the tissue too bulky as this may cause the circular stapler to misfire. When tissue is pulled in toward the shaft of the anvil, it can cause a wrinkle in the colon coming over the edge of the device that crimps over itself, and this can also result in a misfiring.

5. If there are too many diverticula or the diverticula are too large such that pulling them in bulks up the tissue too much, amputate the distal most segment of the colon, and place another purse string, and work with the tissue at that level to exclude any more diverticula. Occasionally, this will need to be repeated until you are satisfied with the quality of the colon going to the anastomosis. Mobilizing the splenic flexure may provide the needed colon length for this maneuver.
6. In cases where too much bulk is pulled in above the purse string around the anvil, using a scissors to remove the excess tissue is acceptable as long as the purse string is intact and tight around the anvil post.
7. In cases where diverticula line up away from the anti-mesenteric wall, consider configuring a side-to-end (Baker type) colorectal anastomosis.
8. In the extremely rare situation of severe diverticulosis not amenable to the above maneuvers, it may be reasonable to create an anastomosis and divert proximally as opposed to performing a completion colectomy with a diverticulum-free ileum to rectal anastomosis. The decision to forego anastomosis and create an end colostomy in this setting is almost always due to the poor quality of the colon coming down to the anastomosis rather than simply the presence of extensive diverticulosis in this segment.

Suggested Reading

1. Feingold D, Steele SR, Lee S, et al. Practice parameters for the treatment of sigmoid diverticulitis. Dis Colon Rectum. 2014;57:284–94.

9 Intraoperatively the Patient Is Found Incidentally to Have Colon or Small Bowel Inflammation

Daniel L. Feingold and Steven A. Lee-Kong

Clinical Scenario

During interval laparoscopic appendectomy in a patient with prior appendicitis treated non-operatively several weeks ago, a Meckel's diverticulum is discovered.

Key Points

1. The treatment for incidentally discovered small bowel or colonic inflammation during an abdominal operation for some other indication depends on the circumstances of the particular patient, and, in many situations, the operative plan is not significantly influenced by these findings. A decision needs to be made whether or not to proceed with the planned operation and what, if anything, should be done in the operating room to address the inflammation. Depending on the extent and severity of the inflammation and the underlying condition of the patient, aborting the planned operation may expedite the needed diagnostic journey and facilitate treatment. Aborting and postponing the operation until the new-found inflammation has been addressed may also improve the surgical outcome.

D. L. Feingold (✉) · S. A. Lee-Kong
Division of Colorectal Surgery, Department of Surgery, Columbia University, New York, NY, USA
e-mail: df347@cumc.columbia.edu

Operative Assessment

1. In a situation where unanticipated bowel inflammation is encountered, the entire abdomen should be carefully surveyed looking for the extent of the problem and any other pathology.
2. Depending on the circumstances and what options are available at that point, consider speaking with the waiting family either to update them regarding the plan or to get their input to help make a plan.

Technical Pearls (Tips and Tricks)

1. The finding of unexpected sigmoid inflammation, ascending colon inflammation, or ileitis can usually be managed similarly, and assessing the anatomy can often point to a plausible diagnosis. For instance, is the inflammation and its distribution consistent with diverticulitis? Are there skip areas with intervening normal bowel or areas of creeping fat consistent with Crohn's disease? Is the appendix normal or is it chronically festering

S. W. Lee et al. (eds.), *Colorectal Surgery Consultation*,
https://doi.org/10.1007/978-3-030-11181-6_9

and secondarily affecting the right colon, a loop of small bowel, or a redundant sweep of the sigmoid colon?

2. Meckel's diverticula, the most common congenital anomaly of the gastrointestinal tract, are due to incomplete obliteration of the vitelline duct. These diverticula may contain ectopic mucosa, most commonly of gastric origin, which secretes acid and can bleed. Meckel's are true diverticula containing all layers of the bowel wall and are asymptomatic in up to 95% of patients. The risks of removing an incidentally found asymptomatic Meckel's diverticulum outweigh the benefits, and prophylactic resection is not supported by the literature. An inflamed appearing Meckel's found during an operation for another indication should be considered symptomatic, and resection is recommended in this situation. While the choice of diverticulectomy versus small bowel resection with anastomosis remains controversial, the chosen operative technique should remove all abnormal tissue, and, in cases of Meckel's diverticulitis, bowel resection will usually be required.

Special Postoperative Care

1. Disclosure to the patient with a plan to address the newly discovered pathology

Suggested Reading

1. Morris G, Kennedy A, Cochran W. Small bowel congenital anomalies: a review and update. Curr Gastroenterol Rep. 2016;18:1–12.
2. Vaos G, Misiakos EP. Congenital anomalies of the gastrointestinal tract diagnosed in adulthood – diagnosis and management. J Gastrointest Surg. 2010;14:916–25.
3. Zani A, Eaton S, Rees CM, Pierro A. Incidentally detected Meckel diverticulum: to resect or not to resect? Ann Surg. 2008;247:276–81.

10 Unexpected Findings: Intraoperatively Suspected Colon Cancer Turns Out to Be Rectal Cancer

Daniel L. Feingold and Steven A. Lee-Kong

Clinical Scenario

A patient undergoes diagnostic colonoscopy as part of an evaluation for bleeding and is found, as per the procedure report, to have a colon cancer "in the sigmoid at 25 cm." The patient's BMI is 37. The CT scans and CEA are noncontributory, and the location of the cancer is difficult to discern on the CT images. At operation, laparoscopy does not demonstrate the tattoo that had been placed, and the cancer site is not readily apparent. On-table CO_2 colonoscopy demonstrates the cancer at the middle valve of Houston.

Key Points

1. Given how the treatment algorithm differs between colon cancer and rectal cancer, it is important to differentiate between these cancers and accurately diagnose patients. If any doubt, perform your own endoscopy to confirm location.
2. If you encounter an unexpected rectal cancer, consider avoiding resection at the time, and ensure the patient is appropriately staged.
3. Patients with proximal third rectal cancers are usually treated similarly to patients with sigmoid colon cancer.
4. Patients with middle and distal third rectal cancers may benefit from neoadjuvant chemoradiotherapy as determined by endo-anal ultrasound or rectal cancer protocol MRI. These patients should have appropriate rectal cancer staging and possibly neoadjuvant therapy before undergoing proctectomy, as circumstances permit.
5. Patients with a colorectal malignancy should be presented at a multidisciplinary tumor board, when possible in advance of surgery, to optimize treatment. This kind of dedicated review can help determine the need for better or more convincing preoperative localization differentiating colon from rectal cancer.

Operative Assessment

1. Accurately determine the location of the cancer endoscopically.
2. Carefully survey the patient looking for evidence of metastasis that may influence the decision to resect at this point.

D. L. Feingold (✉) · S. A. Lee-Kong
Division of Colorectal Surgery, Department of Surgery, Columbia University, New York, NY, USA
e-mail: df347@cumc.columbia.edu

S. W. Lee et al. (eds.), *Colorectal Surgery Consultation*,
https://doi.org/10.1007/978-3-030-11181-6_10

Operative Checklist

1. Additional resources and equipment
   (a) A colonoscope or proctoscope to localize the tumor endoscopically.

Technical Pearls (Tips and Tricks)

1. When performing colonoscopy and assessing the location of a colorectal neoplasm, larger buttocks can artificially increase the length of scope insertion and inaccurately localize the mass in what is presumed to be the sigmoid colon. Avoid the mistake of describing the height of a tumor based on the distance from the buttocks; instead, rely on the distance from the anal verge, rigid proctoscopy evaluation, and/or anatomic landmarks of the proximal, middle, and distal valves of Houston.
2. In general, intraoperatively confirm tumor location before committing to a resection or ligating the main artery to a segment of the colon.
3. Correlate the endoscopy findings with cross-sectional imaging to ensure the correct level of the tumor.

Special Postoperative Care

1. Full disclosure to the patient including the operative findings and facilitate medical/radiation oncology consultation.

Suggested Reading

1. Monson JR, Weiser MR, Buie WD, et al. Practice parameters for the management of rectal cancer. Dis Colon Rectum. 2013;56:535–50.
2. Obias V, Reynolds H. Multidisciplinary teams in the management of rectal cancer. Clin Colon Rectal Surg. 2007;20:143–7.
3. Sauer R, Becker H, Hohenberger W, et al. Preoperative versus postoperative chemoradiotherapy for rectal cancer. N Engl J Med. 2004;351:1731–40.

Unexpected Findings: Can't Find the Colon Lesion

11

Daniel L. Feingold and Steven A. Lee-Kong

Clinical Scenario

During laparoscopic colectomy for what was described as a splenic flexure cancer, no tattoo is found, and the cancer site is not grossly appreciated.

Key Points

1. Confidently localizing lesions preoperatively reaffirms the operative plan and facilitates resection.
2. Under almost all circumstances, blind resection without a confident degree of intraoperative localization should be avoided.
3. Patients with colorectal malignancy should be presented at a multidisciplinary tumor board, when possible in advance of surgery, to optimize treatment. This kind of dedicated review by committee can help determine things like the need for better or more convincing preoperative localization.

D. L. Feingold (✉) · S. A. Lee-Kong
Division of Colorectal Surgery, Department of Surgery, Columbia University, New York, NY, USA
e-mail: df347@cumc.columbia.edu

Operative Assessment

1. Start by looking for the tattoo and/or the cancer in the area that was targeted by preoperative localization. If the target is not localized, evaluate the colon segment by segment looking for the tattoo or lesion. Depending on the redundancy of the colon and the experience of the endoscopist, relying solely on the endoscopy to localize a lesion can carry a high margin of error.

Operative Checklist

1. Additional resources and equipment
   (a) A CO_2 colonoscope to localize the tumor. Using ambient air for the colonoscopy will jeopardize the ability to complete a laparoscopic operation due to distension of the colon.

Technical Pearls (Tips and Tricks)

1. Reliable localization includes colonoscopically visualizing the target in relation to the ileocecal valve preoperatively, locating a previously placed tattoo intraoperatively, identifying the tumor on cross-sectional imaging in advance of surgery and correlating this with

S. W. Lee et al. (eds.), *Colorectal Surgery Consultation*,
https://doi.org/10.1007/978-3-030-11181-6_11

the operative findings, appreciating the mass laparoscopically, or finding the target using on-table intraoperative colonoscopy. Other means of localizing like combining endoscopic clips and x-rays or relying on barium enemas are not commonly used any longer.

2. In cases of absent or questionable localization, on-table CO_2 colonoscopy is the preferred method to localize targets. It may be helpful in this situation to also reach out to the colonoscopist who performed the colonoscopy to begin with for input.
3. In general, intraoperatively confidently confirm tumor location before committing to a resection by ligating the main artery to a segment of the colon.
4. When localizing a lesion during colonoscopy, tattooing the mucosa distal to the target in multiple quadrants facilitates intraoperative localization as some of the tattoo can be obscured by the mesentery, omentum, or epiploica (Fig. 11.1).
5. Move the omentum cephalad out of the way, and manipulate large epiploica to better expose the colon serosa actively looking for a tattoo.
6. When needed, on-table colonoscopy should provide localization. In cases where other methods for localization were unsuccessful, if intraoperative colonoscopic localization fails because of a poor bowel preparation, conversion to an open procedure to manually palpate the colon can be considered but is unlikely to help given the stool burden. In this situation, aborting the procedure may be most prudent.

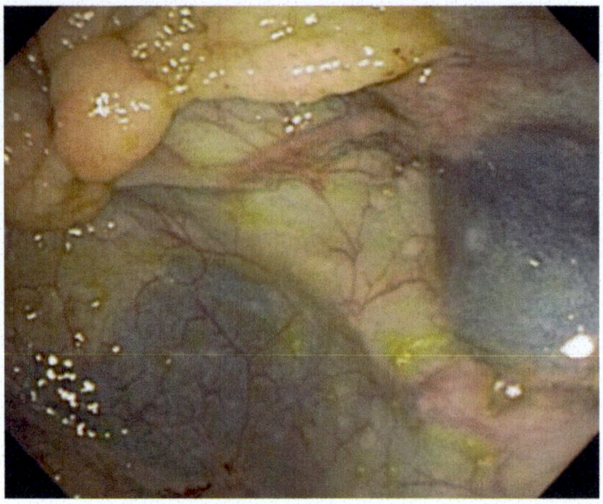

Fig. 11.1 Effective tattooing performed in multiple quadrants just distal to a mass

Suggested Reading

1. Munro A, Brown M, Niblock P, Steele R, Carey F. Do multidisciplinary team processes influence survival in patients with colorectal cancer? A population-based experience. BMC Cancer. 2015;15:686–95.
2. Nakajima K, Lee SW, Sonoda T, Milsom JW. Intraoperative carbon dioxide colonoscopy: a safe insufflation alternative for locating colonic lesions during laparoscopic surgery. Surg Endosc. 2005;19:321–5.

Unexpected Findings: The "Malignant Polyp"

12

Daniel L. Feingold and Steven A. Lee-Kong

Clinical Scenario

A 63-year-old patient at index screening colonoscopy undergoes piecemeal polypectomy of a medium-sized sessile lesion in the descending colon using a snare, and several days later the pathology report reveals adenocarcinoma arising within adenomatous tissue.

Key Points

1. When a patient has unanticipated cancer described in their polypectomy pathology report, it is important to consider whether or not the site of the lesion has been adequately localized. Given the presumed benign nature of the lesion, often the site is not tattooed at the time of polypectomy. Once this situation is recognized, it is important to timely repeat the colonoscopy to accurately localize and tattoo the area of the scar. Ideally, the colonoscopist who performed the polypectomy to begin with should localize the site in this fashion.
2. A malignant polyp contains adenocarcinoma in the submucosa. The assessment in these situations usually centers on the likelihood of mucosal recurrence at the site of polypectomy as well as the risk of having occult nodal disease. Favorable histologic features include malignant polyps removed in one piece, well-differentiated cancer, absent lymphovascular invasion, and negative margins. The pathologic description of tumor budding may be taken as an unfavorable or poor prognostic factor in this situation. As much of the decision-making in these circumstances is based on histopathology, review of the outside pathology slides may influence the recommended treatment plan and should be considered if in-house expertise is available.
3. An assessment of the histologic parameters, usual cancer staging, and the patient's unique medical status allows the surgeon to individualize the recommendation for surgery in these circumstances. In general, patients with an unfavorable histologic factor are recommended to undergo colorectal resection as definitive treatment of their malignant polyp. In terms of setting expectations, it is important that patients who undergo colectomy in the setting of a previously removed malignant polyp understand, in advance of their surgery, the likelihood of having no pathology in their operative specimen and documenting this understanding is advisable.

D. L. Feingold (✉) · S. A. Lee-Kong
Division of Colorectal Surgery, Department of Surgery, Columbia University, New York, NY, USA
e-mail: df347@cumc.columbia.edu

S. W. Lee et al. (eds.), *Colorectal Surgery Consultation*,
https://doi.org/10.1007/978-3-030-11181-6_12

4. Patients with malignant polyps should be evaluated in a multidisciplinary tumor board, when possible in advance of surgery, to optimize treatment.
5. In cases with an unlocalized scar, if repeat colonoscopy fails to localize the polypectomy site and the patient meets criteria for colectomy based on the assessment outlined above, a decision needs to be made whether or not colectomy should be performed based on the information available from the colonoscopy that removed the polyp to begin with. The use of PET-CT to localize under these circumstances is not well established but may be considered. In general, blind resections are not advised.
6. If there are concerns regarding the completeness of the malignant polyp excision, a repeat colonoscopy should be performed to evaluate the site.
7. In cases where colectomy is not performed, patients should typically undergo short-interval surveillance colonoscopy followed by further colorectal surveillance at appropriate intervals. As usual, medical oncology consultation should determine the need for systemic surveillance.
8. Patients with high-grade dysplasia or intramucosal adenocarcinoma described within their adenoma are not classified as having had cancer. As these histologies do not risk nodal metastasis, the treatment in these cases is to remove the lesion completely and perform surveillance.

Suggested Reading

1. Aarons CB, Shanmugan S, Bleier J. Management of malignant colon polyps: current status and controversies. World J Gastroenterol. 2014;20:16178–83.
2. Lieberman DA, Rex DK, Winawer SJ, Giardiello FM, Johnson DA, Levin TR. Guidelines for colonoscopy surveillance after screening and polypectomy: a consensus update by the US Multi-Society Task Force on Colorectal Cancer. Gastroenterology. 2012;143:844–57.
3. Vogel JD, Eskicioglu C, Weiser MR, Feingold DL, Steele SR. The American Society of Colon and Rectal Surgeons clinical practice guidelines for the treatment of colon cancer. Dis Colon Rectum. 2017;60:999–1017.

Unexpected Findings: Positive Air Leak

13

Daniel L. Feingold and Steven A. Lee-Kong

Clinical Scenario

During low anterior resection for a patient with a mid-rectal cancer after neo-adjuvant chemoradiation, an anastomotic leak is found while performing the leak test.

Key Points

1. Patients with a pelvic anastomosis should undergo a leak test to evaluate the integrity of the fresh anastomosis.
2. Patients undergoing low anterior resection should be counseled in advance of surgery regarding the likelihood of stoma creation and should be sited, as well.

Operative Assessment

1. When you realize a leak test is positive, it is helpful to repeat the rectal insufflation, ideally with flexible sigmoidoscopy, to determine the exact location of the leak and the extent of the anastomotic failure.
2. Once the leak is repaired or the anastomosis is redone, the leak test should be repeated to confirm the integrity of the anastomosis.

Operative Checklist

1. Additional resources and equipment
   (a) Pelvic tray including long instruments, lighted pelvic retractors, and EEA sizers.
   (b) Depending on the circumstances (obesity, bleeding, prior radiation, etc.), it is helpful to have an experienced assistant join you.
   (c) A flexible sigmoidoscope or other means to perform a leak test.

Technical Pearls (Tips and Tricks)

1. Leak test the rectal stump before firing the circular stapler as it is easier to expose the linear staple line at that point and address a leak. These leaks are typically repaired with interrupted full-thickness sutures as a running suture may be cut by the circular stapler blade and can result in unravelling recreating the leak. When creating the anastomosis, it may be beneficial to introduce the stapler such that it crowns over the portion of the linear staple line that was suture repaired so

D. L. Feingold (✉) · S. A. Lee-Kong
Division of Colorectal Surgery, Department of Surgery, Columbia University, New York, NY, USA
e-mail: df347@cumc.columbia.edu

S. W. Lee et al. (eds.), *Colorectal Surgery Consultation*,
https://doi.org/10.1007/978-3-030-11181-6_13

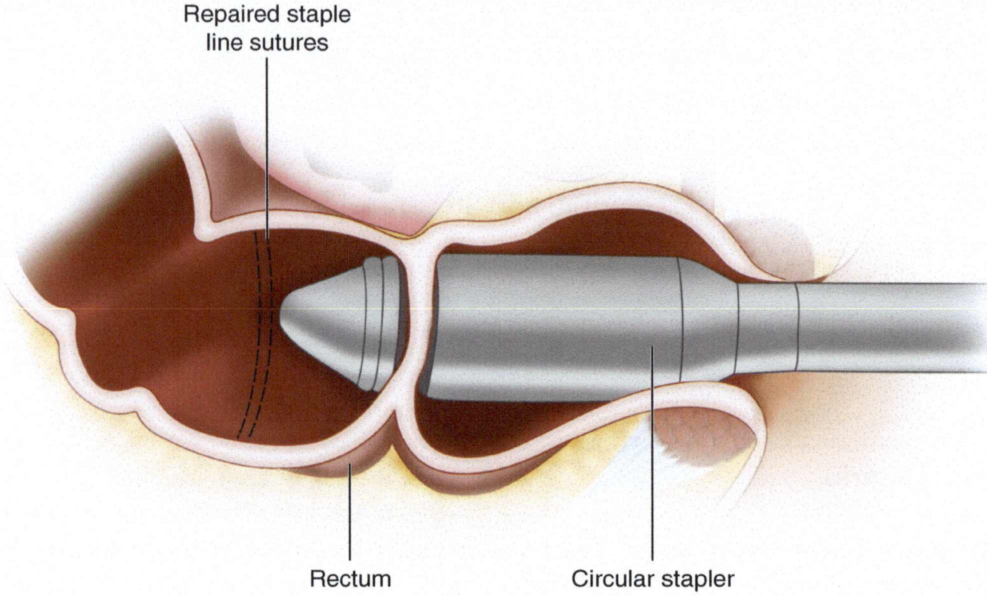

Fig. 13.1 Angling the circular stapler so that the repaired linear staple line is included in the tissue donuts

that portion is excised with the tissue donuts (Fig. 13.1).

2. Using a hand port or an extraction site in a pelvic position allows for direct access to the leaking fresh anastomosis and can facilitate repair.
3. Depending on the circumstances and the patient's anatomy, suture repair of a small defect may be the best option and usually does not require proximal diversion. This is a judgment call that should consider the quality of the tissues and the likelihood that primary repair will prevent a postoperative leak. Suture repair can be a viable option in an irradiated field as these cases will usually be diverted as per the operative plan anyway. Larger or posteriorly located defects that are inaccessible due to the mesentery are not usually addressed in this fashion.
4. Depending on the size and location of the defect, the available colonic reach, and the adequacy of exposure in the pelvis, it may be more prudent to take down the anastomosis and create a new anastomosis. The presence of the colon in the pelvis makes it quite difficult to staple below the leaking anastomosis. Oftentimes manually disrupting the anastomosis and separating the two sides using a finger fracture technique are required after which the rectum will need to be closed to facilitate repeat stapled colorectal anastomosis. The rectum is usually closed in an interrupted full-thickness fashion rather than placing a distal purse-string suture. Given the space constraints of the pelvis, grasping the cut edge of the rectum with stay sutures or long Babcock clamps and negotiating a TA stapler to the level of the open rectum in this situation may not be possible. Depending on the length of the retained rectum and the accessibility of the rectal stump via the abdomen, it may be helpful to use a disposable, fenestrated anoscope from a hemorrhoid stapler kit or more conventional anal retractors to purse string the end of the rectum (Fig. 13.2). An alternative to repeating a stapled approach in some situations is to resect the rectal remnant and hand sew a colo-anal anastomosis.
5. When the leak is small but not readily accessible for repair either transabdominally or trans-anally, especially in cases with questionable additional colon reach or complex pelvic anatomy, it may be appropriate to divert the fecal stream and drain the area rather than

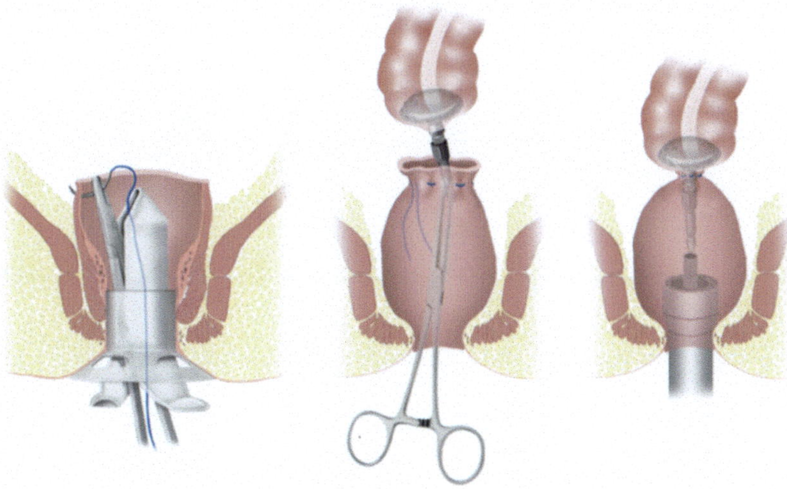

Fig. 13.2 Using a disposable, fenestrated anoscope to place a purse string around the end of the rectum

attempt to create a second anastomosis. This solution should consider what column of stool, if any, lays proximal to the leaking anastomosis.

6. In cases with a significant disruption, an alternative to salvaging a leaking low pelvic anastomosis or remaking an anastomosis is to disrupt the anatomy and create an end colostomy understanding that this stoma will likely be permanent. This decision should incorporate the technical considerations reviewed above as well as the preoperative discussion with the patient regarding the likelihood of colostomy creation.
7. In situations with a more proximal rectal anastomosis (like after sigmoidectomy), it may be best to redo the anastomosis rather than trying to salvage a leaking anastomosis.

Suggested Reading

1. Offodile AC, Feingold DL, Nasar A, Whelan RL, Arnell TD. High incidence of technical errors involving the EEA circular stapler: a single institution experience. J Am Coll Surg. 2010;210:331–5.
2. Ricciardi R, Roberts PL, Marcello PW, Hall JF, Read TE, Schoetz DJ. Anastomotic leak testing after colorectal resection. Arch Surg. 2009;144:407–11.
3. Salvadalena G, Hendren S, McKenna L, et al. WOCN Society and ASCRS position statement on preoperative stoma site marking for patients undergoing colostomy or ileostomy surgery. J Wound Ostomy Continence Nurs. 2015;42:249–52.
4. Sujatha-Bhaskar S, Jafari MD, Hanna M, et al. An endoscopic mucosal grading system is predictive of leak in stapled rectal anastomoses. Surg Endosc. 2017. https://doi.org/10.1007/s00464-017-5860-y.

Unexpected Findings: Anastomotic "Donut" Problems – Incomplete or Missing Donuts with a Negative Leak Test

14

Daniel L. Feingold and Steven A. Lee-Kong

Clinical Scenario

After completing a circular anastomosis during a resection for complicated diverticulitis, the distal donut is observed to be thin or incomplete or is not found on the shaft of the stapler's anvil.

Key Points

1. Ideally, two robust, intact tissue donuts would be retrieved after every firing of a circular stapler. In situations where the distal donut is thin, incomplete, or absent, the leak test and endoscopic assessment of the fresh anastomosis guide further management.

Operative Assessment

1. After firing the circular stapler, routinely assess the tissue donuts, and perform a leak test.

D. L. Feingold (✉) · S. A. Lee-Kong
Division of Colorectal Surgery, Department of Surgery, Columbia University, New York, NY, USA
e-mail: df347@cumc.columbia.edu

S. W. Lee et al. (eds.), *Colorectal Surgery Consultation*,
https://doi.org/10.1007/978-3-030-11181-6_14

Operative Checklist

1. Additional resources and equipment
   (a) A CO_2 flexible sigmoidoscope to evaluate the fresh anastomosis

Technical Pearls (Tips and Tricks)

1. If the distal donut is not found around the shaft of the stapler's anvil, it may be found stuck in the circular groove in the head of the stapler's casing and can be removed and evaluated using a forceps.
2. Regardless of the status of the donuts, a leak test should be performed to evaluate the integrity of the fresh anastomosis. Ideally, a colonoscope is used to directly visualize the anatomy. The distal donut can sometimes be found in the rectum or attached to the circular staple line.
3. If the leak test demonstrates an intact anastomosis, no further intervention is usually needed. Alternatively, a positive leak test will need to be managed as per a previous segment in this chapter.
4. Given how the proximal donut is secured to the anvil with a purse string, an absent or incomplete proximal donut may signify a misfiring of the stapler and should lead to a careful assessment of the integrity of the circular staple line.

5. Tips for using the circular stapler (in addition to Chap. 8 regarding managing patients with diffuse diverticulosis):
   (a) Have the assistant who goes between the legs cut the drapes, so the surgeon can stay sterile while watching how the stapler is being handled; otherwise the assistant works under the drapes, and the stapler is hidden from view.
   (b) In cases where you suspect there may be a stricture at the proximal rectum (from diverticulitis extending distally in the pelvis, radiation, prior pelvic surgery, etc.), it is helpful to pass the EEA sizers before transecting the rectum to confirm that the lumen of the rectum is adequate. If the sizer cannot pass easily due to a stricture or a kink, additional rectum may need to be mobilized and/or resected, and this dissection is easier if the rectum has not yet been transected.
   (c) Insufflating the rectum with a flexible sigmoidoscope or rigid proctoscope may also help the stapler pass from above.
   (d) There may also be a band of tissue on the anterior peritoneal reflection that will need to be divided to allow the passage of the circular stapler to the end of Hartmann's pouch.
   (e) When using a scalpel on a long knife handle to amputate the specimen along the groove of the TA stapler, be careful not to nick the rectum distal to the staple line. Maintaining the TA stapler perpendicular to the field can help prevent this.
   (f) When placing the purse string in the end of the colon, taking larger bites of colon wall will bring more tissue into the stapler mechanism and can cause a misfiring. While larger-sized staplers can accommodate more tissue, smaller staplers cannot.
   (g) Leak test the rectal stump before introducing the circular stapler as it is easier to expose the linear staple line at that point and address a leak.
   (h) When passing sizers and the stapler up to the level of the linear staple line, remember that small movements of the handles of these instruments translate into larger shifts of the heads of the instruments. Fine motions are required to manipulate these instruments taking care not to traumatize the linear staple line.
   (i) Confirm orientation of the colon coming down to the rectum before firing the circular stapler. This is done by following the anti-mesenteric side of the colon and by confirming that there is no colon twisting underneath the cut edge of the colon mesentery.
   (j) Crown the stapler at the linear staple line or at the anterior wall of the rectum, but avoid firing the stapler through a wrinkle of rectal wall as this can cause a mis-firing.
   (k) In low anastomoses, confirm the circular stapler was not mistakenly placed in the vagina by palpating the empty vagina.
   (l) Fire the stapler with a smooth motion without jostling the device.
   (m) Pelvic anastomoses should undergo a leak test to check the integrity of the fresh anastomosis.

Suggested Reading

1. Offodile AC, Feingold DL, Nasar A, Whelan RL, Arnell TD. High incidence of technical errors involving the EEA circular stapler: a single institution experience. J Am Coll Surg. 2010;210:331–5.
2. Ricciardi R, Roberts PL, Marcello PW, Hall JF, Read TE, Schoetz DJ. Anastomotic leak testing after colorectal resection. Arch Surg. 2009;144:407–11.

Unexpected Findings: Locally Advanced Colon Cancer

15

Daniel L. Feingold and Steven A. Lee-Kong

Clinical Scenario

During right colectomy for a large cecal cancer, there is fixation to the retroperitoneum, and as the dissection continues, it becomes clear the right ureter is tethered to the cancer.

Key Points

1. In the setting of colon cancer, staging CT scans of the abdomen and pelvis will typically reveal if the cancer appears to be involving adjacent structures. In general, in the setting of surgery with curative intent and absent distant metastatic disease, en bloc resection of the primary cancer together with the directly involved tissue is indicated.
2. Assessing cross-sectional imaging in advance of operation can reveal the nature of locally advanced colon cancer and permits an upfront discussion with the patient regarding what may be involved in an en bloc resection and allows the surgeon to coordinate with other specialists whose intraoperative expertise may be required.
3. Patients with colon cancer should be evaluated in a multidisciplinary tumor board, when possible in advance of surgery, to optimize treatment. This kind of dedicated review by committee may uncover a concern for a T_4 cancer. A tumor board may also consider intraoperative radiation therapy (IORT) in select complex cases involving the retroperitoneum or pelvis that might risk a positive microscopic margin.

Operative Assessment

1. Carefully assess for any metastatic disease as this may influence the decision to proceed with colectomy involving an en bloc resection of other organs.
2. In cases where the colon cancer directly invades or is adherent to other organs or structures, evaluate the likelihood of complete oncologic resectability (R-0 dissection) before committing to an en bloc resection.

Technical Pearls (Tips and Tricks)

1. While tissue adjacent to the cancer may be adherent through a desmoplastic reaction, the tissues should not be dissected apart out

D. L. Feingold (✉) · S. A. Lee-Kong
Division of Colorectal Surgery, Department of Surgery, Columbia University, New York, NY, USA
e-mail: df347@cumc.columbia.edu

S. W. Lee et al. (eds.), *Colorectal Surgery Consultation*,
https://doi.org/10.1007/978-3-030-11181-6_15

of concern for disrupting a cancer mass and compromising oncologic outcomes.

2. Prior to proceeding with resecting an organ that was otherwise not anticipated in the operative plan, it may be helpful to speak with the waiting family. Engaging the patient's family in a discussion regarding the operative findings before committing to resection rather than surprising them postoperatively can reduce the frustration of the situation and exemplifies effective communication. Depending on the preoperative consent discussion, the complexity of the unanticipated en bloc resection, and the potential for complications of such a resection, it may be prudent to abort the resection.
3. Adequate oncologic resection in cases of T_4 colon cancer is usually based on the surgeon's clinical assessment of the gross margins. In certain situations, obtaining an intraoperative frozen section pathologic analysis may be helpful to establish whether or not the extent of the resection is adequate.
4. When the small bowel is caught up in a colon cancer, en bloc resection requires small bowel resection typically with enteroenterostomy. In colorectal resection cases requiring proximal diversion, it may be prudent to use the two ends of the small bowel resulting from the small bowel resection for the diversion as a divided loop stoma. Cases involving colon cancer invading small bowel mesentery are often more complicated as resecting the mesentery may sacrifice a considerable length of small bowel.
5. A ureter resected for ureteral involvement can be reconstructed in a variety of ways and requires urology service assistance. In cases where there is concern for ureteral involvement or the cancer appears to be in the proximity of the ureter, placing ureteral stents prior to dissecting in the area may facilitate safe dissection.

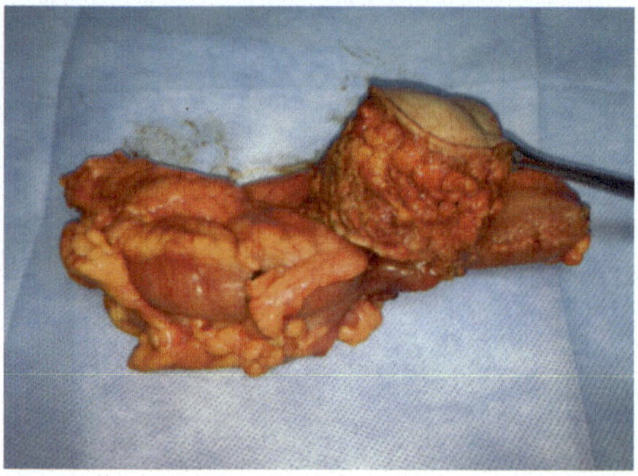

Fig. 15.1 En bloc resection of transverse colon and full-thickness abdominal wall for a T_4 cancer

6. When an area of abdominal wall is excised with the specimen, depending on the site and location of the defect and the local tissue available, the defect may be closed primarily or with a biologic mesh as a bridge (Fig. 15.1). Synthetic mesh is usually avoided in colectomy cases due to infection concerns.
7. Direct extension into the bladder, uterus, or adnexa is usually addressed by a combined resection with urology or gynecology. In these unique situations, the involved bladder can usually be resected allowing for primary repair of the remaining bladder wall. In cases of adnexal involvement, bilateral salpingo-oophorectomy is usually performed.
8. Extension into Gerota's fascia or the perinephric fat is usually addressed by en bloc wide excision. In cases of apparent retroperitoneal involvement, it may be useful to mark the resection site with clips to help localize the area on subsequent imaging studies and to possibly target postoperative radiotherapy, if indicated.
9. The management of duodenal involvement by an ascending or proximal transverse colon cancer depends on the extent of the duodenectomy required. Focal involvement

may be amenable to excising the anti-mesenteric wall of the duodenum en bloc and repairing the small bowel primarily. In situations with more complex duodenal involvement, other reconstructions and more radical duodenectomy may be considered.

10. On occasion, a hepatic flexure or transverse colon cancer will directly invade the edge of the liver. En bloc resection in this situation involves excising a cuff of liver parenchyma with the colectomy specimen.

Special Postoperative Care

1. Disclose to the patient the operative findings and course.

Suggested Reading

1. Vogel JD, Eskicioglu C, Weiser MR, Feingold DL, Steele SR. The American Society of Colon and Rectal Surgeons clinical practice guidelines for the treatment of colon cancer. Dis Colon Rectum. 2017;60:999–1017.

Part III

Technical Tips and Tricks for Difficult Abdominal Cases

16 Difficult to Close Abdomen

Daniel L. Feingold and David A. Kleiman

Clinical Scenario

During an emergency total colectomy for fulminant *Clostridium difficile* colitis, the small bowel becomes quite edematous, and the midline fascia will not close without significant tension.

Key Points

1. A patient with a pre-existing hernia whose operation requires accessing the abdomen through the hernia has a variety of options available in terms of abdominal closure. Depending on the complexity and degree of contamination of the operation being performed, the hernia can be repaired with a variety of synthetic or biologic mesh or using native tissues through a myofascial flap component separation or transversus abdominis release technique. In general, the need to address the hernia should be considered in advance of the surgery, and involving a plastic surgeon or another surgeon with hernia expertise may be warranted to decide on the most appropriate operative plan and to prepare the patient. In some situations it may be best to complete the abdominal operation by closing the skin and leaving the patient with the hernia that they started the operation with in anticipation of a staged hernia repair.
2. In patients with a difficult to close abdomen, closing under significant tension increases the risk of hernia, wound dehiscence, and abdominal compartment syndrome.

Operative Assessment

1. It is usually readily evident when the abdominal wall will not close without undue tension as the small bowel cannot be easily contained within the peritoneal cavity and the fascial edges will not approximate easily. Based on these clinical findings, the patient should undergo temporary abdominal closure (TAC).
2. Engage the anesthesia team, and assess the peak airway pressure, tidal volume, end tidal CO_2, and degree of difficulty ventilating the patient prior to abdominal closure and again during and after fascial closure as these are objective parameters that can reflect abdominal hypertension. Stepwise worsening of these parameters alerts the surgeon to consider temporary abdominal closure.

D. L. Feingold (✉)
Division of Colorectal Surgery, Department of Surgery, Columbia University, New York, NY, USA
e-mail: df347@cumc.columbia.edu

D. A. Kleiman
Lahey Hospital and Medical Center, Department of Colon and Rectal Surgery, Burlington, MA, USA

S. W. Lee et al. (eds.), *Colorectal Surgery Consultation*,
https://doi.org/10.1007/978-3-030-11181-6_16

Operative Checklist

1. Additional resources and equipment
   (a) Access to a variety of temporary abdominal closure products

Technical Pearls (Tips and Tricks)

1. In cases with significant distension due to ongoing bowel obstruction, it may be helpful to evacuate the enteric contents prior to attempting to close the fascia. In cases where there is no bowel injury found or created during the course of the operation, milking the bowel contents retrograde to be aspirated by a nasogastric tube can be helpful. A more effective method to decompress involves aspirating the contents through a defect in the bowel. If the operation requires bowel resection, it is helpful to quarantine the field to contain any spillage and make a controlled enterotomy through which a suction catheter can be passed to evacuate the bowel contents. The small bowel contents can be manually milked toward the enterotomy to be aspirated by the catheter. Given the vegetable matter present and the viscosity of the bowel contents, it may be useful to cut several large side holes in a red rubber catheter and use this to suction (Fig. 16.1). Passing the suction catheter and milking the bowel contents can traumatize the bowel and its mesentery and should be done carefully. Once completed, the bowel injury can be whipstitched and included in the resection.
2. In cases where the abdomen will not close easily, performing a component separation or transversus abdominis release or using a mesh bridge will prolong the operation and may not adequately relieve the abdominal hypertension upon closure. Similarly, relying on retention sutures to buttress a fascial closure under significant tension is not recommended.
3. Temporary abdominal closure can be accomplished using a variety of devices such as Bogota bag or a commercially available negative pressure therapy system (Fig. 16.2). A custom-made negative pressure system can be assembled using two unfolded sterile blue OR towels each encased in a large Ioban-type drape and a nasogastric tube. To temporarily close, one of the wrapped towels is placed in the abdomen, the nasogastric tube is coiled on top of this, and the second towel then covers the wound. The system is then secured to the abdominal skin using another Ioban-type drape with the sump mechanism of the nasogastric tube exposed to air allowing continuous suction. After a temporary closure, patients are usually diuresed in an intensive care setting before undergoing a planned second look and delayed closure.
4. In patients who are expected to have a long course with an open abdomen, using a Wittmann patch or a Gore-tex bridge secured to the fascia may reduce the retraction and lateral displacement of the fascia and help with eventual abdominal closure. These approaches potentially allow for easier reentry into the abdomen and can be trimmed at subsequent reoperations to provide continuous tension across the fascial edges.
5. In cases where there is concern regarding patients developing early postoperative fascial dehiscence (poor quality of the fascia, malnutrition, chronic steroid use, etc.), placing an absorbable mesh underlay to possibly prevent evisceration remains controversial. In certain situations using a biologic mesh as a bridge may facilitate closure.
6. Certain novel devices are available to help close the skin alone, such as the ABRA Surgical Skin Closure (Acell) and DermaClose (Synovis), though are dependent on the extent of the individual wound and awaiting long-term results.

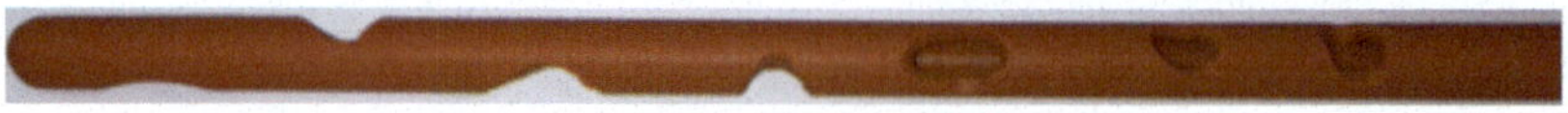

Fig. 16.1 A red rubber catheter with additional side holes cut facilitates bowel decompression

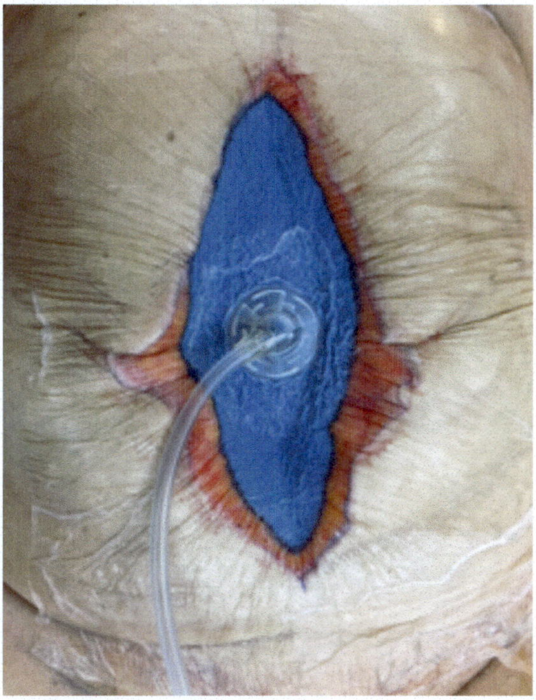

Fig. 16.2 A commercially available negative pressure temporary abdominal closure

Special Postoperative Care

1. Use of a binder may be helpful to reduce tension on the incision.
2. Under the appropriate circumstances, follow for possibly developing abdominal compartment syndrome, and treat the patient accordingly. It is important to recognize that even patients who undergo temporary abdominal closure are still at risk for developing abdominal compartment syndrome.

Suggested Reading

1. Atema JJ, Gans SL, Boermeester MA. Systematic review and meta-analysis of the open abdomen and temporary abdominal closure techniques in non-trauma patients. World J Surg. 2015;39:912–25.
2. Kirkpatrick AW, Roberts DJ, Waele JD, et al. Intra-abdominal hypertension and the abdominal compartment syndrome: updated consensus definitions and clinical practice guidelines from the World Society of the Abdominal Compartment Syndrome. Intensive Care Med. 2013;39:1190–206.
3. Regner JL, Kobayashi L, Coimbra R. Surgical strategies for management of the open abdomen. World J Surg. 2012;36:497–510.
4. Ribeiro MA, Barros EA, de Carvalho SM, et al. Open abdomen in gastrointestinal surgery: which technique is the best for temporary closure during damage control? World J Gastrointest Surg. 2016;8:590–7.
5. Rogers WK, Garcia L. Intra-abdominal hypertension, abdominal compartment syndrome and the open abdomen. Chest. 2017. https://doi.org/10.1016/j.chest.2017.07.023.

17 The Difficult Splenic Flexure

Alison Althans, Deborah S. Keller, and Scott R. Steele

Clinical Scenario

A 60-year-old morbidly obese male with sigmoid diverticulitis is undergoing an anterior resection. During the dissection, the descending colon was mobilized up to the splenic flexure. The distal resection margin was transected using an Endo GIA stapler, and the specimen was exteriorized, resected, and prepared for a double-stapled anastomosis with the end-to-end anastomotic (EEA) stapler. After returning the proximal colon to the peritoneal cavity, the anvil will not reach to the pelvis for the anastomosis. The splenic flexure now needs to be mobilized.

Key Points

1. The splenic flexure takedown is often the most difficult part of the procedure. In patients at high risk for conversion, this can be done first to determine if conversion is needed.
2. Performing the flexure release as the initial step of the operation can minimize incision length if conversion were needed later.
3. The splenic flexure will need to be approached from several directions for successful mobilization.
4. Position changes from Trendelenburg to reverse Trendelenburg during the dissection will assist successful completion.
5. Visualization is better laparoscopically than open, so there is benefit in attempting different approaches and positions before converting to an open procedure.
6. Excess tension on the attachments to the spleen can lead to tearing of the capsule and bleeding.
7. To adequately mobilize the splenic flexure, the omental, splenic, lateral, and retroperitoneal (pancreaticocolic) attachments must all be dissected.

Operative Assessment

1. How much additional length is needed for a tension-free anastomosis?
   (a) Assure the proximal limb can "flop" down into the pelvis.
   (b) Consider using intraoperative fluorescence perfusion testing if there is any

A. Althans
University Hospitals Cleveland Medical Center, Cleveland, OH, USA

D. S. Keller
Department of Surgery, New York-Presbyterian, Columbia University Medical Center, New York, NY, USA

S. R. Steele (✉)
Case Western Reserve University School of Medicine, Cleveland, OH, USA

Department of Colorectal Surgery, Cleveland Clinic, Cleveland, OH, USA

S. W. Lee et al. (eds.), *Colorectal Surgery Consultation*, https://doi.org/10.1007/978-3-030-11181-6_17

question about the viability of the proximal colon.
2. How much mobilization of the splenic flexure was already performed?
   (a) Higher ligation of vessels needed?
   (b) Ensure complete dissection of avascular attachments that tether the colon in multiple directions – including the phrenocolic ligament, pancreaticomesocolic ligaments, lateral retroperitoneal attachments, gastrocolic ligament/omental attachments, and medial retroperitoneal attachments.
3. What can be done to stop splenic capsular bleeding if this occurs?
   (a) Direct pressure: if laparoscopic, use a laparoscopic Kittner or place a sponge.
   (b) Electrocautery: coagulation can be turned up and used as a "spray."
   (c) Topical adjuncts: various hemostatic adjuncts such as Nu-Knit, thrombin, Gelfoam, and fibrin sealants.
   (d) Partial or full splenectomy is rarely needed (see Chap. 45 for further details).

Operative Checklist

1. Additional helpful equipment
   (a) Laparoscopic abdominal set with atraumatic graspers.
   (b) Major abdominal instrument tray with a Bookwalter retractor (if needed to convert to open) – have in the room but do not open initially.
   (c) Good lighting, including a headlight (if needed after conversion).
   (d) Hand-assisted port (if needed to convert to hand-assisted laparoscopy) – have in the room but do not open initially.
2. Positioning
   (a) Patients should be positioned in padded modified lithotomy or on a split-leg table with the legs abducted.
   (b) Initially, the patient is moved into a steep Trendelenburg position, with the left side tilted up. In order to release the splenic flexure, reverse Trendelenburg and tilting the table right side down helps with exposure and facilitates the dissection.
   (c) The surgeon stands between the patient's legs, with the assistant standing on the patient's right side.
   (d) When addressing the left lower quadrant, the surgeon can move to the patient's right with the assistant standing caudal to the surgeon.

Operative Approaches

1. Inferior approach. The transverse colon is placed cephalad, over the stomach. The ligament of Treitz and inferior mesenteric vein (IMV) lateral to the ligament are identified. The IMV is lifted, and the overlying peritoneum is sharply opened (Fig. 17.1). A plane is developed underneath the mesentery and on top of the retroperitoneum (retro-mesenteric plane); dissection continues out to the lateral sidewall, cephalad to the pancreas, and up to the spleen. The retroperitoneal fascia overlying the left kidney is bluntly swept away from the posterior aspect of the left colon mesentery toward the base of the pancreas. When the upper pole of the left kidney is reached, the colon is returned to its original position, and the splenic flexure is approached.
2. Medial-to-lateral dissection. The inferior mesenteric artery (IMA) is isolated, demon-

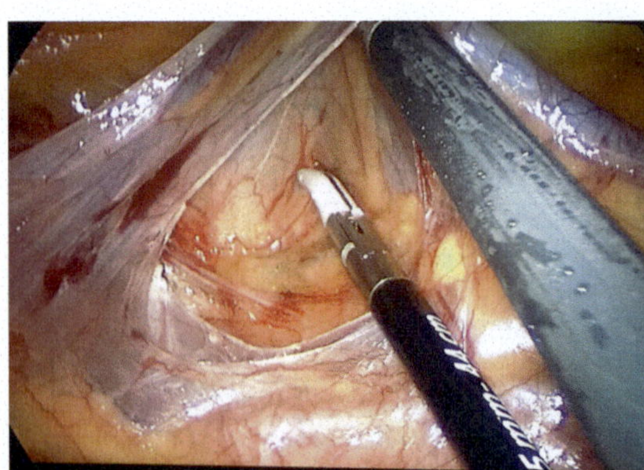

Fig. 17.1 Medial mobilization under the inferior mesenteric vein (IMV)

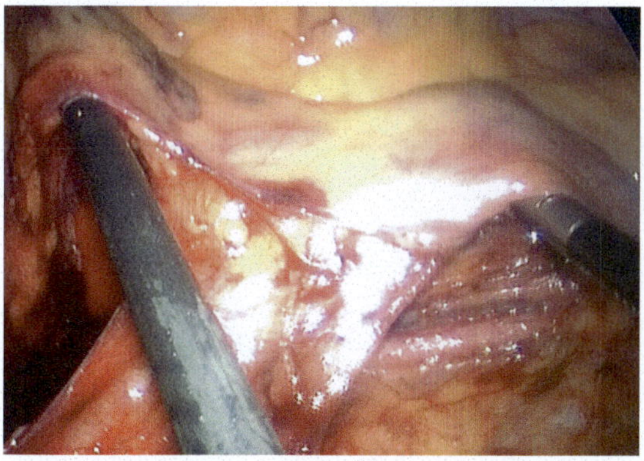

Fig. 17.2 T-shaped IMA pedicle with the left colic artery and IMV in the left part of the image and IMA continuing inferiorly to the right

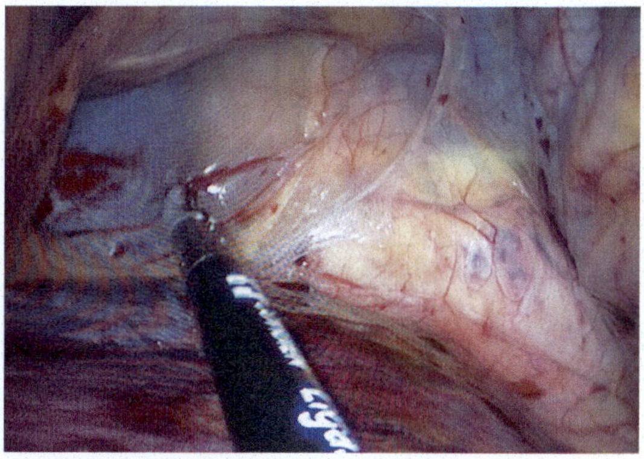

Fig. 17.3 Continued dissection laterally with opening up of the previous dissection

strating a characteristic T shape with the upper wing directed toward the splenic flexure containing the left colic artery/IMV complex and the lower wing directed toward the pelvis containing the superior rectal artery (Fig. 17.2). The IMA is divided, and the dissection plane is extended laterally toward the abdominal wall, separating the mesocolon from Toldt's retroperitoneal fascia and the retroperitoneal structures. The vein is divided. The lateral ligament is divided cephalad, toward the splenic flexure. The splenocolic ligament, the renocolic ligament, and the omental attachments are mobilized. The transverse colon and mesocolon are carefully detached from the inferior border of the pancreas and spleen, and the anterior surface of the pancreas is developed. The greater omentum is dissected off the distal transverse colon from medial to lateral, and the lesser sac is entered. The stomach comes into view after the lesser sac is opened. The mobilization is continued laterally until it meets the previous dissection plane (Fig. 17.3). Any lateral attachments of the descending colon to the left abdominal wall are freed. At this point, the flexure is completely mobilized.

3. Lateral to medial. Complete lateral mobilization of the left colon up to the splenic flexure is performed as the initial step in this approach. The descending colon is pulled medially using an atraumatic bowel grasper. The lateral

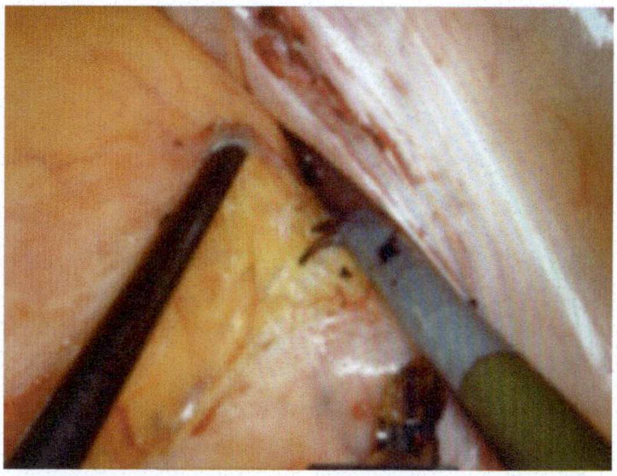

Fig. 17.4 Lateral-to-medial dissecting in the plane to take down the lateral attachments

attachments of the left colon are divided and the colon dissected off Gerota's fascia over the left kidney (Fig. 17.4). With the sigmoid colon retracted anteriorly and superiorly, a broad white line is apparent, delineating the fusion of Toldt's retroperitoneal fascia with the left colon mesentery (the renocolic ligament). The sigmoid colon is retracted medially, and its attachments to the lateral abdominal wall are taken down, staying close to the colon. The lateral ligament is divided cephalad, toward the splenic flexure (Fig. 17.5). The splenocolic ligament, renocolic ligament, and the omental attachments are mobilized. The attachments of between the inferior border of the pancreas and the

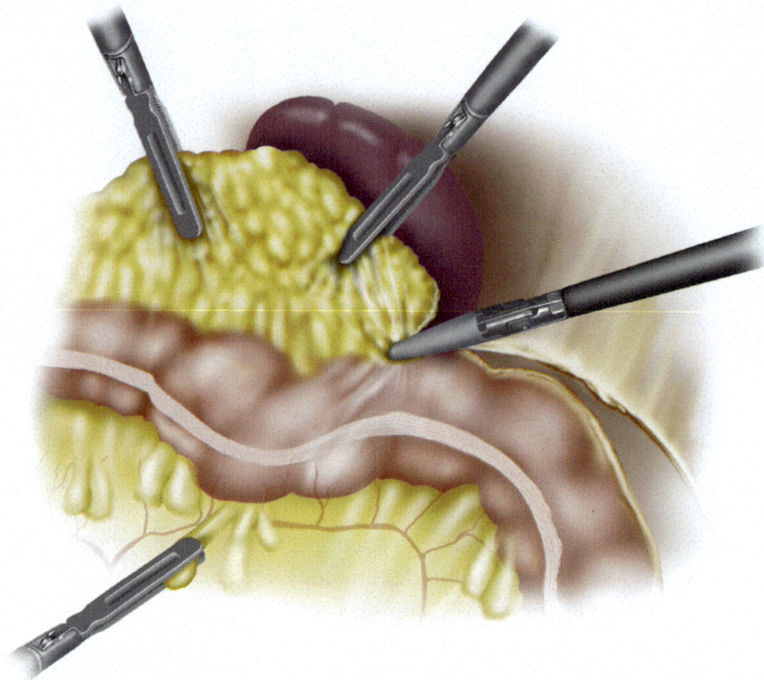

Fig. 17.5 Takedown of the splenic flexure attachments from the colon to the spleen

transverse mesocolon are carefully freed. The greater omentum is dissected off the distal transverse colon from right to left. The lateral attachments of the colon are freed as far proximally as possible, and often this dissection is continued medially over Gerota's fascia to mobilize some of the distal transverse colon. Then it becomes necessary to move medially and enter the lesser sac. To enter the lesser sac, the patient is tilted in reverse Trendelenburg position. The greater omentum is held up, like a cape. Gravity will assist with counter traction by pulling the transverse colon down and to left side, aiding identification of the avascular plane between the greater omentum and the transverse mesocolon. The surgeon grasps the transverse colon toward the left side to aid identification of the avascular plane between the greater omentum and the transverse mesocolon. An energy source is used to dissect this plane and enter the lesser sac, and mobilization is continued laterally toward the splenic flexure. Following separation of the omentum off the left side of the transverse colon, connection to the lateral dissection allows the splenic flexure to be fully mobilized. The colon at the flexure is retracted caudally and medially and any residual restraining attachments divided.

4. Omega maneuver. Takedown of the splenic flexure can be facilitated by approaching the dissection from both the right and the left sides; this effectively makes a knuckle out of whatever is left of the splenic flexure and accentuates where the dissection needs to go in order to make progress with the dissection. The omentum is dissected away from the distal transverse colon in a medial-to-lateral direction as the colon is simultaneously retracted both distal and proximal to the flexure inferiorly, resembling an "omega" formation. Attachments between the splenic flexure and colon can be taken down with the electrocautery or another energy device. While performing this maneuver, care must be taken to avoid excessive tension on the spleen, which can tear the splenic capsule and cause bleeding.
5. Anterior/supramesocolic approach. Approaching the splenic flexure anteriorly along the mid-transverse colon is an alternate approach to access the lesser sac. The trans-

verse colon is held on tension inferiorly, and the gastrocolic ligament is opened just distal to the falciform ligament to enter the lesser sac. In the lesser sac, the stomach can be reflected cephalad to expose the posterior gastric wall and the pancreas. The dissection is continued in this plane between the colon and the omentum, staying close to the colon wall, out toward the inferior pole of the spleen. The splenocolic ligament is taken down to free the colon from the spleen. The colon is then retracted inferomedially, and the mobilization is continued laterally to fully mobilize the descending colon from the lateral sidewall and release the splenic flexure.

6. Right lateral position. In cases where the lesser sac is tethered by adhesions, placing the patient in the right lateral position has been described to complete the mobilization. While this approach requires repositioning and redraping the patient, it provides excellent visualization of the splenic flexure, as the small bowel, stomach, and greater omentum fall away from the descending colon with minimal assistance or retraction. Three trocars are used: a 5-mm trocar in the left upper quadrant 2–3 cm below the costal margin at the midclavicular line, a 10-mm trocar at the umbilicus, and a 10-mm trocar in the left iliac fossa 2–3 cm medial to the anterior superior iliac spine. The camera is placed through the umbilical port. The lateral attachments of the descending colon are divided up to the splenic flexure, dissecting the mesocolon from Gerota's fascia. The tail of the pancreas and inferior mesenteric vein are identified, and the lesser sac is opened. The pancreas is separated from the transverse mesocolon, and the inferior mesenteric vein is fully mobilized to the inferior border of the pancreas. Splenic flexure mobilization is completed with high division of the inferior mesenteric vein just below the pancreas.
7. Change the patient position. While the procedure may be initiated in Trendelenburg, changing to reverse Trendelenburg is preferred when entering the lesser sac through the gastrocolic ligament. This positioning allows the transverse colon to fall away from the spleen from gravity without applying additional tension. Alternating between Trendelenburg and reverse Trendelenburg at any point when progress of the dissection slows may give a fresh approach and facilitate successfully completing the mobilization without converting to a HALS or open approach.
8. Hand assistance. Converting to hand-assisted laparoscopic surgery (HALS) or open surgery may provide additional retraction required to complete the mobilization. There may also be a need for finger dissection or palpation that cannot be achieved by a pure laparoscopic approach, and opening completely maybe necessary in the case injury to or bleeding from the surrounding anatomical structures. The hand-access port should be placed based on the location of the pathology and where you expect to exteriorize the colon.

Technical Pearls (Tips and Tricks)

1. Early mobilization of the splenic flexure posteriorly allows the flexure to drop down, increasing the distance between it and the capsule of the spleen in most cases.
2. Standing between the patient's legs and working through supraumbilical ports in the epigastrium can be a helpful approach.
3. An additional 5-mm port in the left upper quadrant port may be helpful, particularly in those with a very high splenic flexure, the very tall, or obese individuals.
4. In cases of difficult splenic flexure release, using multiple different approaches to the left upper quadrant and moving back and forth from one approach and back to another approach help release the attachments tethering the colon.
5. An energy device works well for limiting blood loss during takedown of the splenic flexure.
6. Consider leaving the omentum on the distal transverse colon.

7. Change the patient position (alternate between reverse Trendelenburg and Trendelenburg) for a fresh approach.
8. Adding a hand-assisted port can help overcome some of the most difficult splenic flexure releases. During a difficult hand-assisted splenic flexure release, the operating surgeon should be standing between the legs with their left hand in the abdomen and should use a left-sided instrument port. Placing the patient in steeper reverse Trendelenburg is helpful in hand-assisted cases as this delivers the field closer to the hand port.
9. Converting to an open procedure is not a sign of failure; converting to open surgery may be the safest way to complete the operation. Consider converting if the operation does not progress despite trying the available maneuvers. It is important to recognize that, in experienced hands, a difficult splenic flexure release will still be very difficult after converting to an open approach. In this situation, having a dedicated assistant retracting the left upper quadrant abdominal wall is very helpful as the retraction needed is dynamic and changes as the flexure is approached from any number of directions. A self-retaining body wall retractor can also be used but is not as helpful as an assistant.
10. To completely release the splenic flexure, the base of the transverse mesocolon needs to be dissected free from the inferior edge of the pancreas. This release should extend to the level of the ligament of Treitz in order to fully release the flexure and provide the needed distal reach to the pelvis.

Suggested Reading

1. Frame RJ, Wahed S, Mohiuddin MK, Katory M. Right lateral position for laparoscopic splenic flexure mobilization. Color Dis. 2011;13(7):e178–80.
2. Kye BH, Kim HJ, Kim HS, Kim JG, Cho HM. How much colonic redundancy could be obtained by splenic flexure mobilization in laparoscopic anterior or low anterior resection? Int J Med Sci. 2014;11(9):857–62.
3. Reddy SH, Gupta V, Yadav TD, Singh G, Sahni D. Lengthening of left colon after rectal resection: what all is adequate? A prospective cohort study. Int J Surg. 2016;31:27–32.
4. Ross HM, Lee SW, Mutch MG, Rivadeneira DE, Steele SR. Laparoscopic sigmoidectomy/left colectomy. In: Minimally invasive approaches to colon and rectal disease technique and best practices. New York: Springer; 2015. p. 71–80.
5. Schlussel AT, Wiseman JT, Kelly JF, Davids JS, Maykel JA, Sturrock PR, Sweeney WB, Alavi K. Location is everything: the role of splenic flexure mobilization during colon resection for diverticulitis. Int J Surg. 2017;40:124–9.

Hartmann Takedown: Managing the Hard to Reach or Devascularized Left Colon

18

Christine Hsieh and Sang W. Lee

Clinical Scenario

A 55-year-old male underwent a Hartmann procedure for perforated sigmoid diverticulitis. After 6 months, the patient underwent an unsuccessful attempt at reversing the colostomy during which the left and the distal two-thirds of the transverse colon were removed due to intraoperative devascularization. The patient has now has a proximal transverse colon end colostomy and presents for another attempt at stoma reversal.

Key Points

1. Preoperative planning is critically important when performing a Hartmann takedown. In many cases, patients have undergone the index procedure elsewhere, and documentation may be variable. In addition to understanding the indications for the patient's initial operation, any operative reports and images should be reviewed with the following in mind.
   (a) Length and location of resected colon
   (b) Length of the rectal stump and its relation to the pelvic viscera
   (c) Remaining vascular pedicles and collateral blood supply
2. Success of a pelvic colorectal anastomosis depends upon the creation of a tension-free anastomosis and maintenance of adequate blood supply to the proximal and distal aspects of the fashioned anastomosis.
   (a) This is facilitated by mobilization of the proximal colon as well as the rectal stump, at times.
   (b) Obtaining adequate exposure is required in order to perform a safe anastomosis free of surrounding structures and tissues.
3. In some cases, the proximal transverse colon to rectal anastomosis has to be performed as the transverse and left colon were previously removed or need to be resected because of devascularization.
   (a) A retroileal pull-through of the transverse colon whereby the transverse colon is delivered into the pelvis behind the ileocolic pedicle.
   (b) The Deloyers procedure is a salvage maneuver in which the right colon is completely mobilized and rotated counterclockwise into the pelvis to perform an anastomosis between the right colon and rectal stump.

C. Hsieh
Keck School of Medicine – University of Southern California, Los Angeles, CA, USA

S. W. Lee (✉)
Department of Surgery – Colon and Rectal Surgery, Keck School of Medicine of University of Southern California, Los Angeles, CA, USA

S. W. Lee et al. (eds.), *Colorectal Surgery Consultation*,
https://doi.org/10.1007/978-3-030-11181-6_18

Operative Assessment

1. How much of the colon is remaining?
   (a) Sigmoid colostomy.
      (i) Mobilize flexure.
      (ii) High ligation of vessels.
      (iii) Side-to-end anastomosis.
      (iv) Rectal mobilization.
   (b) Distal transverse colostomy.
      (i) Mobilize colon proximally.
      (ii) Rectal mobilization.
      (iii) Retroileal pass.
   (c) Proximal transverse colostomy.
      (i) Deloyers procedure.
      (ii) Ileorectal procedure.
2. Is the colon fully mobilized?
   (a) Takedown splenic flexure.
   (b) High ligation of inferior mesenteric artery (IMA) and inferior mesenteric vein (IMV).
3. Is the rectal stump fully mobilized?
   (a) Depending on the patient's circumstances at the time of initial operation, the rectal stump may vary significantly in regard to length and positioning within the pelvis.
4. Does the anastomosis itself require reconfiguration?
   (a) A side-to-end Baker-style anastomosis may reach more easily into the pelvis than an end-to-end anastomosis (Fig. 18.1).
   (b) An ileorectal anastomosis or ileal pouch-anal anastomosis (IPAA) may need to be entertained in the rare circumstance that the colon will not reach into the pelvis at all.

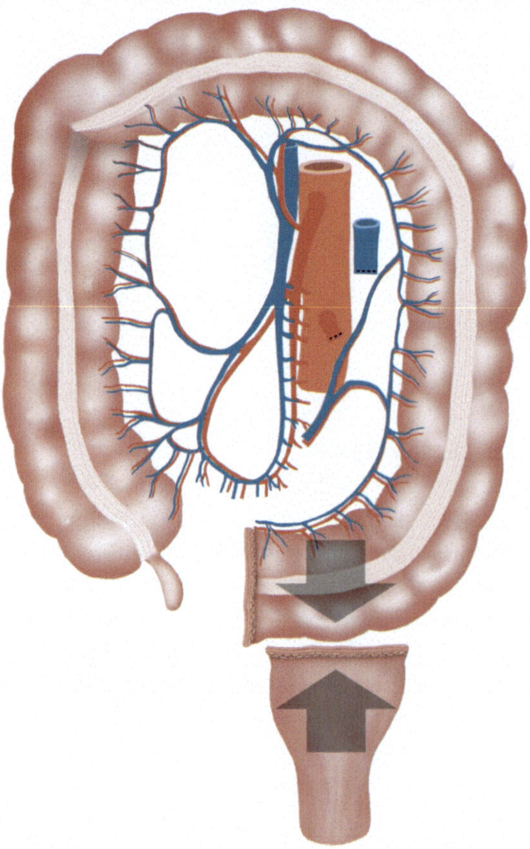

Fig. 18.1 A Baker-type side-to-end anastomosis will allow greater reach down into the pelvis for a tension-free colorectal anastomosis

Operative Checklist

1. Additional helpful equipment
   (a) Long pelvic instrument tray
   (b) Long continuous sutures
   (c) Pelvic retractors (lighted retractors if available)
   (d) Good lighting (headlights)
   (e) Rigid proctoscope or flexible sigmoidoscope
2. Positioning
   (a) Patients are typically positioned in lithotomy or on a split-leg table for access to the rectum.

Operative Techniques

1. Splenic flexure mobilization
   (a) Perform splenic flexure mobilization by dividing the lateral peritoneal attachments in the left upper quadrant, separating the omentum from the distal transverse colon, dividing attachments to Gerota's fascia of the left kidney, and lysing adhesions between the transverse colon mesentery and the posterior wall of the stomach (Fig. 18.2).

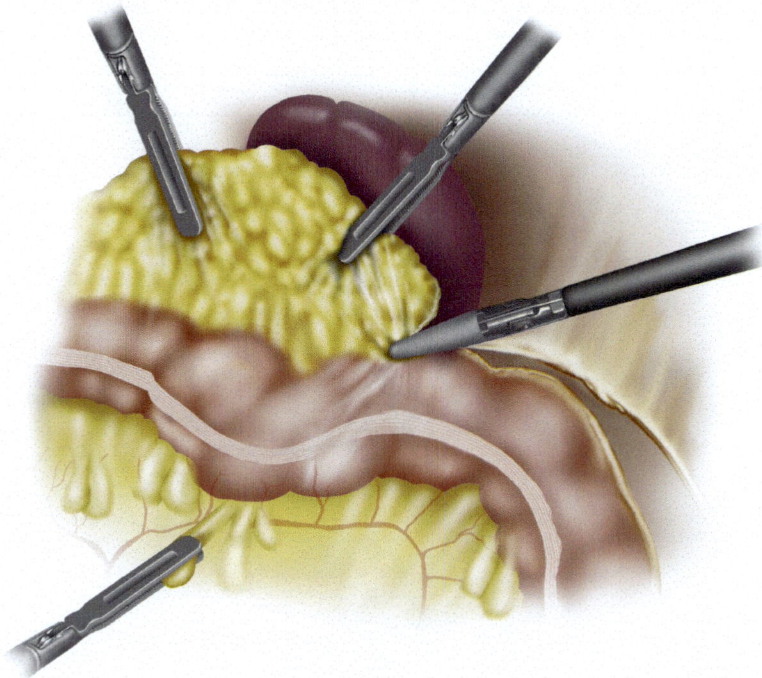

Fig. 18.2 Splenic flexure mobilization: If left colon to rectal mobilization, splenic flexure mobilization will provide additional reach

2. High vessel ligation
   (a) Additional length can be attained by high vessel ligation. Ligate the IMA at its origin, and disconnect the left colic artery. Dividing the IMV at the inferior edge of the pancreas also allows for further mobilization (Fig. 18.3). In the event that the descending colon becomes devascularized and resection of the splenic flexure is necessary, the mobility of the transverse colon will become limited by the tethering of the middle colic vessels. Serial ligation of the middle colic vessels from left to right can provide more length, thus relying on the marginal artery to perfuse the anastomosis. Careful assessment of perfusion must be performed and additional colon resected until adequate arterial inflow and venous drainage are confirmed.
3. Rectal stump mobilization
   (a) "If the mountain will not come to Muhammad, then Muhammad must go to the mountain." Mobilizing the rectum will provide significant additional length. Dissect circumferentially around the rectal stump in the mesorectal fascial plane, and proceed with sharp dissection distally into the presacral space. It is important not to devascularize the rectum as dissection proceeds. An end-to-end anastomotic (EEA) sizer inserted into the rectal stump helps to elucidate planes and demonstrate mobility of the stump.
4. Side-to-end anastomosis
   (a) The limiting factor in distal reach of the left colon is often the vasculature and not the colon. The portion of the left colon with the longest reach is usually not the end of the left colon but the colon proximal to it in line with either IMA or superior hemorrhoidals. A Baker-type side-to-end anastomosis will allow greater reach down into the pelvis for a tension-free colorectal anastomosis (Fig. 18.1).
5. Retroileal pull-through (Fig. 18.4)
   (a) When a transverse colon to rectum anastomosis must be performed, rotating the colon along the left gutter and into the pelvis may become difficult. A direct

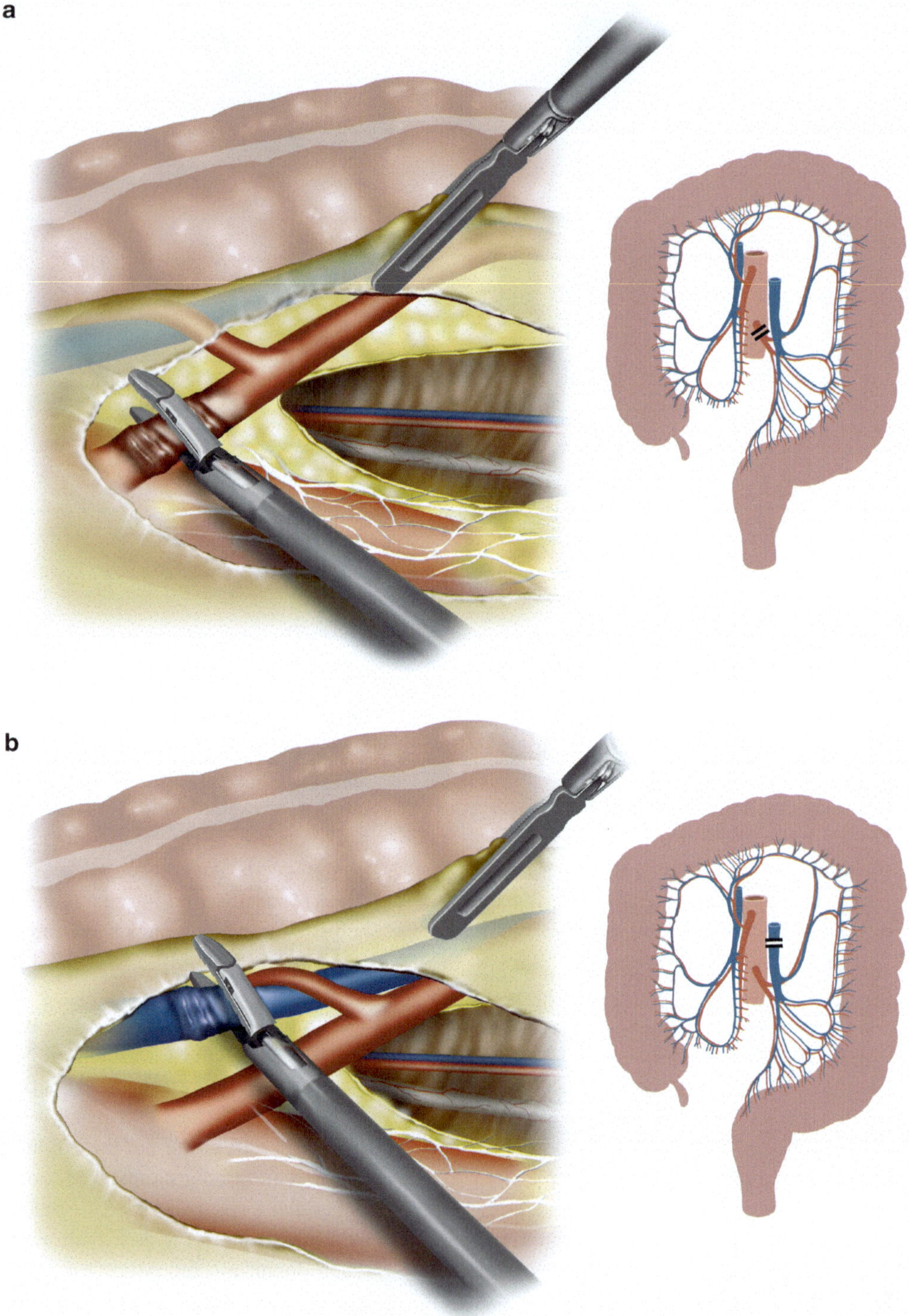

Fig. 18.3 Additional length can be attained by high vessel ligation. Ligate the inferior mesenteric artery (IMA) at its origin (**a**), and disconnect the left colic artery. Dividing the inferior mesenteric vein (IMV) at the inferior edge of the pancreas (**b**) also allows for further mobilization

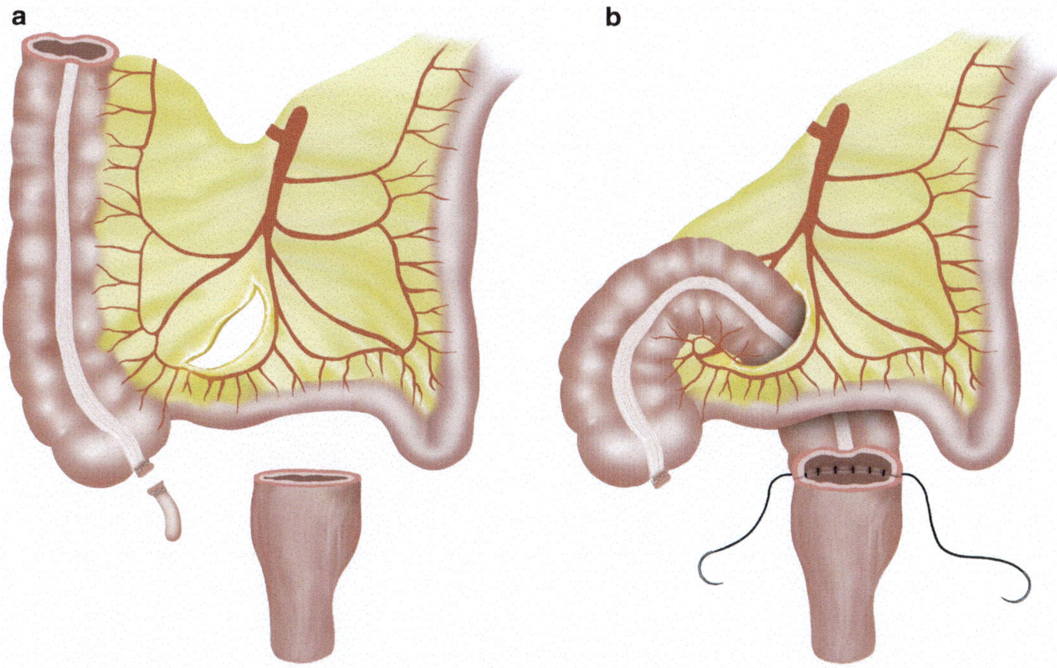

Fig. 18.4 Retroileal pull-through. Take down the hepatic flexure (**a**), and pass the end of the colon through the opening toward the pelvis (**b**)

path from the midline of the body into the pelvis is not advisable as this may entrap small bowel underneath the mesentery and create tension upon the anastomosis. To circumvent these problems, create a window caudal to the ileocolic pedicle in the terminal ileal mesentery that will accommodate the transverse colon and mesentery. Take down the hepatic flexure, and pass the end of the colon through the opening and into the pelvis.

6. Deloyers procedure (Fig. 18.5)
   (a) Failure to reach through a retroileal window may occur if a proximal transverse colon to rectum anastomosis is attempted. The Deloyers procedure entails mobilizing the hepatic flexure and right colon off the retroperitoneum before rotating the colon counterclockwise into the pelvis. The middle colic pedicle must be sacrificed in this case, and perfusion thus relies on the ileocolic pedicle. Appendectomy should be performed.

Technical Pearls (Tips and Tricks)

1. Bowel perfusion may be assessed visually, by palpation of the mesentery or by handheld Doppler ultrasound, but newer technologies such as ICG fluorescence may be a very helpful adjunct.
2. Be wary of creating a high-risk anastomosis – in some cases, recreating a stoma will be the necessary, safe procedure for the patient.
3. Having ureteral stents can facilitate this reoperative dissection.

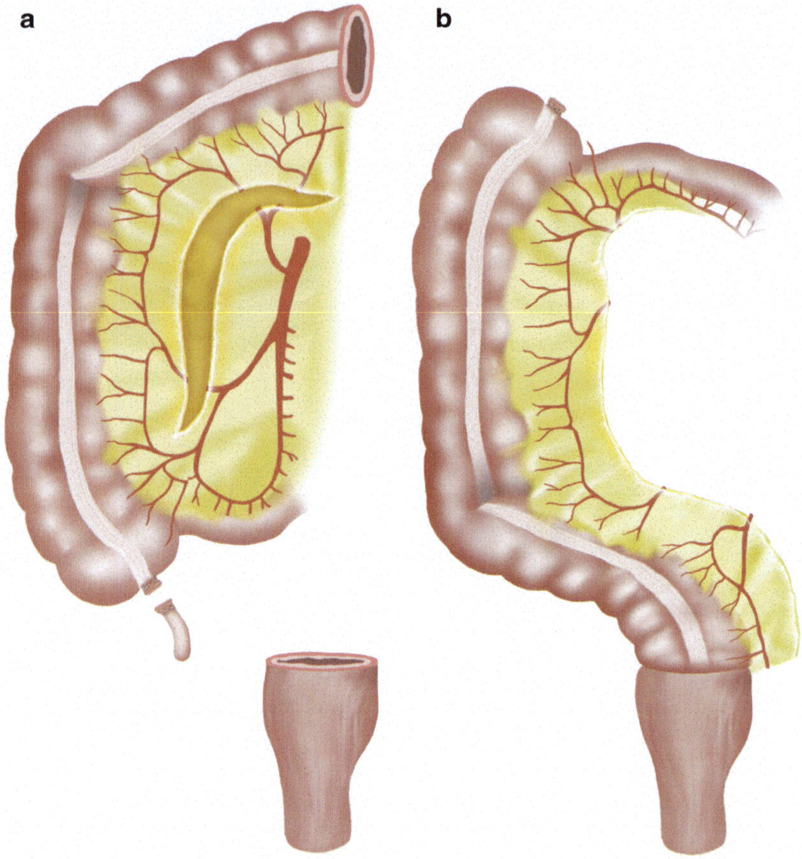

Fig. 18.5 The Deloyers procedure entails mobilizing the hepatic flexure and right colon off the retroperitoneum before rotating the colon counterclockwise into the pelvis (**a**). The middle colic pedicle must be sacrificed in this case, and perfusion thus relies on the ileocolic pedicle. Appendectomy should be performed (**b**)

Special Postoperative Care

1. Diet can be advanced as usual.
2. Drain placement may be advisable, especially after low pelvic dissection.

Suggested Reading

1. Dunlavy P, Allan L, Raman S. Totally laparoscopic retroileal transverse colon to rectal anastomosis following extended left colectomy. Dis Colon Rectum. 2017;60(11):1224.
2. Hunt SR, Silviera ML. Anastomotic construction. In: Steele SR, Hull TL, Read TE, Saclarides TJ, Senagore AJ, Whitlow CB, editors. The ASCRS textbook of colon and rectal surgery. 3rd ed. New York: Springer; 2016. p. 141–60.
3. Manceau G, Karoui M, et al. Right colon to rectal anastomosis (Deloyers Procedure) as a salvage technique for low colorectal or coloanal anastomosis: postoperative and long-term outcomes. Dis Colon Rectum. 2012;55(3):363–8.
4. Rombeau JL, Collins JP, Turnbull RB. Left-sided colectomy with retroileal colorectal anastomosis. Arch Surg. 1978;113(8):1004–5.
5. Shariff US, Kullar N, Dorudi S. Right colonic transposition technique: when the left colon is unavailable for achieving a pelvic anastomosis. Dis Colon Rectum. 2011;54(3):360–2.

Cannot Find the Rectal Stump During Hartmann Reversal

19

David E. Rivadeneira

Clinical Scenario

You are in the operating room attempting to reverse a prior open Hartmann procedure done for perforated diverticulitis 3 months ago by another surgeon from another hospital in a 56-year-old male with a body mass index (BMI) of 40 kg/m^2. You attempt a laparoscopic approach; however, it becomes very apparent that he has significant dense adhesions and you convert. After several hours of lysing adhesions and disconnecting the colostomy from mucocutaneous junction and left abdominal wall, you look for the rectal stump, and you are unable to find it.

Key Points

1. Use caution in reversing a colostomy in a patient in whom you did not do the original Hartmann procedure. These situations are filled with many unknowns that can often cause significant angst for the surgeon and potential complications for the patient.
2. Review prior operative reports and pathology. These will often indicate how extensive the prior surgery was and how much of the sigmoid colon and, possibly, rectum was removed. The prior operative report may indicate how they dealt with the stump. Was it stapled off? Was a suture tag placed for future identification? Was it tacked to the abdominal wall?
3. Imaging studies with rectal contrast should be performed preoperatively as this will demonstrate the length and contour of the rectal stump and may demonstrate the presence of retained sigmoid diverticula that may need to be addressed. Imaging studies such as a CT scan with rectal contrast or a gastrografin enema study through the rectal stump and colostomy are very useful in providing a "road map" and are recommended.
4. Preoperative endoscopy through the rectal stump will also reveal the condition and the length of the rectal stump and can be used to evacuate any retained contrast medium or inspissated mucus balls that can interfere with passing up an end-to-end anastomotic (EEA) stapler at the time of the reversal surgery.
5. Avoid taking down the colostomy or committing to the operation until you have identified the rectal stump and have inserted an EEA sizer (Ethicon Endo-Surgery, Inc.) or stapler to assure patency of the stump. In certain situations, however, it may make sense to start the

D. E. Rivadeneira (✉)
Surgical Strategic Initiatives, Northwell Health, New Hyde Park, NY, USA

Surgical Services and Colorectal Surgery, Huntington Hospital, Huntington, NY, USA

Hofstra University-Northwell School of Medicine, Hempstead, NY, USA
e-mail: DRivadeneira@northwell.edu

S. W. Lee et al. (eds.), *Colorectal Surgery Consultation*,
https://doi.org/10.1007/978-3-030-11181-6_19

operation by taking down the end colostomy, closing the fascia here and placing a port at this site to insufflate the abdomen and insert a camera to start a laparoscopic stoma reversal.

6. Accurate preoperative assessment of the height of the rectal stump is critical. Very short rectal stump would indicate that the operation will be difficult and proper preparation should be made accordingly.
7. Preoperative discussion with the patient should include a possibility that Hartmann takedown may not be feasible or that, even if is possible, a second protective ileostomy may be needed.

Operative Assessment

1. Will you be able to perform the operation safely laparoscopic? Will you need a hand-assisted technique or open approach?
2. After performing a thorough assessment of the abdomen and pelvis, is the rectal stump visible?
3. Will you need additional help and/or an assistant with an experience?
4. Will you need stents for the ureters?
5. It is more common that a long Hartmann stump including some retained sigmoid colon be present well above the peritoneal reflection and usually can be identified quickly. However, if the first surgery resulted in an overly aggressive distal resection, then the rectal stump may be well below the peritoneal reflection and may not be easily identifiable.

Operative Checklist

1. Instrumentation
   (a) Extra-long instruments
   (b) St. Mark's Retractor, preferably lighted
   (c) EEA sizers/dilators.
   (d) Rigid proctoscope/flexible sigmoidoscope
   (e) Proper laparoscopic graspers
2. Positioning
   A. Lithotomy/split leg

Operative Technique

1. Survey the abdomen.
2. Perform thorough lysis of adhesions. Clear the pelvis of any adherent loops of small bowel. Often a loop of small bowel will adhere itself to the rectal stump suture or staple line. Let the small bowel loops in the pelvis lead you to the stump.
3. If a distal resection was performed at the original operation, then the stump will be situated in the low pelvis, often below the peritoneal reflection.
4. Manipulating an EEA sizer in the rectum will aid in identifying the Hartmann stump.
5. A lighted rigid proctoscope or flexible sigmoidoscope can be used to trans-illuminate the stump.
6. In female patients, placing a dilator or sponge on a stick into the vagina can help delineate the posterior wall of vagina and facilitate dissection from the anterior wall of the rectal stump.
7. Start the dissection in the posterior midline after palpating the sacral promontory. This will avoid injury to the lateral neurovascular structures and the ureters. This dissection usually starts by scoring the peritoneum and gaining access to the underlying tissues that have been scarred over. Once the peritoneum is incised, a plane can be developed posteriorly and then laterally.
8. Proceed with rectal stump posterior midline dissection, and then advance to more lateral wall dissection and finally with an anterior dissection.

Technical Pearls (Tips and Tricks)

1. At the time of the Hartmann's procedure, placing guide sutures at each corner of the rectal staple line can aid in identifying the rectal stump at the time of the reversal (Fig. 19.1).
2. Don't hesitate to insert an EEA dilator (Fig. 19.2) or an EEA sizer into the rectal stump. This will help delineate the contour of the stump.

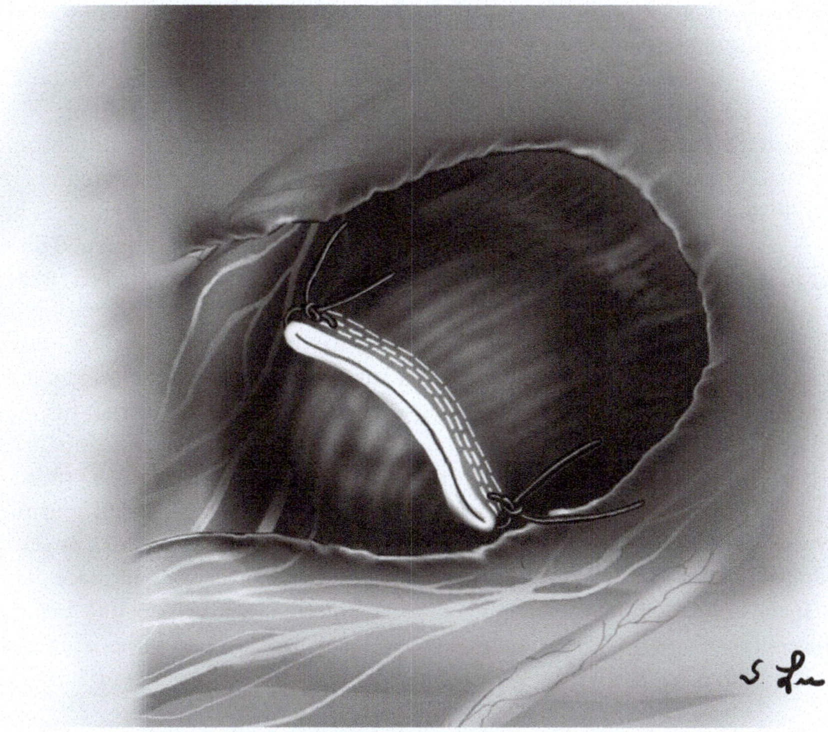

Fig. 19.1 At the time of Hartmann's procedure, placing guide sutures at each corner of the rectal staple line can aid in identifying the rectal stump at the time of the reversal

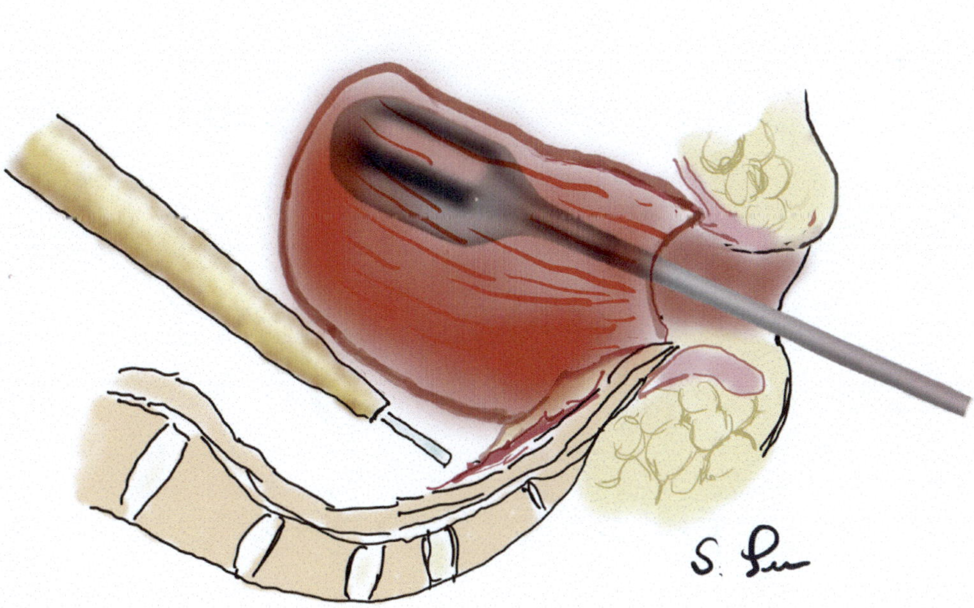

Fig. 19.2 Inserting an end-to-end anastomotic (EEA) sizer into the rectal stump can help delineate the contour of the stump

3. In women, placing a dilator into the vagina will aid in dissecting the vaginal wall from the rectal stump.
4. Do not disconnect the colostomy site until you have identified the stump.
5. Use a lighted rigid proctoscope or flexible sigmoidoscopy to help trans-illuminate the rectal stump.
6. If the stump is in the mid to low pelvis, then start the pelvic dissection in the midline, as this will often be the easiest and safest place to start looking for the stump. Use the sacral promontory as a marker of the midline, and palpate the aortic bifurcation and the common iliac arteries to appreciate the anatomy.
7. If a relatively short rectal stump is remaining, simultaneous digital manipulation of the rectal stump from below while dissecting from above may delineate the anatomy better (Fig. 19.3).
8. Remember loops of small bowel often will adhere themselves to the rectal stump. Follow the small bowel into the pelvis, and it will often lead you to the stump.
9. In the event that the lumen of the end of the retained sigmoid or of the proximal rectum is entered during the dissection, it is helpful to use this as a guide for continued dissection.
10. In cases of a scarred pelvis that has re-peritonealized over the rectal stump, it is easy to veer off midline. It is important to identify and preserve the ureters during this dissection as they are at risk for injury, and having ureteral stents can facilitate this.
11. In many emergent Hartmann procedures, the sigmoid mesentery is taken mid-mesentery leaving the main sigmoidal artery and the superior hemorrhoidals in place. This tissue can interfere with dissecting out the rectal cuff and would need to be addressed at the time of attempted reversal.

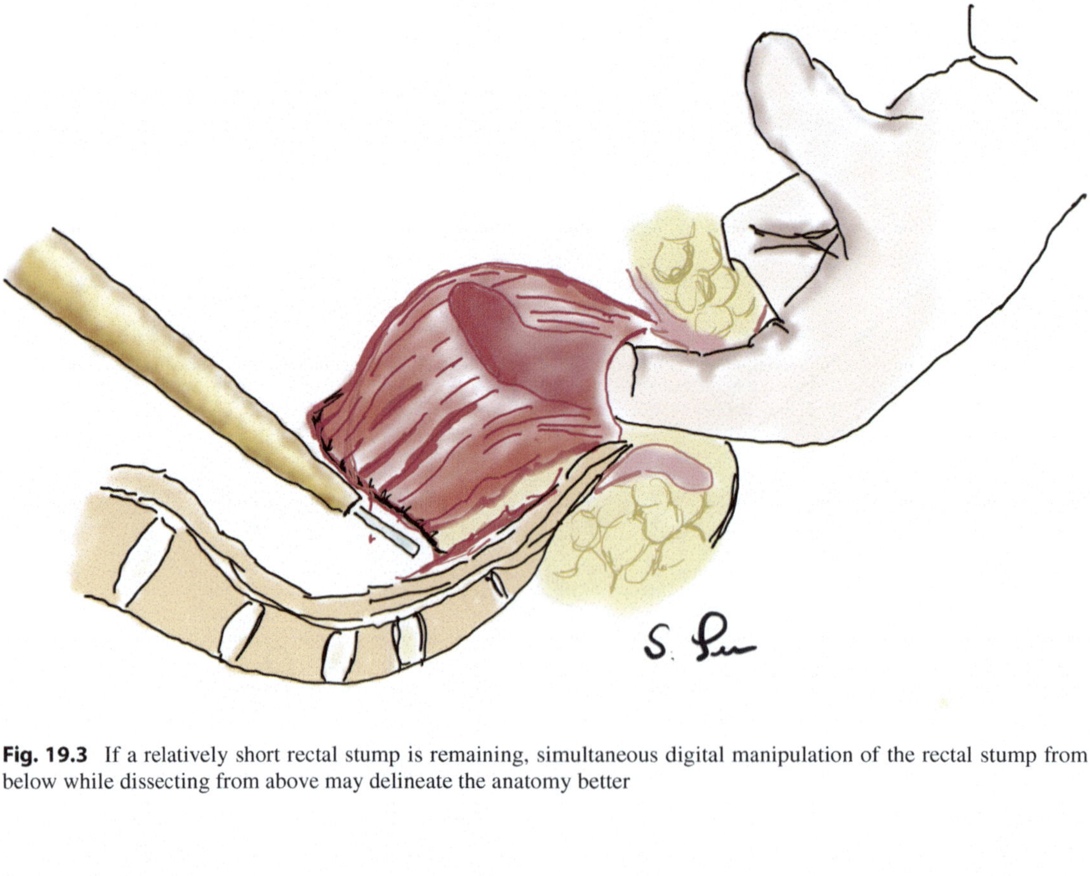

Fig. 19.3 If a relatively short rectal stump is remaining, simultaneous digital manipulation of the rectal stump from below while dissecting from above may delineate the anatomy better

Special Postoperative Care

1. There are no special considerations per se, and standard postoperative care should be followed.

Suggested Reading

1. Gorgun E. Laparoscopic stoma reversal. In: Ross, Lee, Mutch, Rivadeneira, Steele, editors. Minimally invasive approaches to colon and rectal disease: technique and best practice. New York: Springer; 2015.

Rectal Stump Perforation Stump While Passing an End-to-End Anastomotic Stapler

20

Sang W. Lee

Clinical Scenario

A 60-year-old male with rectal cancer is undergoing a low anterior resection. The distal resection margin was transected using a TA stapler, and the specimen was removed. While performing a double-stapled end-to-end anastomosis (EEA), the rectal staple line was inadvertently disrupted due to forceful passage of the stapler.

Key Points

1. Try to prevent this complication by effectively communicating with your assistant who is passing the stapler.
   (a) Remind him/her that it is a low anastomosis.
   (b) Dilate the anal canal prior to passing the stapler.
   (c) Consider using a smaller stapler with a smaller diameter than usual.
2. Upper rectal stump disruption should be approached from above.
3. Distal rectal stump disruption may be repaired from below.
4. After repairing a disrupted staple line, even if the anastomosis is complete and no air leak is detected, it may be prudent to consider diverting the patient.
5. Even in diverted patients, chronic pelvis sepsis can occur if the anastomosis is inadequately healed. The best time to deal with a TA staple line disruption is when it occurs.

Operative Assessment

1. How much of the rectal staple line is disrupted?
   (a) A small, limited disruption may be amenable to local repair followed by EEA anastomosis.
   (b) A complete or major disruption of the staple line will require reclosure of the staple line (Fig. 20.1).
2. Where is the level of the rectal staple line?
   (a) Upper rectal staple line disruption is usually amenable to an abdominal approach.
   (b) Distal rectal disruption may be more easily approached using a transanal repair.

Operative Checklist

1. Additional helpful equipment
   (a) Abdominal approach
      (i) Long pelvic instrument tray
      (ii) Long continuous sutures
      (iii) Pelvic retractors (lighted retractors, if available)

S. W. Lee (✉)
Department of Surgery – Colon and Rectal Surgery, Keck School of Medicine of University of Southern California, Los Angeles, CA, USA

S. W. Lee et al. (eds.), *Colorectal Surgery Consultation*,
https://doi.org/10.1007/978-3-030-11181-6_20

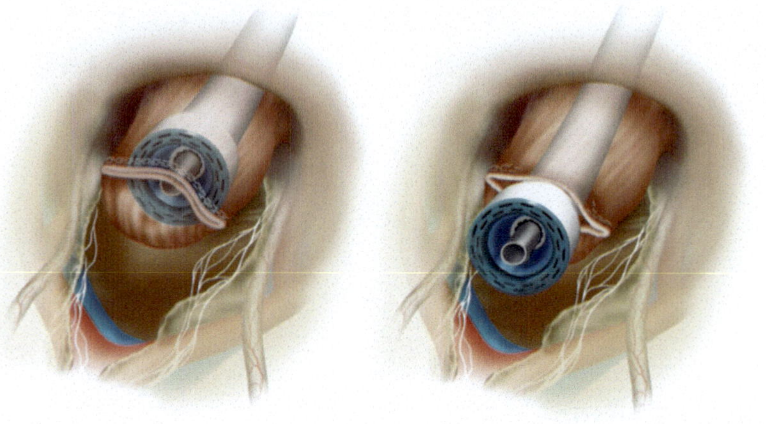

Fig. 20.1 Complete disruption of the staple line will require either re-stapling or purse-string placement

(iv) Good lighting (headlights)

(b) Transanal approach

(i) Anoscopes: Hill-Ferguson, Pratt bivalve, or purse-string suture. Anoscope from a stapled hemorrhoidopexy kit

2. Exposure
   (a) If occurred during a laparoscopic procedure, consider making either a low midline incision or Pfannenstiel incision.
3. Positioning
   (a) Patients who are undergoing low anterior resections are already in lithotomy position. For the abdominal approach, there is no need for repositioning.
   (b) For transanal approaches, patients need to be placed in the exaggerated lithotomy position.

Operative Techniques

1. Abdominal approach suture repair
   (a) Limited disruption of TA staple line can be suture repaired primarily. Interrupted rather than continuous suture repair should be done since the EEA stapler knife can cut and undo the entire running suture. If possible, try to incorporate the repaired TA staple line in the donuts of the EEA stapler.
2. Abdominal approach reapproximation using a TA stapler
   (a) For sigmoid and upper rectal staple line disruptions, it is often feasible to dissect the distal stump further distally. The disrupted staple line is reapproximated using a series of long Allis clamps to prevent contamination and further disruption of the staple line. These clamps are also very helpful in applying traction during the rectal mobilization. Once enough of the rectal or sigmoid stump is mobilized, a TA stapler is fired distal to the disrupted area creating a fresh, closed rectal cuff (Fig. 20.2).
3. Abdominal approach reapproximation using a purse-string suture placement
   (a) Alternatively, the disrupted TA staple line can be excised, and a full-thickness purse-string suture can be placed around the circumference of the opened rectal stump. Guide sutures or Allis clamps placed at the corners can be helpful in placing the purse string. The EEA stapler is introduced into the rectum, and the purse-string suture is then tied after full extension of the center rod spike of the EEA stapler (Fig. 20.3).
4. Transanal placement of full-thickness purse-string placement
   (a) In the case of a very distal rectal stump staple line dehiscence, it may not be possible to re-staple from above, and transabdominal purse-string suture placement in

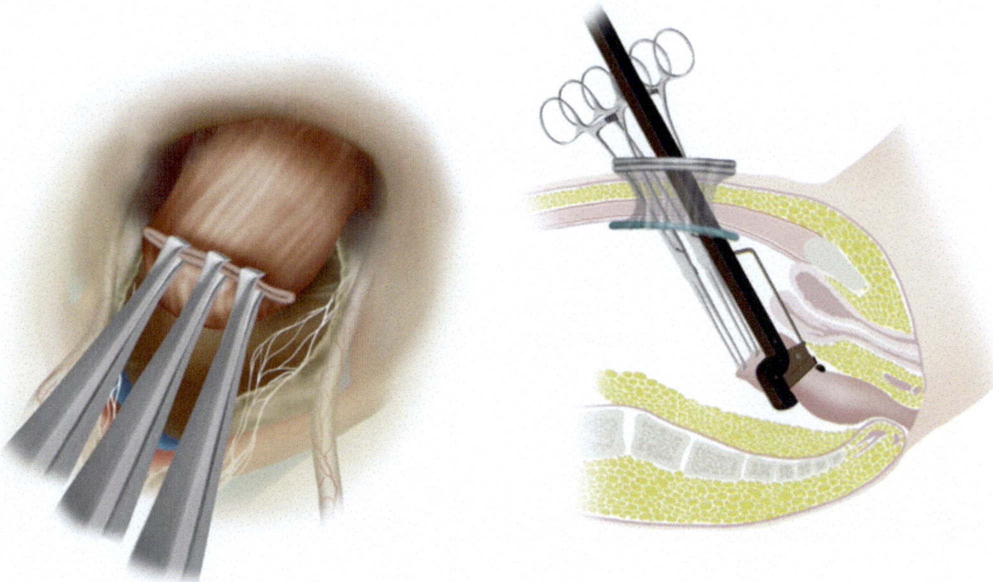

Fig. 20.2 Abdominal approach reapproximation using a TA stapler. For upper to mid-rectal stump staple line disruption, further rectal dissection followed by re-stapling can be performed

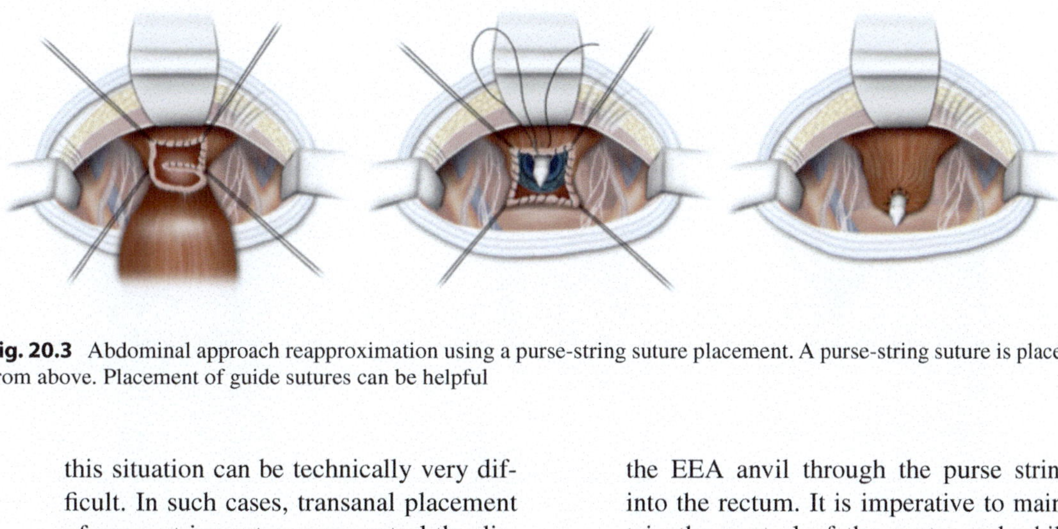

Fig. 20.3 Abdominal approach reapproximation using a purse-string suture placement. A purse-string suture is placed from above. Placement of guide sutures can be helpful

this situation can be technically very difficult. In such cases, transanal placement of purse-string suture can control the disrupted rectal cuff. A Hill-Ferguson or Pratt bivalve anoscope can be used for this purpose. Alternatively, the purse-string suture anoscope from a stapled hemorrhoidopexy kit can be used. In this approach, the purse-string suture has to be tied from the anal side, and, because of it, it is important to deliver the center rod of the EEA anvil through the purse string into the rectum. It is imperative to maintain the control of the center rod while tying down the purse-string suture (Fig. 20.4).

5. Mucosectomy and hand-sewn coloanal anastomosis
   (a) If none of the options listed above are feasible, transanal mucosectomy followed by hand-sewn coloanal anastomosis may be required (Figs. 20.5 and 20.6).

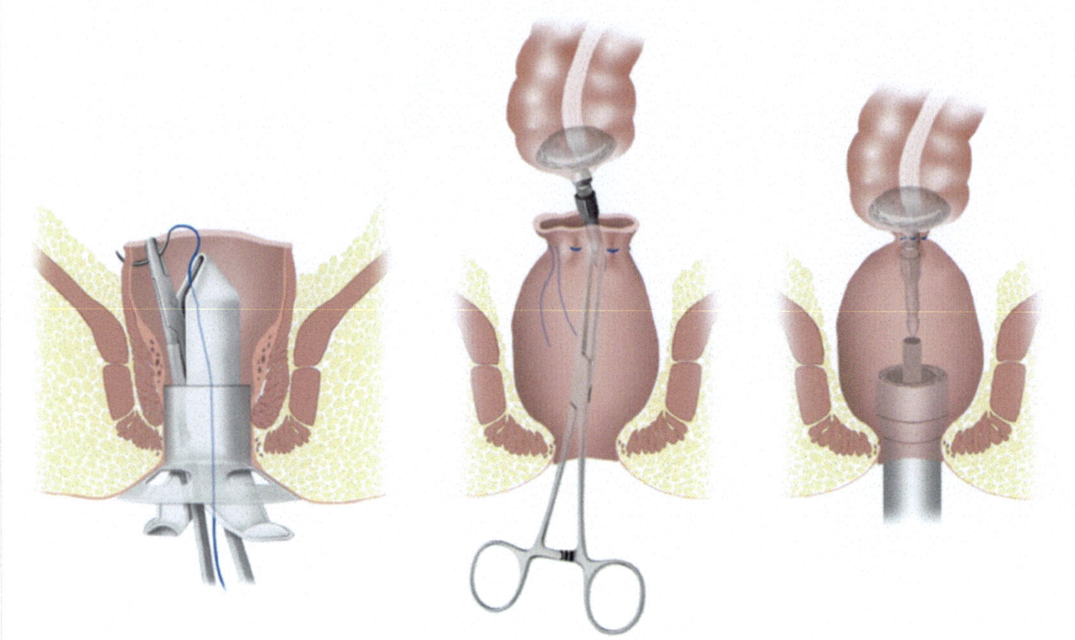

Fig. 20.4 Transanal placement of full-thickness purse-string placement. The purse-string anoscope from the stapled hemorrhoidectomy kit can be used to perform transanal full-thickness purse-string sutures

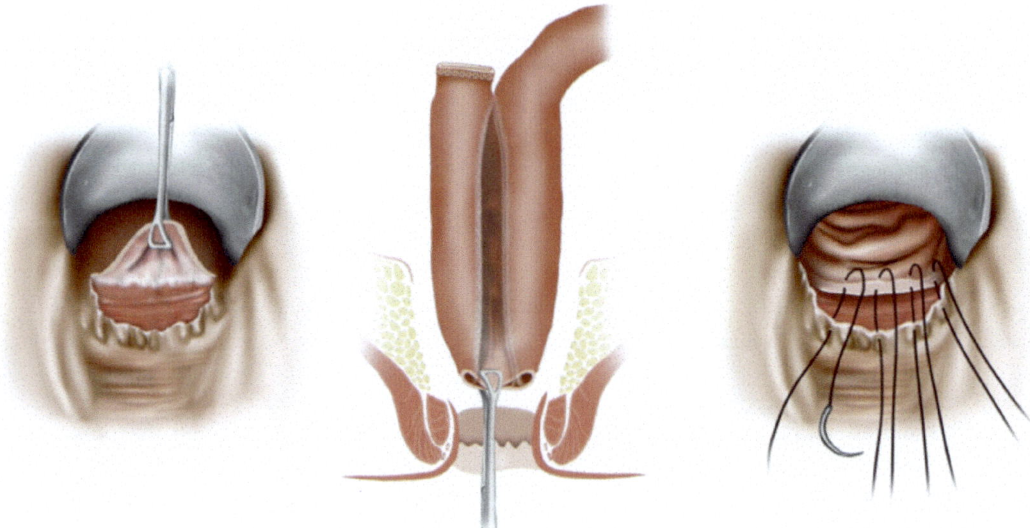

Fig. 20.5 Mucosectomy and hand-sewn pouch anal anastomosis. Mucosectomy is performed starting at the dentate line. The J pouch is delivered through the anus and circumferential interrupted hand-sewn anastomosis performed

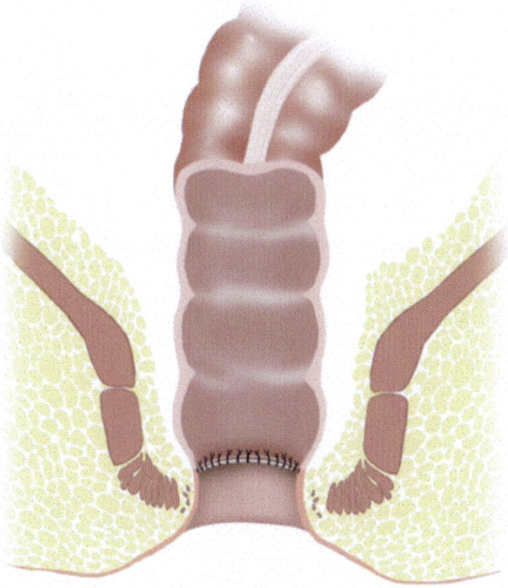

Fig. 20.6 Mucosectomy and hand-sewn coloanal anastomosis

Technical Pearls (Tips and Tricks)

1. For the abdominal approach, it is helpful to assess the integrity of the reapproximated distal colon/rectal stump prior to performing an anastomosis. Preferably, flexible endoscopy should be performed to accomplish this. At minimum, an air leak test should be performed.
2. For primary suture repair of small staple line disruptions, interrupted rather than continuous suture repair should be done since EEA stapler knife can undo the entire running suture.
3. Try to incorporate the repaired TA staple line in the donuts of the EEA stapler.
4. Even if the anastomosis is complete and no air leak is detected, it may be prudent to consider diverting the patient.
5. Distal rectal dissection can be facilitated by having an assistant push up the anorectum from the perineal side.
6. For the transanal purse-string placement technique, using the purse-string suture anoscope from a stapled hemorrhoidopexy kit may be very helpful. Maintaining control of the center rod of the anvil while tying down the purse suture from below is essential.

Special Postoperative Care

1. Diet can be advanced as usual.
2. If there is significant contamination, 24 hours of IV antibiotics can be considered.
3. It is my preference to leave a drain in the pelvis if dissection is performed below the peritoneal reflection.

Suggested Reading

1. Smallwood N, Mutch MG, Fleshman JW. The failed anastomosis. In: Steele SR, Maykel JA, Champagne BJ, Orangio GR, editors. Complexities in colorectal surgery. New York: Springer Publ; 2014. p. 447–62.

Inabilty to Pass End-to-End Anastomotic Stapler

21

Howard M. Ross

Clinical Scenario

For 2.5 hours, you perform a hand-assisted laparoscopic sigmoid colon resection on Mrs. R. She is morbidly obese and had a nearly complete, symptomatic large bowel obstruction due to a diverticular stricture. After complete splenic flexure mobilization, the phlegmon was freed from the pelvic sidewall and posterior uterus. The distal sigmoid colon was divided with a stapler, and the main sigmoid artery was divided with a tissue sealing device. All is good. You make a colotomy proximal to the phlegmon and place the EEA anvil through the colotomy and feed it proximally. The left colon is then stapled proximal to the colotomy, and the specimen is passed off the field. The anvil's trocar is brought out through the colon staple line, and you begin thinking about lunch. Your partner goes below to pass the EEA stapler via the anus, but it simply won't make it to the rectal transection line.

H. M. Ross (✉)
Division of Colon and Rectal Surgery,
Lewis Katz School of Medicine at Temple University and the Temple University Health System,
Philadelphia, PA, USA
e-mail: Howard.Ross@tuhs.temple.edu

Key Points

1. There is little more frustrating in colon and rectal surgery than having difficulty passing the end-to-end anastomotic (EEA) stapler.
2. The inability to pass the stapler often occurs at the end of a case when the entire surgical team may be tired and hopeful for the prompt conclusion of the operation.
3. Knowledge of options and management of the team is essential.
4. Surgical maneuvers to pass an EEA stapler that seemingly won't advance include further distal rectal mobilization, further distal rectal dissection and then additional resection of the proximal rectum, end left colon to side proximal rectal stapler anastomosis, and gentle dilation of the rectum with sequentially larger rectal dilators.

Operative Assessment

1. Evaluate where the stapler gets caught and why the stapler is not advancing.
2. Ensure visualization of the pelvis is optimized.
3. Review checklist of options with entire team.
4. Use well-lubricated EEA sizers to evaluate the anatomy. Do not force the stapler or EEA sizers against resistance as this will split the rectal wall.

S. W. Lee et al. (eds.), *Colorectal Surgery Consultation*,
https://doi.org/10.1007/978-3-030-11181-6_21

Operative Checklist

1. Additional helpful equipment to facilitate exposure:
   (a) An additional 5 mm port
   (b) A fan extractor to lift floppy bladder or uterus
   (c) A Keith needle to lift the uterus
2. Exposure:
   (a) A need for complete visualization of both sides of the rectum down to deep pelvis is mandatory
   (b) All maneuvers to gain exposure should be readily employed
3. Positioning:
   (a) Steep Trendelenburg to deliver small bowel from pelvis and keep all intestines away from field
4. Operative techniques:
   (a) Mobilize both lateral sides of the rectum and also anteriorly by scoring the peritoneum. The enhanced mobility of the rectum may allow the stapler to now pass.
   (b) Mobilize the proximal rectum down to the point where the stapler does not advance. Resect the additional proximal rectum at this point (Fig. 21.1). At times the proximal rectum lacks the luminal diameter of the more capacious distal rectum. Resection at this point allows end-to-end anastomosis.
   (c) Create a stapled anastomosis from the side of the rectum distal to the stapled rectal cuff to the end of the left colon (Fig. 21.2). This technique allows safe anastomosis. Adequate mobilization of left colon is mandatory. This author demands a 2 cm "gap" between the transection line at the most proximal rectum and the edge of the EEA circular staple line edge in order to prevent ischemia to the intervening rectal wall.
   (d) Utilize sequentially larger rectal dilators passed via the anus to the rectal transection line (Fig. 21.3). This allows not only physical dilation of the rectum but also

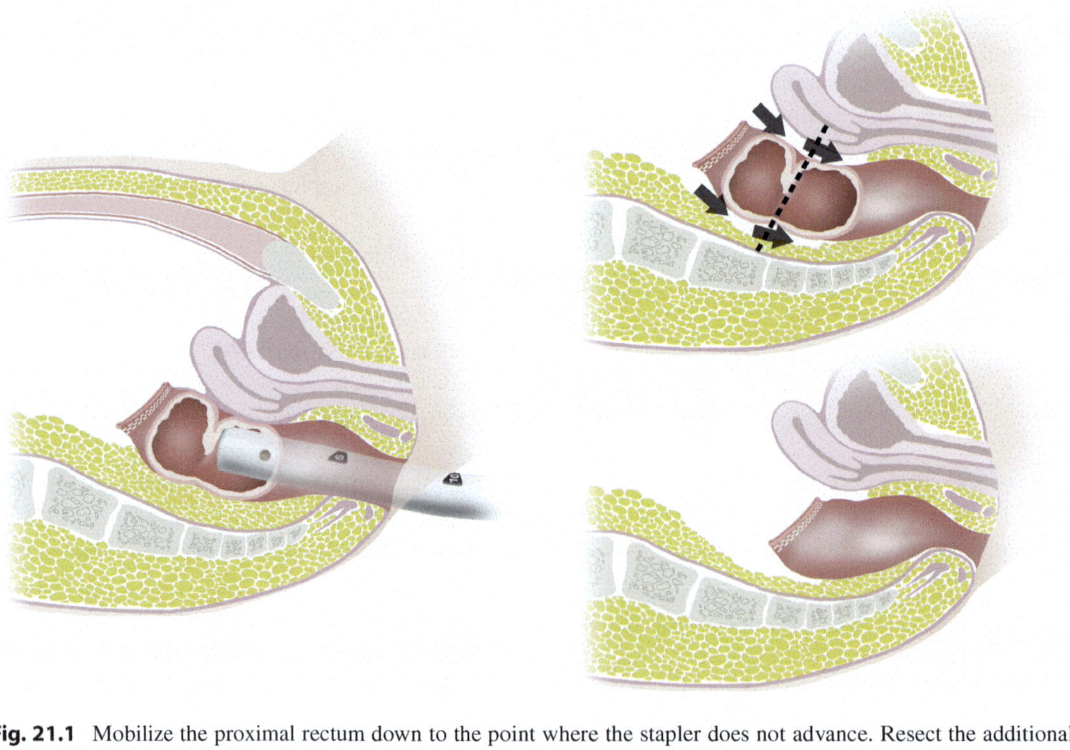

Fig. 21.1 Mobilize the proximal rectum down to the point where the stapler does not advance. Resect the additional proximal rectum at this point

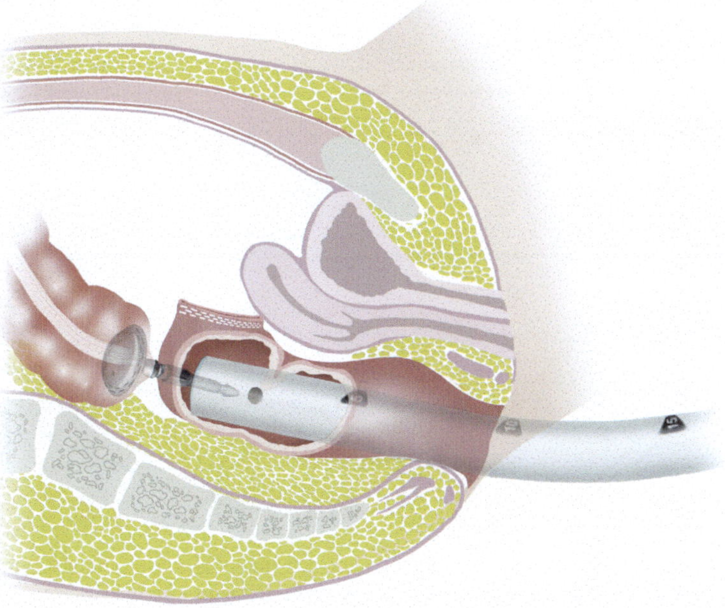

Fig. 21.2 Create a stapled anastomosis from the side of the rectum distal to the stapled rectal cuff to the end of the left colon

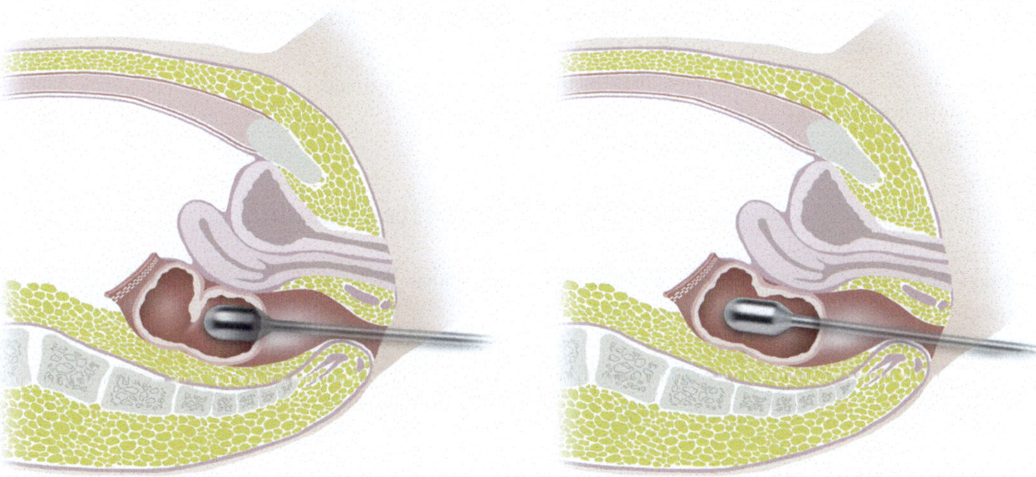

Fig. 21.3 Utilize sequentially larger rectal dilators passed via the anus to the rectal transection line

allows the surgeon placing the stapler to better understand the curvature of the rectum.

(e) Place a purse-string suture around the rectal stump, and tie around the center rod of the anvil. Pass the EEA circular stapler through a transverse colotomy created proximal to the left colon (Fig. 21.4).

Technical Pearls (Tips and Tricks)

1. Be prepared for this troubling, though solvable, technical dilemma.
2. Never force the stapler against resistance.
3. In cases where there has been significant pelvic inflammation, it is helpful to pass EEA sizers up to the rectum before transecting the

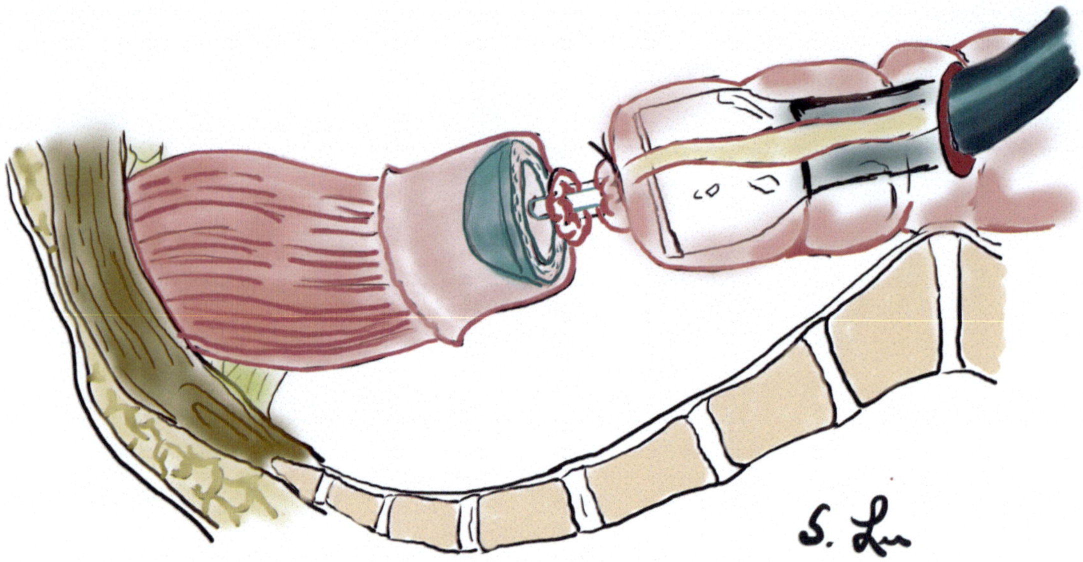

Fig. 21.4 Place a purse-string suture around the rectal stump, and tie around the center rod of the anvil. Pass the EEA circular stapler through a transverse colotomy created proximal to the left colon

distal margin in order to confirm the rectum is not structured and will accommodate the stapler when the operation calls for this. If the sizers will not pass, it is easier to mobilize more the rectum before transecting the rectum.

4. A combination of the above operative techniques may be required.
5. Air test the completed anastomosis. Thoroughly inspect any potential rectal damage. In room fiber-optic endoscopy is valuable.

Special Postoperative Care

1. None required.

Suggested Reading

1. Schoegz DJ Jr, et al. Low anterior resection: alternative anastomotic techniques. Am Surg Oncol Clin N Am. 2010;19:761–75.

The J Pouch Does Not Reach

22

Deborah S. Keller, Richard Cohen,
and Scott R. Steele

Clinical Scenario

An obese, 45-year-old woman is undergoing total proctocolectomy with ileal pouch-anal anastomosis (IPAA) for ulcerative colitis refractory to medical management. After completing the resection, it becomes apparent that the terminal ileum mesentery will not allow for a J pouch to reach the pelvic floor.

Key Points

1. Restorative proctocolectomy with ileal pouch-anal anastomosis in the J pouch configuration is the procedure of choice for patients with ulcerative colitis requiring surgery. A tension-free IPAA is one of the critical portions of the procedure.
2. Assess reach by pulling the intended apex of the J pouch to approximately 5–6 cm past the pubic symphysis, and evaluate tension on the tissue.
3. If additional reach is needed, there is a stepwise algorithm of operative maneuvers that can be used that affords several additional centimeters.
4. If there is difficulty with reach despite attempting the maneuvers in your armamentarium, ask for help from another surgeon. If experienced help is not available or you are still not able to achieve a tension-free anastomosis, divert the patient, and plan to come back in 3–6 months for another attempt at restorative ileal pouch-anal anastomosis. This is not a failure – this may be the best option for the patient.

Operative Assessment

1. Was the rectum/rectal stump completely mobilized?
   (a) For the proctectomy, an anterior dissection is done to the lower border of the prostate gland in men or lower one-third of the vagina in women.
   (b) A transanal digital evaluation is done to assess the level of transection.
2. Was the small bowel mesentery mobilized as proximally as possible?

D. S. Keller
Department of Surgery, New York-Presbyterian, Columbia University Medical Center, New York, NY, USA

R. Cohen
University College London Hospitals, NHS Foundation Trusts, Department of Surgery and Interventional Sciences, London, UK

S. R. Steele (✉)
Case Western Reserve University School of Medicine, Cleveland, OH, USA

Department of Colorectal Surgery, Cleveland Clinic, Cleveland, OH, USA

S. W. Lee et al. (eds.), *Colorectal Surgery Consultation*,
https://doi.org/10.1007/978-3-030-11181-6_22

   (a) Completely mobilize the cut edge of the ileal mesentery up to the level of the duodenum (D3). This should be done routinely in these cases to help the ileal pouch reach to the level of the levator plate without tension.
3. Does the J pouch reach?
   (a) Perform the "plop test," where the anticipated apex of the J pouch is tested for reach beyond the pubic symphysis.
   (b) If there is not adequate length to reach, additional operative maneuvers can help.

Operative Checklist

1. A headlight for transillumination through the mesentery and improved visualization in the pelvis.
2. Basic laparoscopic tray with atraumatic graspers.
3. Open laparotomy tray with pelvic retractors (lighted retractors, if available) and long pelvic instrument tray if performing open; if performing laparoscopically, have these trays available in case of conversion.
4. GIA stapler for constructing the pouch (the authors prefer to use two firings of the 100-size stapler) and transecting the bowel, as well as an intraluminal (29 mm) stapler for creating the ileoanal anastomosis.

Operative Techniques

1. Simulate the J pouch, and deliver the proposed apex of the pouch with a clamp into the pelvis using a Babcock clamp. Visualizing the clamp at the top of the levators or palpating the clamp using an index finger in the anus can verify whether there is appropriate reach to the pelvis (Fig. 22.1).
2. Assure the small bowel mesentery is mobilized adequately. Sharply mobilize the cut edge of the small bowel mesentery up to the level of the most proximal level duodenum in the right upper quadrant (Fig. 22.2).

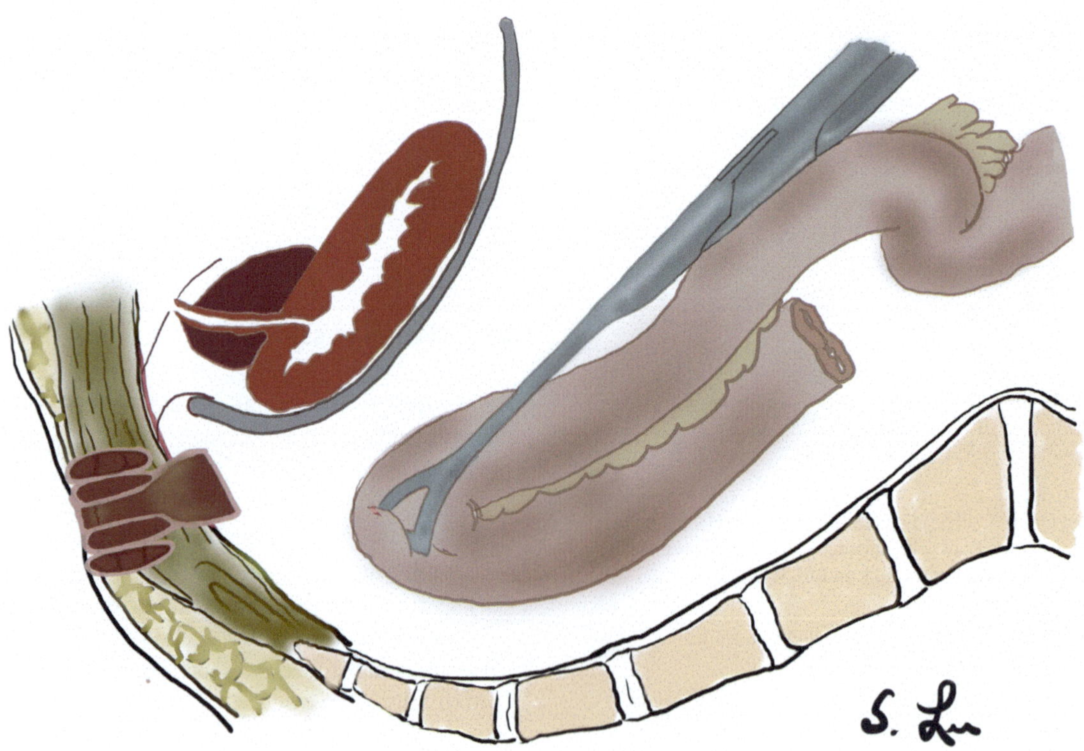

Fig. 22.1 Using a Babcock clamp to initially determine if appropriate length is present

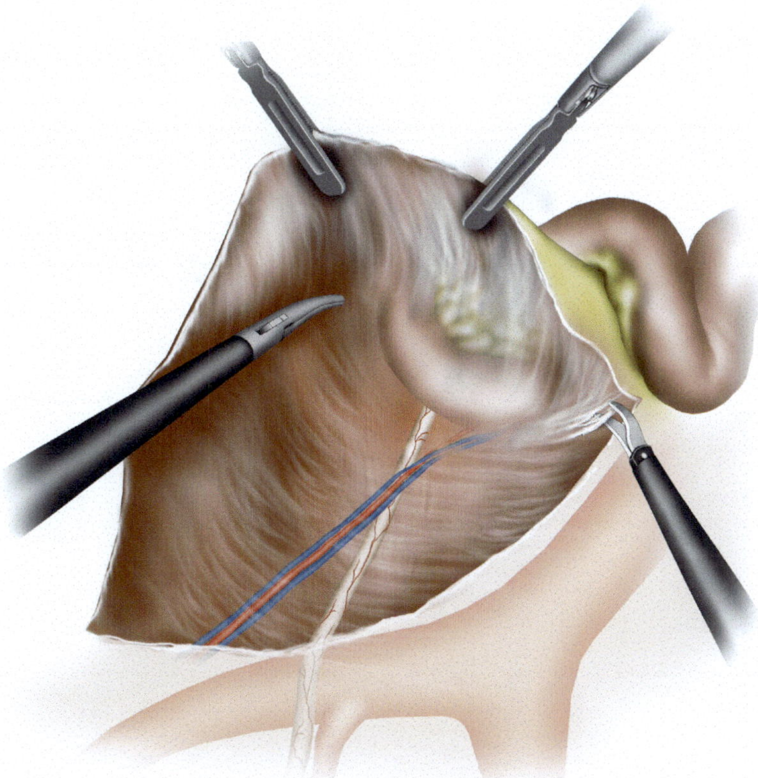

Fig. 22.2 Mobilizing the small bowel mesentery

3. Perform a Kocher maneuver to formally mobilize the duodenum. Incise the peritoneum at the right edge of the duodenum, and reflect the duodenum and the head of pancreas toward the left to provide additional reach.
4. Release the peritoneum around the superior mesenteric vessels: Transilluminate and incise the peritoneal tissue to the right of the superior mesenteric vessels leaving a very small edge of peritoneum lateral to the vessels.
5. Create rents in the peritoneum over the superior mesenteric vessels: Score a series of 1–2 cm transverse incisions in the peritoneum along the length of the SMA; assure both the anterior and posterior leaflets are incised for maximal release (Fig. 22.3).
6. Divide the ileocolic pedicle. Ligation of the ileocolic pedicle at its origin from the superior mesenteric artery can extend the ileum 1–2 cm. Start by transilluminating the mesentery to better identify the ileocolic artery and assure preservation of the superior mesenteric artery, the terminal arcade, and the collateral flow.
7. Create a window in the ileal mesentery. Open the mesentery by dividing the proximal ileal arcades individually; create the window at the point of maximal tension of the small bowel under transillumination of the mesentery. Again, with vascular division, assure preservation of the terminal arcade and collateral flow.
8. Create a shorter pouch. The classic teaching is to create a 15–20 cm pouch (18 cm is the author's preference). However, the pouch will naturally dilate over time, and use of any efferent limb length greater than 12 cm will allow for an adequate reservoir.
9. Consider a different pouch configuration (Fig. 22.4). Because a J pouch is the easiest to create, it is the most commonly used pouch configuration. The S pouch can reach up to

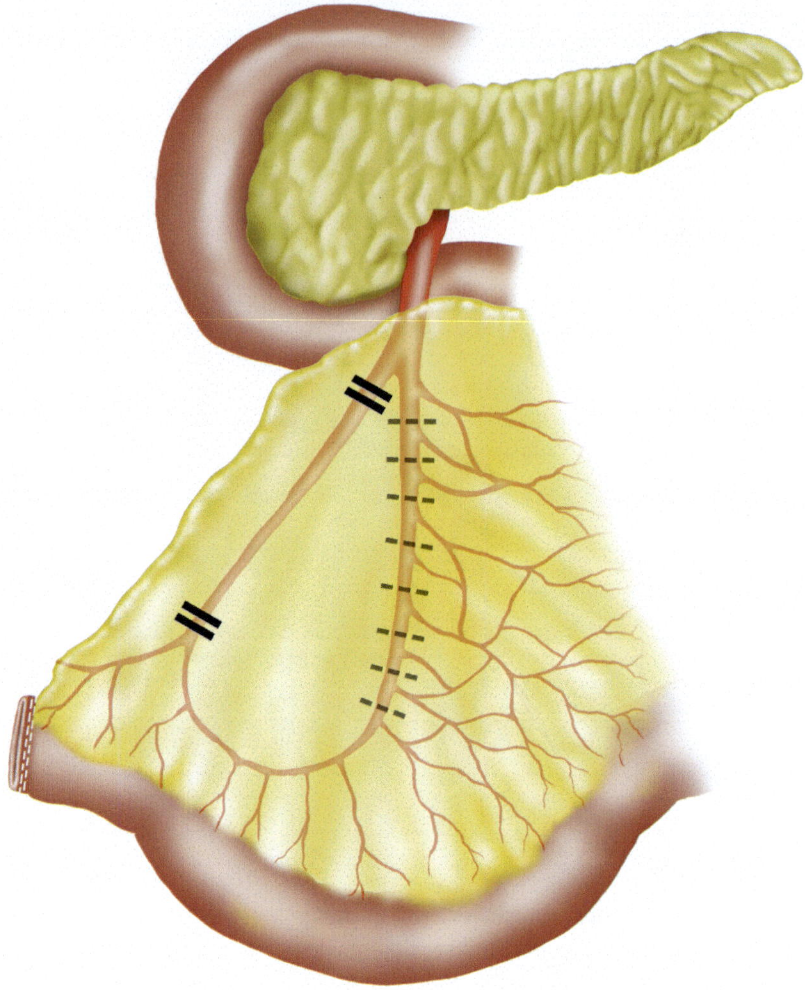

Fig. 22.3 Scoring the mesentery along the vascular arcades to gain additional length

2–4 cm further than a J pouch and is an option if there is excessive tension in the IPAA (Fig. 22.5). An S pouch is constructed using three limbs of 12–15 cm of terminal ileum with a 2 cm exit on the distal limb. The folded ileum segments are approximated with two rows of continuous seromuscular sutures. Then, an enterotomy is created in the front wall of in an "S" shape to expose the back wall of the pouch. Continuous running full-thickness sutures are applied to approximate the two posterior anastomotic lines. The anterior wall is closed with continuous seromuscular sutures (Fig. 22.6). If you try to overcome a reach issue and create too long of an efferent limb, this can lead to pouch outlet obstruction and a dysfunctional pouch. Another alternative is to create a W pouch; there the terminal small bowel is folded into four loops, each 10–12 cm long, forming a W-shaped configuration. The creation is similar to the S pouch, but the reservoir is hand sewn with three posterior suture lines and a long anterior suture line to form the pouch.

Technical Pearls (Tips and Tricks)

1. Optimize patients before surgery. If obese or overweight, encourage weight loss to reduce visceral and mesenteric fat. Consult a nutritionist, if the service is available, for a multidisciplinary approach.

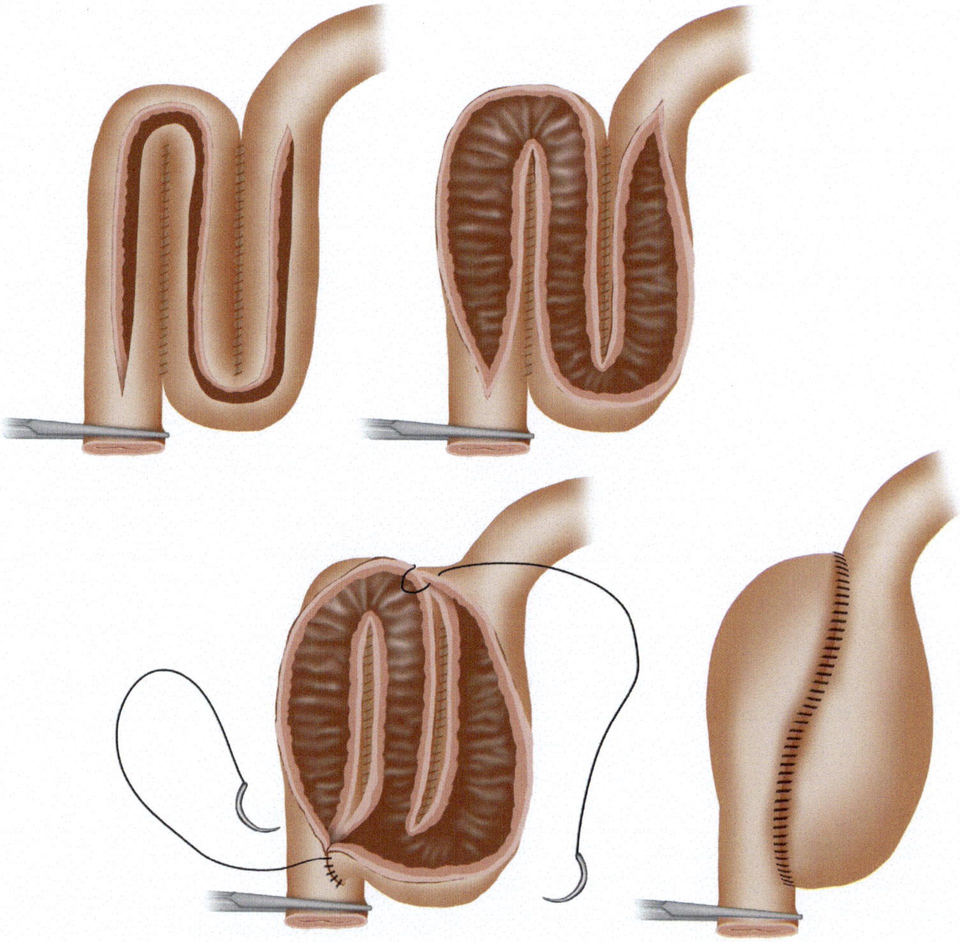

Fig. 22.4 Construction of an S pouch

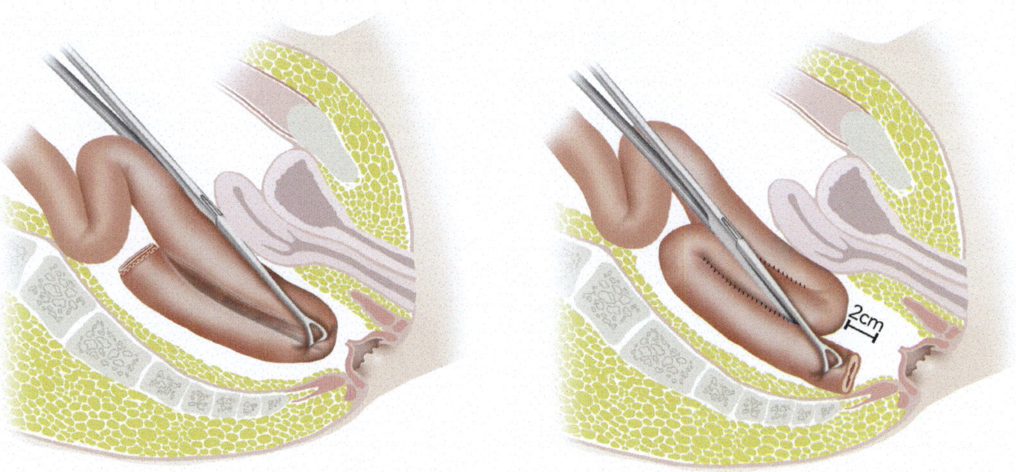

Fig. 22.5 The S pouch can provide a few extra centimeters in the pelvis compared to the J pouch

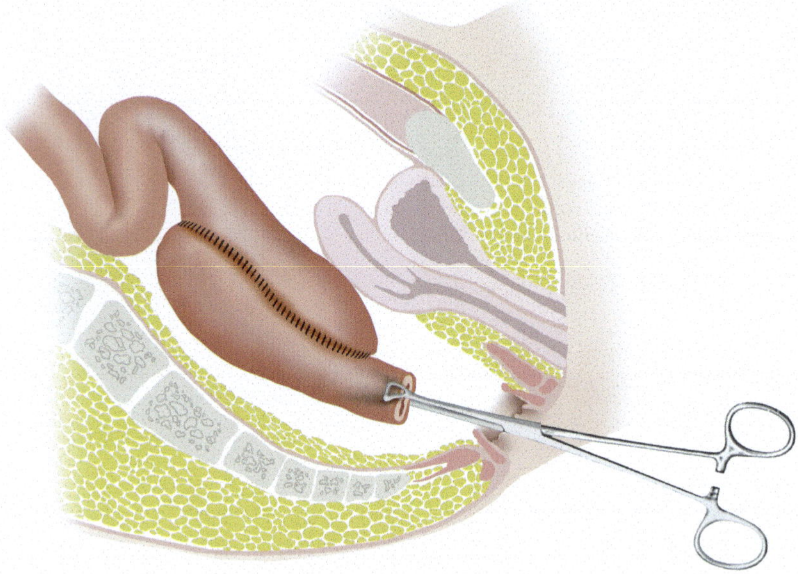

Fig. 22.6 Bringing the completed S pouch down for anastomosis

2. Check for reach prior to transecting distal rectum. In certain situations where all maneuvers fail to provide the needed length, preserving some rectum may allow a tension-free anastomosis.
3. Fluorescence angiography can be used to confirm a well-perfused pouch and anastomosis intraoperatively, especially in cases where the ileocolic pedicle or ileocolic arcade was ligated.

Postoperative Care

1. Routine postoperative care along an enhanced recovery protocol is recommended.
2. If an IPAA anastomosis is created, a transanal drain may be placed to vent the pouch.
3. If a stoma is created, routine stoma care and teaching should be performed.

Suggested Reading

1. Davis B, Rafferty JF. Technical aspects. In: Steele SR, Maykel JA, Champagne BJ, Orangio GR, editors. Complexities in colorectal surgery. New York: Springer; 2014.
2. Kirat HT, Remzi FH. Technical aspects of ileoanal pouch surgery in patients with ulcerative colitis. Clin Colon Rectal Surg. 2010;23(4):239–47.
3. Nivatvongs S. Ulcerative colitis. In: Gordon PH, Nivatvongs S, editors. Principles and practice of surgery for the colon, rectum, and anus. 3rd ed. Boca Raton: Taylor and Francis Group; 2007.
4. Uraiqat AA, Byrne CM, Phillips RK. Gaining length in ileal-anal pouch reconstruction: a review. Color Dis. 2007;9(7):657–61.

23 Intraoperative Management of Bleeding at Stapled Side-to-Side Anastomosis

Nivedh V. Paluvoi and Sang W. Lee

Clinical Scenario

A 55-year-old male with cecal cancer is undergoing laparoscopic right colectomy. After exteriorization and removal of the specimen, a side-to-side functional end-to-end anastomosis is performed. Brisk endoluminal bleeding from the linear staple line is identified after the inspection from the common enterotomy/colotomy.

Key Points

1. Postoperative anastomotic hemorrhage may be as high as 5% after colorectal resection. The best method to manage anastomotic bleeding is prevention.
   (a) Maintain closure of the stapler for 30 seconds prior to firing to decrease tissue edema.
   (b) Take care not to include any mesentery within the stapler prior to firing.
2. Direct visualization of the staple line is a must for evaluation of hemostasis.
   (a) Visual inspection of the entire staple line should be performed prior to closure of the common enterotomy/colotomy in a side-to-side anastomosis.
   (b) Routine colonoscopic visualization and inspection should be performed after the creation of an end-to-end anastomosis.
3. If bleeding is identified, immediate hemostasis must be achieved to reduce postoperative morbidity including transfusion requirement and increased length hospital stay. Management is based on the type of anastomosis created.
   (a) Side-to-side anastomosis. Adequate exposure for direct suture repair.
      (i) Bleeding at the crotch of the staple line may be difficult to visualize and necessitates optimizing exposure.
   (b) End-to-end anastomosis.
      (i) Endoscopic visualization during direct suture repair.
      (ii) Endoscopic modalities including coagulation, placement of clips, and epinephrine injection.
4. If hemostasis cannot be achieved with endoscopic maneuvers or direct suture repair, takedown and revision of the anastomosis must be performed.

N. V. Paluvoi
University of Miami, Department of Surgery, Division of Colorectal Surgery, Pasadena, CA, USA

S. W. Lee (✉)
Department of Surgery – Colon and Rectal Surgery, Keck School of Medicine of University of Southern California, Los Angeles, CA, USA

S. W. Lee et al. (eds.), *Colorectal Surgery Consultation*, https://doi.org/10.1007/978-3-030-11181-6_23

Operative Assessment

1. Can the entire length of the staple line be seen?
   (a) Visualization of the entire staple line must be performed prior to attempting to obtain hemostasis as the staple line near the crotch may also be bleeding.
2. Where is the location of bleeding?
   (a) Proximal bleeding near the opening of the enterotomy/colotomy can be exposed with handheld retractors.
   (b) Distal bleeding near the crotch of the staple line may require the use of clamps to elevate and expose the staple line.

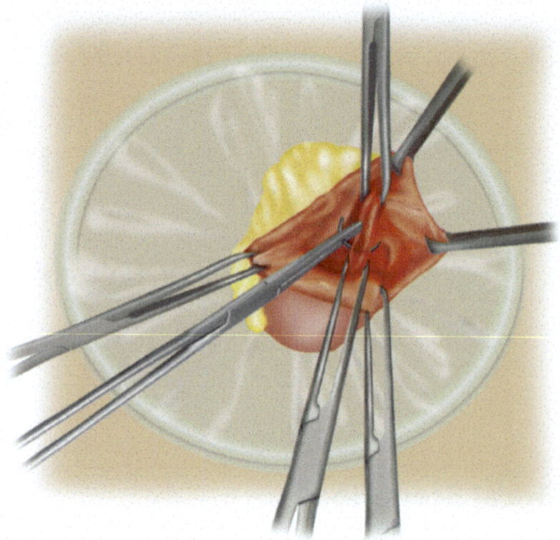

Fig. 23.1 Long Allis clamps may be used to grasp and elevate the staple line to allow for direct suture repair

Operative Checklist

1. Additional helpful equipment.
   (a) Long instrument tray for longer clamps.
   (b) Right angle handheld retractors (lighted retractors, if available).
   (c) Good lighting (headlights).

Operative Techniques

1. Direct suture repair of proximal bleeding.
   (a) When persistent bleeding is noted from the staple line after attempts with direct coagulation, suture repair should be performed. Exposure with either ring forceps or handheld retractors should be maintained to allow for placement of a polyfilament absorbable suture through the bleeding staple line from within the lumen. After placement and tying of the suture, re-evaluation of the staple line should be performed. If need be, additional sutures can be placed to achieve hemostasis.
2. Direct suture repair of distal bleeding.
   (a) If the source of bleeding is identified in the distal portion of the staple line, adequate exposure is key prior to attempting to obtain hemostasis. Long Allis clamps may be used to grasp and elevate the staple line to allow for direct suture repair (Fig. 23.1). Polyfilament absorbable suture should be used through the staple line. If difficulty is encountered in placing the sutures from within the lumen, sutures may be placed through the staple line exteriorly while looking into the lumen to confirm placement of suture into the desired location. Alternatively, placing interrupted sutures across the staple line and using these as a stay suture to elevate the next segment of the staple line allow the surgeon to march down the staple line and place further sutures, as needed. The staple line should once again be inspected to ensure that hemostasis is obtained. If need be, another suture can be placed either intra- or extraluminally to aid in obtaining hemostasis. After sutures are placed and prior to closing the common enterotomy/colotomy, it is important to confirm the lumen of the anastomosis was not compromised or "back walled." This can be done by using a ring forceps to expose the lumen.
3. Direct coagulation of proximal bleeding.
   (a) If the source of bleeding is identified in the proximal portion of the staple line, direct monopolar coagulation can be performed. Adequate exposure must be created by either using ringed forceps to gently retract and elevate adjacent to the staple line or by

placing a lighted handheld retractor to optimize both exposure and visualization. Care must be taken to not coagulate the normal appearing staple line or adjacent mucosa when using monopolar electrocautery. This can be prevented with the use of the protected cautery tip. Aggressive use of electrocautery to the staple line has been associated with increased anastomotic fistulae, likely due to dissipation of energy along the staple line. As such, if persistent bleeding is noted, we recommend direct suture repair. It is the authors' preference to perform suture repair rather than direct coagulation of the staple line.

Operative Assessment

1. Can the location of bleeding be clearly visualized at the anastomosis?
   (a) Clear visualization of the site of bleeding must be identified prior to attempts at obtaining hemostasis. The area should be thoroughly irrigated with saline with use of the endoscope.
2. The anatomic position of bleeding should be identified under endoscopic visualization.
   (a) A DeBakey forceps (or bowel grasper when doing laparoscopy) can be used to press on the bowel wall with direct endoscopic visualization identifying compression of the lumen, which will aid in determining anatomic location of the bleeding site.

Technical Pearls (Tips and Tricks)

1. The tissue should be compressed for 30 seconds prior to firing the stapler.
2. Confirm that no mesentery is included within the stapler prior to firing.

Special Postoperative Care

1. One should maintain a low threshold for concern for recurrent bleeding postoperatively with any signs of hypotension or tachycardia.
2. Chemical thromboprophylaxis can be continued postoperatively if no further concern for bleeding is raised after obtaining hemostasis.
3. Placement of a drain is unnecessary in this scenario.
4. Diet can be advanced as usual.

Suggested Reading

1. Golda T, Zerpa C, Kreisler E, Trenti L, Biondo S. Incidence and management of anastomotic bleeding after ileocolic anastomosis. Color Dis. 2013;15:1301–8.
2. Malik JH, East JE, Buchanan GN, Kennedy RH. Endoscopic haemostasis of staple-line haemorrhage following colorectal resection. Color Dis. 2008;1:616–8.
3. Martinez-Serrano M-A, Pares D, et al. Management of lower gastrointestinal bleeding after colorectal resection and stapled anastomosis. Tech Coloproctol. 2009;13:49–53.

24 Postoperative End-to-End Anastomotic Bleeding

Christine Hsieh and Sang W. Lee

Clinical Scenario

A 65-year-old man underwent elective sigmoid resection for diverticulitis. On postoperative day 3, the patient becomes hypotensive and oliguric despite several boluses of crystalloid. He has multiple episodes of passing a large volume of dark clot mixed with fresh blood.

Key Points

1. Passage of a small amount of blood is common after an end-to-end anastomosis (EEA), often occurs with or before the first bowel movement, and is typically self-limited. Only rarely do patients require intervention, and returning to the operating room to control bleeding in this situation is an uncommon occurrence given the availability and effectiveness of endoscopic therapies.
2. Patients should be counseled about this in the preop setting to avoid undue anxiety or alarm.
3. Anastomotic bleeding may be evident immediately post-op, and as late as 9 days or later.
   (a) Patients may describe repeated evacuation of blood or clots, tenesmus, liquid stools mixed with variable amounts of blood, or perceived incontinence and soilage from dripping blood.
4. A step-up approach is reasonable for management of postoperative hematochezia given that most patients stop bleeding spontaneously or are successfully managed with non-operative techniques.
   (a) Observation: Hemodynamic monitoring, cessation of nonessential anticoagulant or antiplatelet medications, and close attention to the quality and quantity of blood passed per rectum. Trending blood levels and correcting coagulopathy should be done per institutional practice.
   (b) Resuscitation: If the patient manifests clinical signs or symptoms of acute blood loss hypovolemia, appropriate resuscitative measures with crystalloid infusion or blood product transfusion should be commenced.
   (c) Localization: Ongoing bleeding should be considered anastomotic bleeding until proven otherwise. Flexible or rigid sigmoidoscopy is the diagnostic modality of choice and poses minimal stress to patient. Other sources should be ruled out based on the patient's clinical condition and medical comorbidities.
   (d) Treatment: Endoscopic interventions are highly effective. Surgical interventions

C. Hsieh
Keck School of Medicine – University of Southern California, Los Angeles, CA, USA

S. W. Lee (✉)
Department of Surgery – Colon and Rectal Surgery, Keck School of Medicine of University of Southern California, Los Angeles, CA, USA

S. W. Lee et al. (eds.), *Colorectal Surgery Consultation*,
https://doi.org/10.1007/978-3-030-11181-6_24

are rarely necessary but must be performed if endoscopic interventions are not effective.

Operative Assessment

1. Standard investigative and resuscitative measures should be employed.
2. Report should be obtained from the surgeon about any intraoperative events as well as the anastomotic level and technique.

Operative Techniques

1. Flexible endoscopy.
   (a) This is a highly effective strategy for obtaining hemostasis. No bowel preparation is necessary given the cathartic effect of intraluminal blood. Depending on the patient's clinical condition, many endoscopic interventions can be safely delivered under monitored anesthesia care rather than general anesthesia.
      (i) Identify then thoroughly irrigate the area of the anastomosis to clear away adherent clot to identify the bleeding point(s). Filling the lumen with cold water can aid this as well, and, in many cases, cold irrigation alone is sufficient to stop the bleeding.
      (ii) Active arterial bleeding can be controlled with endoscopic clips (Fig. 24.1).
      (iii) Mucosal oozing is often amenable to cautery.
      (iv) Submucosal injection with dilute epinephrine solution (1:100,000 saline) is also effective but may require repeated attempts to ensure durable hemostasis.
      (v) Avoid colonoscope trauma, torqueing, or looping in these settings to prevent secondary injury.
2. Rigid sigmoidoscopy.
   (a) If flexible sigmoidoscopy is not available, rigid sigmoidoscopy can be performed. The typical length of a rigid sigmoidoscope is 25 cm, and distal rectosigmoid anastomoses can be easily visualized. A long metal suction device is necessary for hemostasis.
      (i) With caution, advance the rigid scope to the anastomotic site. Circumferentially inspect the entire anastomosis to localize the bleeding site (Fig. 24.2).
      (ii) Once identified, advance the scope gently against the anastomosis while centering the bleeding site in the channel of the scope. A long metal suction device is inserted through the scope and advanced until the bleeding site comes in contact with the suction device. While suctioning out blood using the metal suction device, apply monopolar electrocoagu-

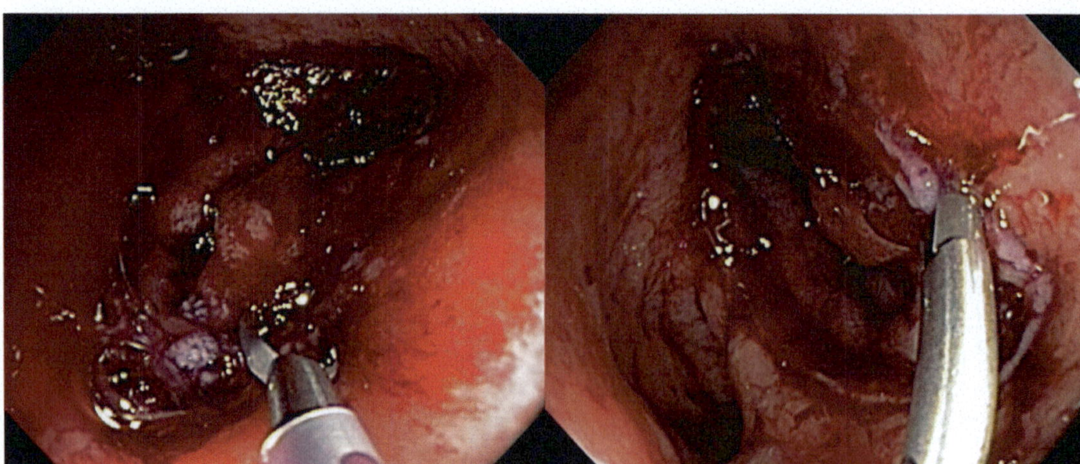

Fig. 24.1 Active arterial bleeding can be controlled with endoscopic clips

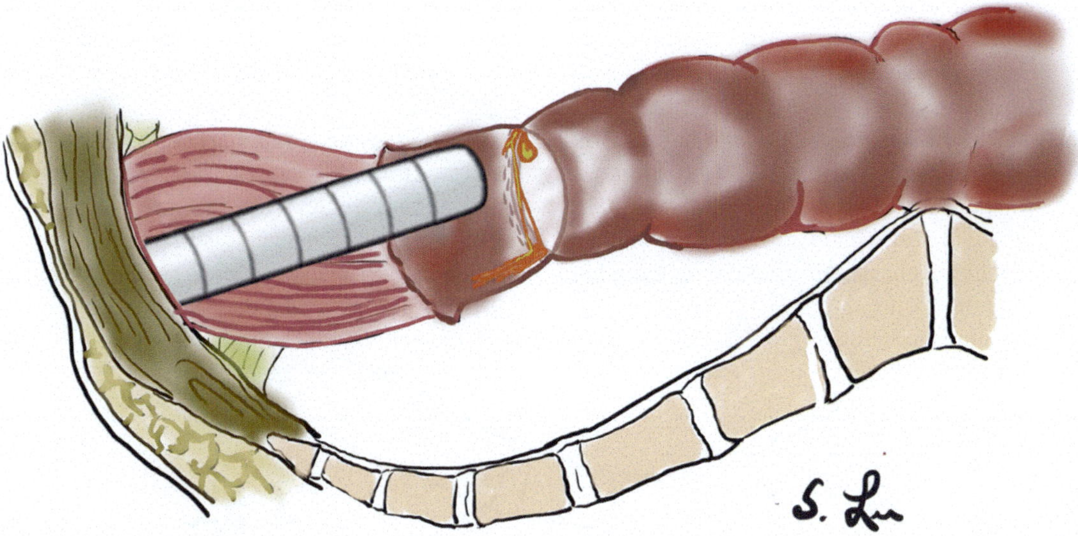

Fig. 24.2 With caution, advance the rigid scope to the anastomotic site. Circumferentially inspect the entire anastomosis to localize the bleeding site

lation by contacting the suction device with Bovie (Fig. 24.3). This is a technically challenging maneuver, and care must be taken to not coagulate the normal appearing staple line or adjacent mucosa when using monopolar electrocautery. Aggressive use of electrocautery to the staple line has been associated with increased anastomotic fistulae, likely due to dissipation of energy along the length of the staple line.

3. Surgery.
   (a) A transanal approach with the patient in lithotomy position may be feasible in patients with a low pelvic anastomosis.
      (i) Placement of sutures at the anastomosis can be very effective if exposure is adequate.
      (ii) Insertion of a hemostatic plug can also be an effective maneuver.
   (b) Exploratory laparotomy in the bleeding, unstable patient, or one who fails conservative measures can prove difficult due to adhesions, inflammation, and anatomic constraints. This should be undertaken with caution.
      (i) The anastomosis can be oversewn and reinforced or entirely redone depending on the situation.
      (ii) This can be done with increased precision with the aid of an endoscopic view provided by an assistant working from below.

Technical Pearls (Tips and Tricks)

1. Prevention of anastomotic bleeding starts in the operating room.
   (a) Clear any mesentery from anastomotic sites prior to joining with a stapling device. Compression of the tissues may induce temporary hemostasis, but this may not be a durable affect.
2. Perform an endoscopic examination of the anastomosis intraoperatively in patients at high risk of bleeding.
   (a) It may be useful to request flexible sigmoidoscopy equipment for all cases employing stapled colorectal or colocolonic anastomoses, if the resources are available (Fig. 24.4).
3. Consider performing interventions for post-op anastomotic bleeding in the OR, even for initial endoscopic attempts, in the event that general anesthesia for operative intervention becomes necessary.

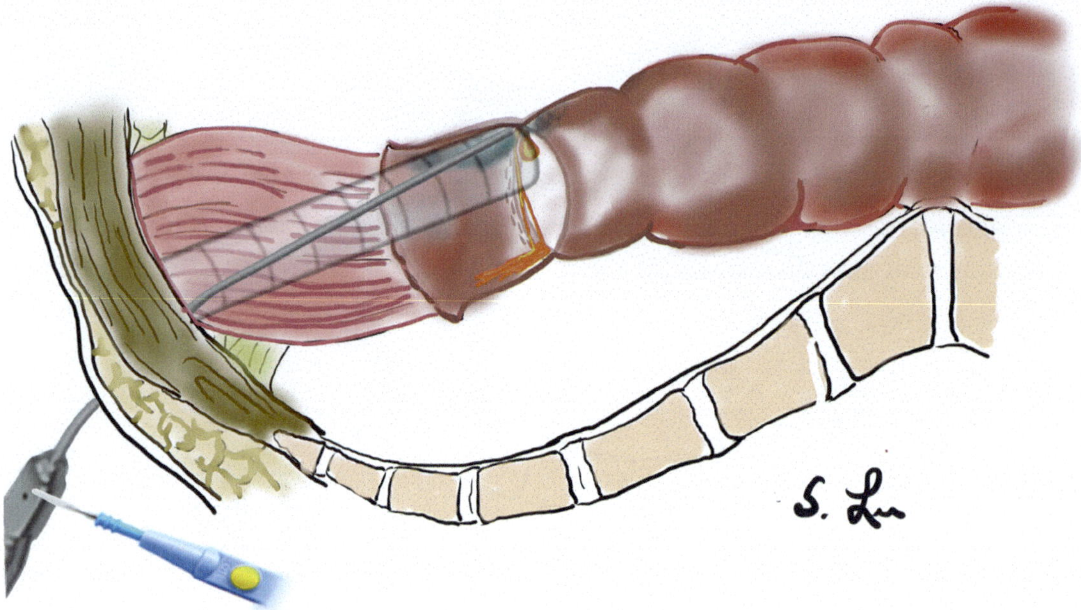

Fig. 24.3 Once bleeding source is identified, advance the scope gently against the anastomosis while centering the bleeding site in the channel of the scope. A long metal suction device is inserted through the scope and advanced until the bleeding site comes in contact with the suction device. While suctioning out blood using the metal suction device, apply monopolar electrocoagulation by contacting the suction device with electrocautery

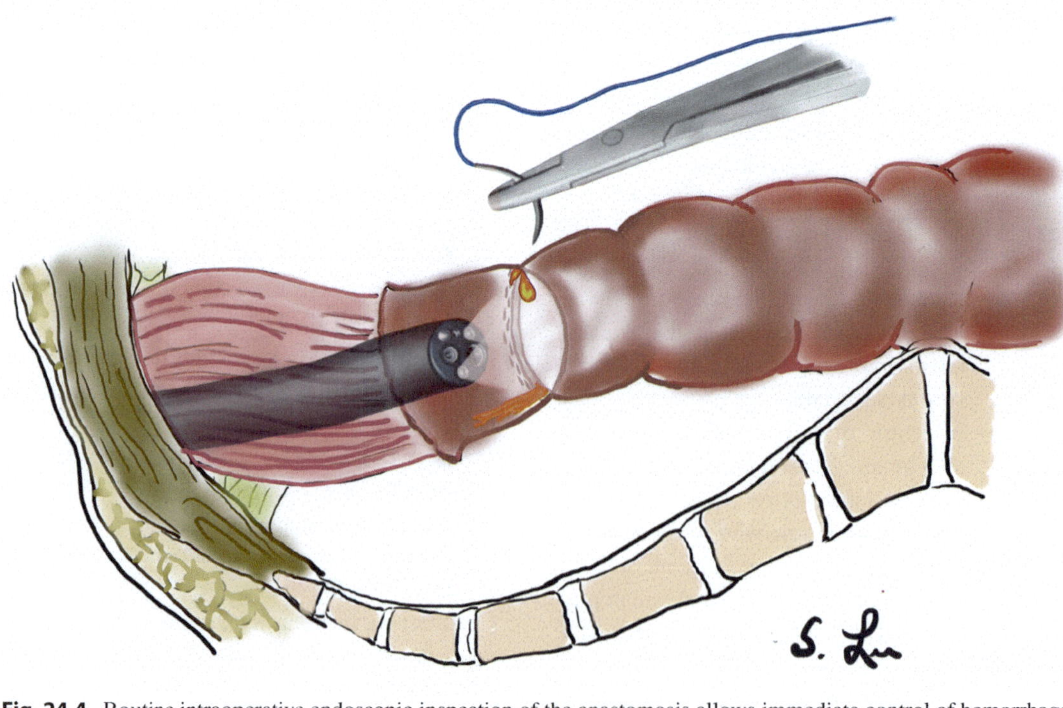

Fig. 24.4 Routine intraoperative endoscopic inspection of the anastomosis allows immediate control of hemorrhage

Special Postoperative Care

1. The patient should be closely monitored after any intervention. Repeated endoscopic interventions may be indicated, and in the case of refractory hemorrhage, operative intervention may be a necessary last resort.
2. The possibility of disrupting the anastomosis with hemostatic techniques and leading to ischemia/necrosis of the tissue is a concern. There is also a risk of dissipating energy along a staple line in unpredictable fashion causing local tissue damage.
3. Consider individualizing the use of NSAIDS or prophylactic anticoagulation.

Suggested Reading

1. Davis B, Rivadeneira DE. Complications of colorectal anastomoses: leaks, strictures, and bleeding. Surg Clin N Am. 2013;93:61–87.
2. Lou Z, Zhang W, et al. Colonoscopy is the first choice for early postoperative rectal anastomotic bleeding. World J Surg Oncol. 2014;12:376.
3. Malik AH, East JE, et al. Endoscopic haemostasis of staple-line haemorrhage following colorectal resection. Color Dis. 2008;10:616–8.
4. Martinez-Serrano M-A, Pares D, et al. Management of lower gastrointestinal bleeding after colorectal resection and stapled anastomosis. Tech Coloproctol. 2009;13:49–53.
5. Perez RO, Sousa A, et al. Endoscopic management of postoperative stapled colorectal anastomosis hemorrhage. Tech Coloproctol. 2007;11:64–6.

Postoperative Anastomotic Leak After Low Anterior Resection

25

Matthew M. Philp and Howard M. Ross

Clinical Scenario

A 65-year-old female undergoes a robotic LAR for a mid-rectal cancer. Preoperative staging revealed a T2N0 tumor, and no neoadjuvant treatment was given. Total mesorectal excision with colonic J-pouch reconstruction was performed, and the leak test was negative. The patient discharged on POD #4 but returned 1 week later. She is febrile to 102 F, heart rate is 120, and blood pressure is 90/50. After IV fluid resuscitation and IV broad-spectrum antibiotics, abdominal CT scan demonstrates a 6 cm pelvic fluid collection with air adjacent to the anastomosis. Physical examination reveals a diffusely tender and peritoneal abdomen. Vital signs are not improving.

M. M. Philp
Division of Colon and Rectal Surgery, Temple University School of Medicine, Philadelphia, PA, USA

H. M. Ross (✉)
Division of Colon and Rectal Surgery, Lewis Katz School of Medicine at Temple University and the Temple University Health System, Philadelphia, PA, USA
e-mail: Howard.Ross@tuhs.temple.edu

S. W. Lee et al. (eds.), *Colorectal Surgery Consultation*, https://doi.org/10.1007/978-3-030-11181-6_25

Key Points

1. Anastomotic leaks happen to the best surgeons and are very stressful events. They require sound surgical decision-making for the best possible outcomes. Communicate with your patient and their families. Do not be afraid to ask a colleague or trusted mentor for an opinion or assistance.
2. Anastomotic leak after LAR presents the surgeon with a unique set of challenges. Causes of leaks are multifactorial and, in addition to traditional risk factors, which impact tissue healing, preoperative chemoradiotherapy and low colorectal or coloanal anastomoses are compounding factors.
3. The diagnosis of anastomotic leak is made by a combination of history, physical exam, and imaging. Oral or rectal contrast extravasation is not required to diagnose a leak, and, very commonly, extravasation will not be seen on imaging even in the presence of a leak.
4. Leaks can masquerade as a cardiopulmonary event. Patients may present with a picture consistent with a cardiac complication or a pulmonary embolism, and only after a negative evaluation is an anastomotic leak entertained as the underlying etiology for the patient's decompensation. It is important to consider that patients with pulmonary or hemodynamic deterioration after a recent anastomosis may have a leak secondarily

causing the cardiopulmonary findings. Under these circumstances, the order in which a patient is evaluated, in terms of ruling in or out different possible diagnoses, is based on the surgeon's judgment.

5. First and foremost, assess the stability of the patient. The unstable patient with sepsis and diffuse peritonitis requires immediate resuscitation and prompt operative management with washout and fecal diversion.
6. Proximal fecal diversion will minimize the clinical consequences of anastomotic leak (though it won't prevent them unfortunately). Many patients who are already diverted and develop clinical signs of leak can be managed nonoperatively. Though fecal diversion can present its own set of challenges and complications, there should be thoughtful consideration about which low pelvic anastomoses should be protected.
7. For the stable patient with leak (especially if there is a covering stoma in place), nonoperative management techniques can be attempted and are often successful. Percutaneous drainage can be used to drain sizable collections. Transanal closure of small anastomotic defects is possible. Depending on the level of the anastomosis, this can be done with endoscopic clips (through or over-the-scope), TEM/TAMIS, or conventional transanal techniques.
8. Broad-spectrum antibiotic therapy should be started as soon as possible. There should be a strong coverage of both gram-negative enteric and anaerobic flora. As patients re-present after discharge from the hospital and the events unfold, there is a tendency to focus on getting lab work and imaging done, and, many times, antibiotics are not started for several hours or longer until all the studies have been completed and the diagnosis of leak is definitively made. When patients present with a concern for anastomotic leak, it makes sense to order the antibiotics as early as possible. Ordering "the first dose STAT" is a useful practice to get patients their needed antibacterial coverage.

Operative Assessment

1. Has the patient had a diverting ileostomy (or colostomy)? If not, preoperative stoma marking is always a good idea, if possible. Emergency stomas are often permanent, and poorly chosen sites will only cause more problems down the road.
2. What is the level of the anastomosis? Intra-abdominal anastomoses may allow for resection and revision (if early and not significantly inflamed). For extraperitoneal anastomoses, unless there is complete dehiscence, often drainage and diversion is the best option, as exposure or dissection in the inflamed deep pelvis is often futile.
3. How big is the leak and what caused it? Small pinhole leaks might be best managed by simple repair, drainage, and diversion. Sometimes the omentum can be used to buttress these repairs. A large, near complete dehiscence might require complete takedown and conversion to end colostomy. Although most leaks won't have a clear etiology, one important distinction to make is the ischemic anastomosis. Bowel that has vascular compromise should be resected, as simply diverting these patients will leave behind a source of ongoing sepsis. Endoscopic evaluation of the anastomosis may be very useful in situations where the blood supply is in question. If available, technology like ICG immunofluorescence may be useful to confirm a well-perfused rectum and colonic conduit.

Operative Checklist

1. Abdominal wall self-contained retraction devices.
2. Good suction and irrigation sources.
3. Adequate lighting. Headlamps are very useful.
4. Tools for pelvic surgery: long instruments, St. Mark's retractors.
5. Patients should be positioned in lithotomy, or variation of, to allow transanal access.

6. If attempting laparoscopic management, prepare for steep Trendelenburg position to expose the pelvis. Skilled assistants will be necessary to aide in exposure. Tuck arms to allow for access. Make sure there has been adequate IV volume resuscitation, as pneumoperitoneum will precipitate hypotension if not.
7. A flexible endoscope.
8. Stoma marking. If the patient does not already have a stoma, they will most likely require one. A poorly placed stoma will make the postoperative recovery all the more miserable for the patient. For an obtunded patient or if there is a large pannus, place the stoma as cephalad as possible.

Operative Approaches

1. Although minimally invasive approaches to the management of anastomotic leaks are well described in the literature, unless you are very experienced, this is probably the time for open exploration and treatment. If you attempt laparoscopic exploration, have a low threshold for conversion if you can't get adequate exposure or perform satisfactory washout.
2. Lithotomy position is very useful to allow for transanal or endoscopic techniques.
3. Open or laparoscopic exposure of all abdominal quadrants to assess for contamination and allow for washout.
4. Widely drain the pelvis with closed suction drains.
5. In almost all situations, fecal diversion is warranted. Unstable patients with intraperitoneal anastomoses should have anastomotic takedown and conversion to end colostomy. Lower, extraperitoneal anastomoses most often can be diverted proximally, if the area of leak is small. Loop ileostomy is the easiest diversion to perform and is also easier to reverse; however, it does have the potential to leave a column of stool above the leaking anastomosis. Anterograde on-table lavage can be performed to clear the stool burden. Transverse loop colostomies tend to have higher complication rates but can be useful in some situations.
6. If there is available omentum, it can be mobilized into a vascularized pedicle to reach the pelvis and facilitate coverage.

Technical Pearls (Tips and Tricks)

1. Though tempting as it may be, suture closure of an anastomosis defect by itself is unlikely to be successful. With the ongoing infection and inflammation, the sutures can tear through the tissue.
2. Endoscopic clips can be useful to close small defects in these situations as the mucosal side tissue is often soft, pliable, and healthy.
3. Avoid closing the skin in grossly contaminated or infected cases. Instead, pack the wounds and consider vacuum-assisted closure later.

Special Postoperative Care

1. Approximately a quarter of patients with stomas created for an anastomotic leak will never have them reversed. Have good enterostomal education and support for your patients.
2. Patients who develop an anastomotic leak are at risk of developing further complications. Meticulous attention to postoperative care is required in order to try to prevent further complications from occurring. Wound care, appropriate antibiotic coverage, DVT prophylaxis, and nutrition are a few of the areas that warrant special consideration in this group of patients.
3. Many patients after leak treatment, or even in asymptomatic patients having interrogation for elective diverting stoma closure, will be found to have an anastomotic leak or sinus noted.
4. Time will allow for many of these sinus cavities to close. Although it can be difficult to wait, allowing several months to pass may let smaller cavities close and prevent longer-term problems associated with premature stoma

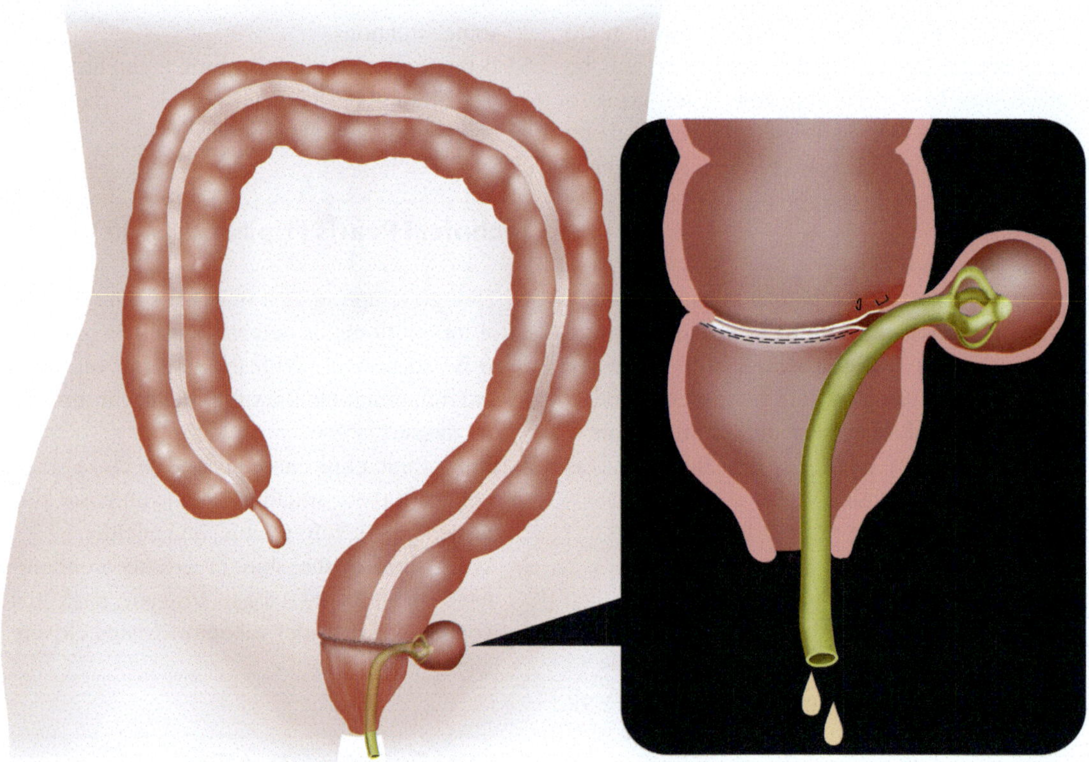

Fig. 25.1 Transanal catheter drainage using a Foley or Malecot catheter can promote sinus cavity emptying and closure

closure. If 6 months has passed and the sinus remains, as long as there is no communication with the peritoneal cavity, most patients can have stoma closure done safely. In one series though, 16% of similar patients developed sepsis after restoration of continuity and required more extensive reconstruction.

5. Transanal catheter drainage using a Foley or Malecot catheter can promote sinus cavity emptying and closure (Fig. 25.1). In addition to promoting drainage from the sinus cavity back into the rectum, the catheter "stents" the anus open. This further promotes drainage externally and away from the leak cavity, thus promoting the chance of spontaneous closure. In one series, 93% of patients with leak were able to have ileostomy closure after transanal catheter drainage. Endoscopic sponge devices have also been described. There appears to be greater benefit when patients started treatment sooner after surgery (75% healing within 6 weeks vs. 38% after that time period). Patients with large presacral cavities can be managed with linear stapler application to marsupialize the cavity and broaden communication with rectal lumen.
6. Strictures are very possible after the healing of an anastomotic leak, and patients with obstructive symptoms should be evaluated accordingly. Poor functional results from local pelvic fibrosis and loss of compliance are also common.

Suggested Reading

1. Blumetti J, Abcarian H. Management of low colorectal anastomotic leak: preserving the anastomosis. World J Gastrointest Surg. 2015;7(12):378–83.
2. Blumetti J, Chaudhry V, Prasad L, Abcarian H. Delayed transanal repair of persistent coloanal anastomotic

leak in diverted patients after resection for rectal cancer. Colorectal Dis Off J Assoc Coloproctol G B Irel. 2012;14(10):1238–41.
3. Chadi SA, Fingerhut A, Berho M, DeMeester SR, Fleshman JW, Hyman NH, et al. Emerging trends in the etiology, prevention, and treatment of gastrointestinal anastomotic leakage. J Gastrointest Surg. 2016;20(12):2035–51.
4. Dapri G, Guta D, Grozdev K, Antolino L, Bachir N, Jottard K, et al. Colorectal anastomotic leakage corrected by transanal laparoscopy. Colorectal Dis Off J Assoc Coloproctol G B Irel. 2016;18(6):O210–3.
5. Güenaga KF, Lustosa SAS, Saad SS, Saconato H, Matos D. Ileostomy or colostomy for temporary decompression of colorectal anastomosis. Cochrane Database Syst Rev. 2007;(1):CD004647.
6. Hain E, Maggiori L, Manceau G, Zappa M, Prost à la Denise J, Panis Y. Persistent asymptomatic anastomotic leakage after laparoscopic sphincter-saving surgery for rectal cancer: can diverting stoma be reversed safely at 6 months? Dis Colon Rectum. 2016;59(5):369–76.
7. Haito-Chavez Y, Law JK, Kratt T, Arezzo A, Verra M, Morino M, et al. International multicenter experience with an over-the-scope clipping device for endoscopic management of GI defects (with video). Gastrointest Endosc. 2014;80(4):610–22.
8. Matthiessen P, Hallböök O, Rutegård J, Simert G, Sjödahl R. Defunctioning stoma reduces symptomatic anastomotic leakage after low anterior resection of the rectum for cancer: a randomized multicenter trial. Ann Surg. 2007;246(2):207–14.
9. Sirois-Giguère E, Boulanger-Gobeil C, Bouchard A, Gagné J-P, Grégoire RC, Thibault C, et al. Transanal drainage to treat anastomotic leaks after low anterior resection for rectal cancer: a valuable option. Dis Colon Rectum. 2013;56(5):586–92.
10. Stewart BT, Stitz RW. Marsupialization of presacral collections with use of an endoscopic stapler. Dis Colon Rectum. 1999;42(2):264–5.
11. van Koperen PJ, van Berge Henegouwen MI, Rosman C, Bakker CM, Heres P, Slors JFM, et al. The Dutch multicenter experience of the Endo-Sponge treatment for anastomotic leakage after colorectal surgery. Surg Endosc. 2009;23(6):1379–83.

Colon Does Not Reach for a Coloanal Anastomosis

26

Shirley Shih and David E. Rivadeneira

Clinical Scenario

You are operating on a 55-year-old obese man with foreshortened mesentery undergoing low anterior resection for a low rectal cancer approximately 2 cm from anorectal ring. As you prepare the colon for a hand-sewn anal anastomosis, you realize the colon gets stuck in the pelvis and does not reach the anus.

Key Points

1. Mobilize the avascular embryonic planes.
   (a) Complete mobilization of all lateral/white line of Toldt and retroperitoneal attachments, those adherent to Gerota's fascia. Dissection medially should allow for clear visualization of the major vasculature, that's the inferior mesenteric vein, left colic artery, and inferior mesenteric artery.
2. Mobilize the entire splenic flexure.
   (a) Must mobilize the complete splenic flexure, this is accomplished by dissecting the tethering attachments to the gastrocolic, phrenicocolic, renalcolic, and splenocolic ligaments.
3. Ligation of inferior mesenteric vein (IMV).
   (a) Appropriate tension-free distal colorectal and coloanal anastomosis often require ligation of the IMV.
4. Break the pelvic air seal.
   (a) Sweep with fingers around the colon from below to release the vacuum.
      (i) Placing a plastic Ferguson Retractor or a Alexis wound protector in through the anus will aid in lessening the friction of the thick colon.
5. Exposure and Retraction from below
   (a) Place either effacing sutures or lone star retractors and place interrupted guide sutures.
   (b) Remove the effacing sutures or lone stars as you do the anastomosis so that the anus will recoil back into the pelvis.

Operative Assessment

1. Almost all circumstances the splenic flexure will need to be mobilized completely. Releasing the splenic flexure, whether

S. Shih
Northwell Health, Department of Colorectal Surgery, Woodbury, NY, USA

D. E. Rivadeneira (✉)
Surgical Strategic Initiatives, Northwell Health, New Hyde Park, NY, USA

Surgical Services and Colorectal Surgery, Huntington Hospital, Huntington, NY, USA

Hofstra University-Northwell School of Medicine, Hempstead, NY, USA
e-mail: DRivadeneira@northwell.edu

S. W. Lee et al. (eds.), *Colorectal Surgery Consultation*,
https://doi.org/10.1007/978-3-030-11181-6_26

performed open or laparoscopically, adds 10–28 cm of colon length.
2. Proper identification of the vascular supply is mandatory, clear identification of the inferior mesenteric artery and vein, left colic artery, and marginal artery.
3. If the case starts either robotic or laparoscopic and unable to mobilize the colon appropriately, then conversion to hand-assisted or open technique should be considered.

Operative Checklist

1. Extra-long laparoscopic bowel graspers are often useful for laparoscopic mobilization of splenic flexure.
2. Angled laparoscopic such as a 30° or a flexible tip laparoscope can provide additional visualization particularly of the flexure.
3. Increasing use of fluorescence imaging has been used particularly to map out the vascular supply of the colon to be anastomosed.

Operative Technique

1. Incise the gastrocolic ligament to separate the transverse colon from the omentum in order to gain entrance into the lesser sac. Another option if the splenic flexure is very high or in the splenic hilum is to get into the lesser sac along greater curvature of the stomach and leave the omentum attached to colon. Ensure your incision is long enough to gain access to left upper quadrant (LUQ) and that retraction is positioned so that LUQ is maximally exposed.
2. Laparoscopic surgery allows for excellent visualization of the flexure and is our preferred approach. Continue the medial to lateral dissection that was already initiated at the IMA level up toward the splenic flexure so that only a thin layer of peritoneum needs to be incised on the lateral aspect to fully take down the flexure.
3. The purpose of taking down the splenic flexure is to afford reach of the colon end to the pelvis. In some patients there are splenic flexure adhesions between the distal transverse colon and the proximal descending colon that cause a corner or a kink in the colon. This may be due to adherent epiploica, scarred omentum from prior inflammation, or congenital adhesions along the leaflets of the mesentery. By releasing these adhesions, the colon is straightened and allows for better reach to the pelvis. Similarly, an avascular area of mesentery just lateral to the IMV can be incised allowing the mobilized colon to reach further caudal. Palpating the vessels and transillumination may be particularly helpful in these situations. It is important to understand that it is the mesentery of the colon that limits reach.
   (a) High ligation of IMA 1 cm distal to takeoff from aorta
   (b) Ligation of IMV at base of pancreas
   (c) Blood supply to remaining colon, after ligation of IMA and IMV is provided by middle colic artery through marginal artery.
4. In cases where the above maneuvers do not provide adequate reach, a more proximal colon resection may be necessary. This is particularly true in cases of a short, fatty mesentery. As more mesentery is mobilized from left to right of the patient, the colon end invariably becomes ischemic and needs to be sacrificed. In these cases, it may be prudent to leave the patient with an end colostomy or consider a Deloyers procedure or a retroileal dissection (see Chap. 18).

Technical Pearls (Tips and Tricks)

1. Understanding of vascular anatomy and embryonic planes.
2. Complete mobilization of the splenic flexure is mandatory.
3. Ligation of the inferior mesenteric vein will add considerable length to the colon to be anastomosed.
4. Sweep with fingers around the colon from below to release the pelvic air-vacuum.

5. Placing a plastic Ferguson Retractor or a self-expanding wound protector in through the anus will aid in lessening the friction of the thick colon.
6. Place either effacing sutures or lone star retractors and place interrupted guide sutures.
7. Remove the effacing sutures or lone stars as you do the anastomosis so that the anus will recoil back into the pelvis.
8. Plan in advance and counsel patient on potential for additional colon resection and even possibility of a permanent colostomy should all above maneuvers fail to allow for tension free anastomosis. This is especially important in patients seen preoperatively who are obese and the potentially for foreshortened mesentery is greater. Also caution with patients with prior colon resections as their blood supply maybe compromised and increase ischemia of the mobilized colon.

Suggested Reading

1. Davis B, Rafferty JF. Technical aspects. In: Steele SR, Maykel JA, Champagne BJ, Orangio GR, editors. Complexities in colorectal surgery. New York: Springer Publ; 2014. p. 508–10.
2. Lee S, Ross H, Rivadeneira DE, Steele S, Feingold D. Advanced colonoscopy and endoluminal surgery. Cham: Springer; 2017.
3. Ross H, Lee S, Champagne B, Pigazzi A, Rivadeneira DE, editors. Robotic colorectal surgery. New York: Springer Publishing; 2015.
4. Ross H, Lee S, Mutch M, Rivadeneira D, Steele SR, editors. Minimally invasive approaches to colon and rectal disease: technique and best practices. New York: Springer Publishing; 2015.

27 Cannot Find Internal Opening of Fistula-in-Ano

Daniel L. Feingold and J. Mark Kiely

Clinical Scenario

A 30-year-old woman who had an abscess incised and drained in the emergency room 3 months ago, presents with continuing minimal daily drainage through an opening in the I and D scar consistent with fistula in ano. During exam under anesthesia, the probe tracts toward the anal canal but no internal opening is found.

Key Points

1. Accurately identifying the internal opening is critical to the successful treatment of fistula in ano. Where there is a high suspicion of having a fistula but the internal opening is not readily discernable, it is important not to over aggressively probe the external opening looking for the internal opening as this can create a false passage. In this situation, the "recurrence" after the subsequent fistula operation may, in reality, be a "persistence" of the original fistula tract.
2. Goodsall's rule predicts the location of the internal opening based on the location of the external opening and has a higher predictive value for fistulas with posterior external openings (Fig. 27.1). According to this rule of thumb, fistulas with an external opening posterior to the transverse anal line are curved with internal openings in the posterior midline, while fistulas with external opening anterior to the transverse anal line have internal openings that track in a radial fashion. Fistulas that are longer, due to non-cryptoglandular etiologies or anterior, are less likely to follow Goodsall's rule.

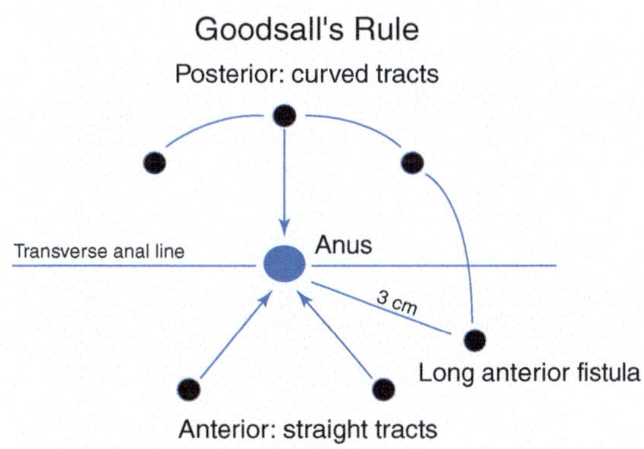

Fig. 27.1 Goodsall's rule

D. L. Feingold (✉) · J. M. Kiely
Division of Colorectal Surgery, Department of Surgery, Columbia University, New York, NY, USA
e-mail: df347@cumc.columbia.edu

S. W. Lee et al. (eds.), *Colorectal Surgery Consultation*,
https://doi.org/10.1007/978-3-030-11181-6_27

Operative Checklist

1. Additional resources and equipment.
   (a) A dedicated anorectal surgery instrument tray with a variety of "S" probes, malleable probes, and fine lacrimal duct probes as well as a syringe with a 14 gauge angiocatheter and hydrogen peroxide and a sigmoidoscope.

Technical Pearls (Tips and Tricks)

1. Review prior operative reports, if available, as these may give insight into the location of the internal opening.
2. Careful digital exam feeling for a cord or induration combined with anoscopy can often determine the site of the internal opening. Manual pressure on a residual abscess can discharge through the internal opening demonstrating the internal opening.
3. Inject the external opening with hydrogen peroxide through a 14-gauge angio-catheter while performing anoscopy to determine the location of the internal opening. If the peroxide does not pass, move the anoscope to another location and repeat the injection looking for the internal opening (Fig. 27.2). A smaller anal retractor works better as a larger retractor can actually occlude the fistula tract.

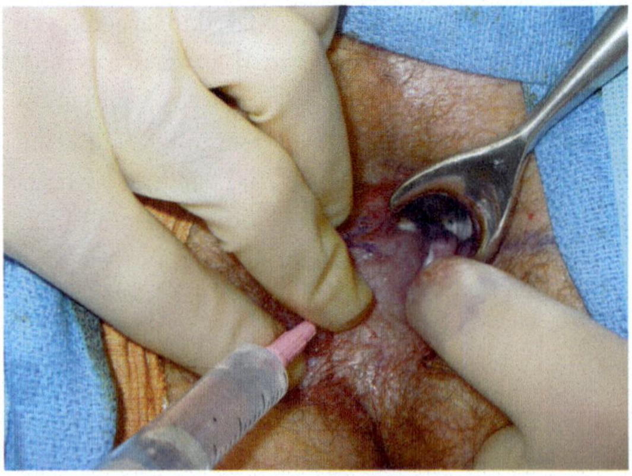

Fig. 27.2 Inject the external opening with hydrogen peroxide through a 14-gauge angio-catheter while performing anoscopy to determine the location of the internal opening. (Courtesy of Dr. Adrian Ortega)

4. Carefully probe the external opening with an "S" shaped rigid probe or a malleable probe using an index finger in the canal as a guide. Ideally, the probe should drop into the internal opening relatively effortlessly. Fine lacrimal duct probes may be helpful to negotiate tracts.
5. Fishhook-shaped probes can be used transanally to evaluate possible internal openings.
6. Avoid excessive retraction on the buttocks as this can distort the fistula anatomy and make it difficult to pass a probe.
7. Evaluate the rectum with a sigmoidoscope and with careful anoscopic examination looking for an extra-sphincteric internal opening.
8. If an internal opening is not found despite the above maneuvers, unroof and debride the external opening to provide wider drainage, curette the chronic abscess cavity and marsupialize the wound. Alternatively, a drain can be placed in the external opening to provide drainage and to potentially use for postoperative fistulography, though MRI has supplanted this modality in most circumstances.

Special Postoperative Care

1. Disclose to the patient that no internal fistula opening was found at the exam under anesthesia. It is important that patients understand that just because no internal opening was found does not mean there is no fistula. Patients should be counseled about the risks for recurrent infection and continued drainage, which may require repeat exam under anesthesia.
2. Consider cross-sectional imaging with MRI and counsel the patient that the yield from this study may be low and that any apparent tract visualized will still need to be found during repeat exam under anesthesia. Other ancillary imaging modalities like CT or ultrasonography (endoanal or trans-perineal) may be used depending on available expertise.

Suggested Reading

1. Garg P, Singh P, Kaur B. Magnetic resonance imaging: operative findings correlation in 229 fistula-in-ano patients. World J Surg. 2017;41:1618–24.
2. Vogel JD, Johnson EK, Morris AM, Paquette IM, Saclarides TJ, Feingold DL, Steele SR. Clinical practice guideline for the management of anorectal abscess, fistula-in-ano, and rectovaginal fistula. Dis Colon Rectum. 2016;59:1117–33.

How to Deal with Crohn's Friable and Fragile Mesentery

28

Anuradha R. Bhama and Scott R. Steele

Clinical Scenario

A 28-year-old male is undergoing an ileocolic resection for medically refractory Crohn's disease. The segment of bowel to be resected has been identified. When taking the mesentery to this segment, there is profuse bleeding from the mesentery.

Key Points

1. Crohn's mesentery can range in thickness and inflammation leading to bleeding intraoperatively and postoperatively (Fig. 28.1). Controlling the mesentery is often the most difficult part of this kind of operation.
2. Gentle traction should be used when handling the bowel to avoid unnecessary troublesome bleeding.
3. It is necessary to know several techniques to control fragile mesentery.
4. Controlling bleeding intraoperatively and preventing postoperative bleeding are mandatory in these operations.
5. It may be necessary to utilize several different techniques in the same operation to control bleeding in Crohn's mesentery.

Operative Assessment

1. How inflamed and thick is the mesentery?
   (a) When there is greater inflammation, the mesentery is more friable and bleeding is harder to control.
   (b) Prepare for bleeding before it starts.
2. Does the bleeding continue with the currently employed method?
   (a) Surgical staplers
   (b) Suture ligation (ties versus ligature)
   (c) Energy devices for hemostasis
3. If laparoscopic, it may be necessary to convert to an open procedure to control hemorrhage.

Operative Checklist

1. Additional helpful equipment.
   (a) Surgical stapler (Fig. 28.2).
      (i) White vascular loads on GIA stapler (use 60 mm or 75 mm stapler).
      (ii) Can use open or laparoscopic staplers.

A. R. Bhama
Department of Colorectal Surgery, Cleveland Clinic, Cleveland, OH, USA

S. R. Steele (✉)
Case Western Reserve University School of Medicine, Cleveland, OH, USA

Department of Colorectal Surgery, Cleveland Clinic, Cleveland, OH, USA

S. W. Lee et al. (eds.), *Colorectal Surgery Consultation*,
https://doi.org/10.1007/978-3-030-11181-6_28

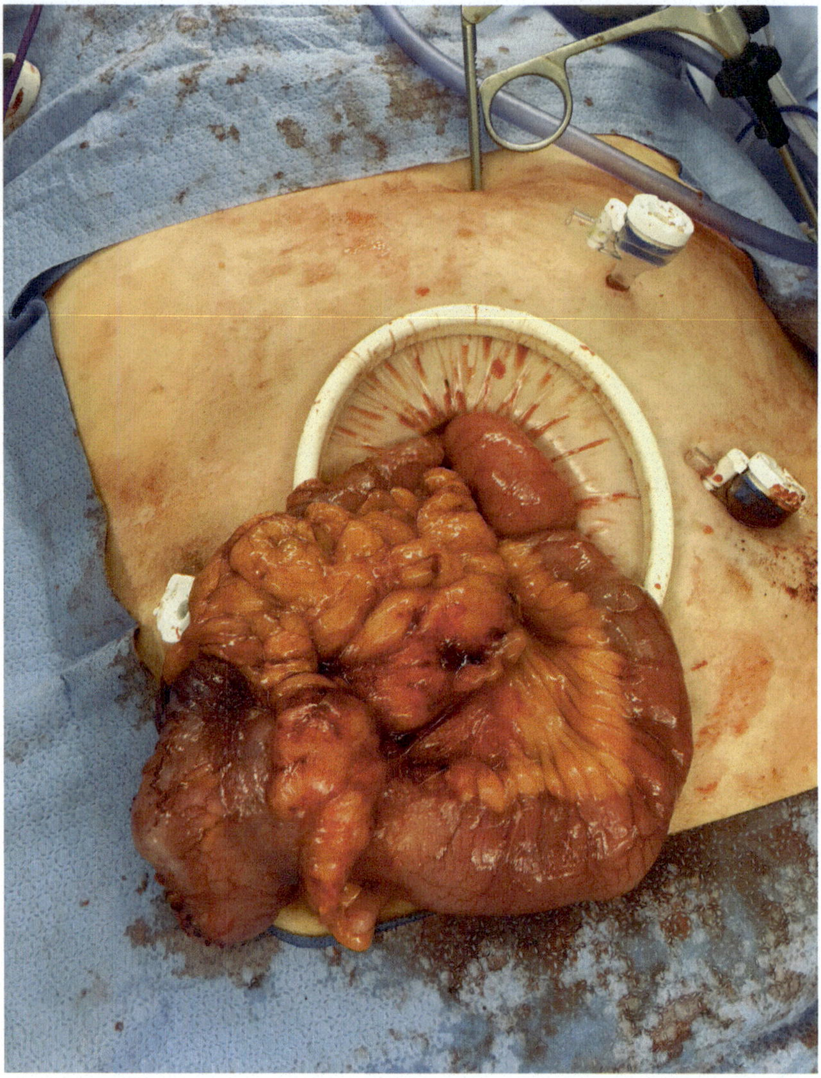

Fig. 28.1 Assessment of mesenteric thickness in Crohn's disease

(b) Suture ligation.
   (i) Larger-caliber ties (0 or #1 suture).
   (ii) Larger-caliber suture on large needle (0 or #1 on CT-1).
   (iii) Large clamps (i.e., Pean, Kelly, Crawford).
(c) Energy devices.
   (i) LigaSure, Harmonic, Enseal, Thunderbeat, Sonovision, etc.
   (ii) Can use open or laparoscopic devices: may need to take in layers.
      (a) Five millimeter devices can be difficult.
      (b) May need to "fire" several times prior to dividing.
(d) Converting to open.
   (i) Retractor of choice (Bookwalter, Balfour, Omni, Thompson, etc.).
   (ii) Wound protector.

2. Exposure.
   (a) If performing a laparoscopic procedure and unable to obtain hemostasis with laparoscopic energy devices or laparoscopic staplers, convert to an open procedure with an incision generous enough to visualize and control the bleeding. Place a

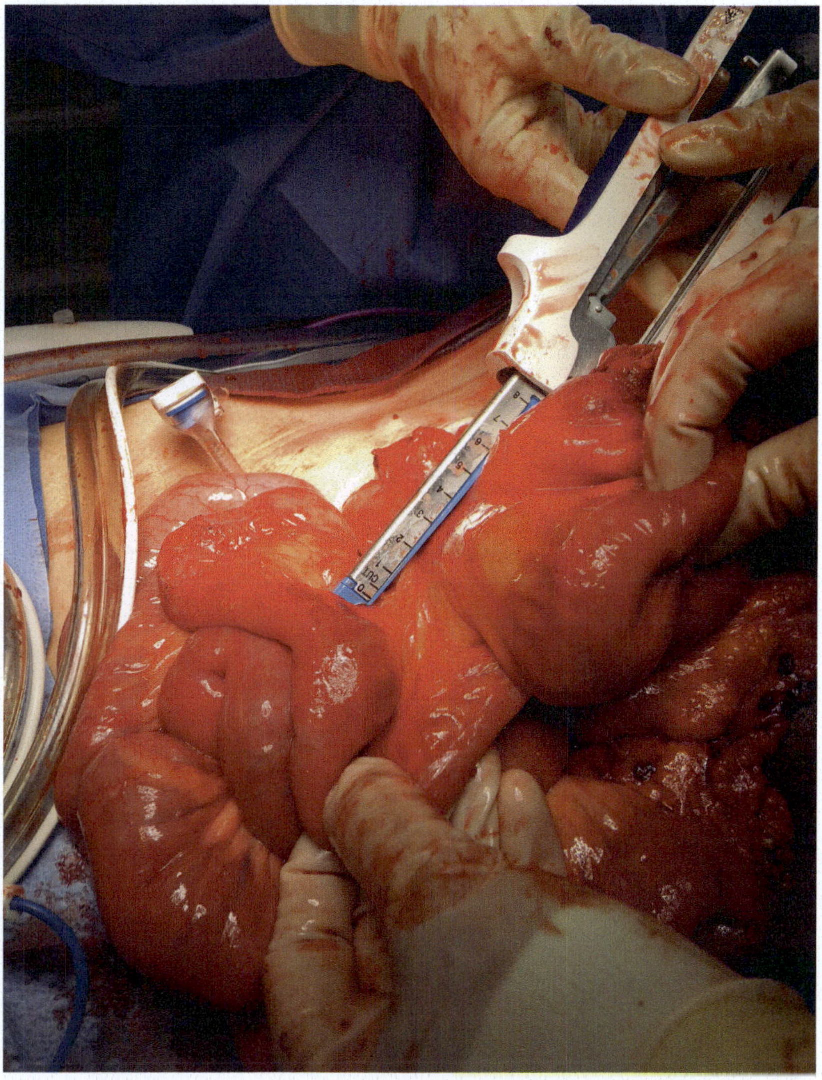

Fig. 28.2 Surgical stapler transection of mesentery

wound protector and body wall retractor, if needed.

3. Positioning.
   (a) Patients typically do not require repositioning unless converting from laparoscopic to open, in which case the operating table can be leveled.

Operative Techniques

1. Surgical staplers.
   (a) Surgical staplers can provide both compression of the tissues and hemostasis. It is necessary to use a stapler with the proper size staples to ensure hemostasis (i.e., white vascular load). Hold the stapler clamped for a period of time to compress tissue prior to dividing (Fig. 28.2).
2. Clamps and ties.
   (a) If possible, using a larger clamp, such as a Kocher, Pean, or Kelly clamp, will be more effective than using a smaller clamp, such as a hemostat or tonsil. Smaller clamps cause more bleeding from the inflamed mesentery. Ensure that the clamp is all the way across the mesentery that is to be ligated. Using larger-caliber ties will provide better hemostasis than thinner suture, which may saw through the

mesentery causing more bleeding or may simply break (Figs. 28.3 and 28.4).

3. Suture ligature.
   (a) In some situations, simply clamping and tying will not adequately control the bleeding. In these situations, it is necessary to perform a formal suture ligature. If the mesentery is quite thick, preferentially use a larger needle, as a standard SH needle will not be long enough to pass through to the other side of the mesentery. If bleeding continues, re-clamp the mesentery with another clamp and place another stitch (Fig. 28.5). In many cases it is possible to use overlapping clamps, and the clamp may need to be a Kocher-type to have adequate tissue holding ability.
4. Vessel-sealing energy devices.
   (a) There are several different commercially available energy devices. For thinner mesentery, it is possible to use these in the standard fashion (Fig. 28.6). When the mesentery is thicker and friable, one may have to adjust the technique of using the device in order to achieve hemostasis. This may include taking the mesentery in two layers or activating the device while closing the jaws. It may be necessary to forgo using the energy device and utilize suture ties or ligatures, instead.

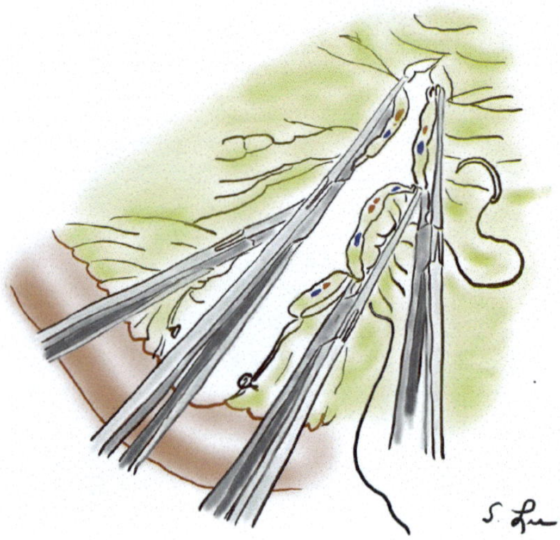

Fig. 28.3 Kocher clamps and suture ligation of the mesentery

Technical Pearls (Tips and Tricks)

1. For surgical staplers. Clamp down the stapler on the mesentery, and wait 30 seconds for tissue compression. This will help compress the edema, and allow the staples to penetrate the thickness of the tissue. Use 60 or 75 mm loads, and ensure that the stapler is completely across the segment of tissue to be transected

Fig. 28.4 Completed closure of the mesentery after suture ligation

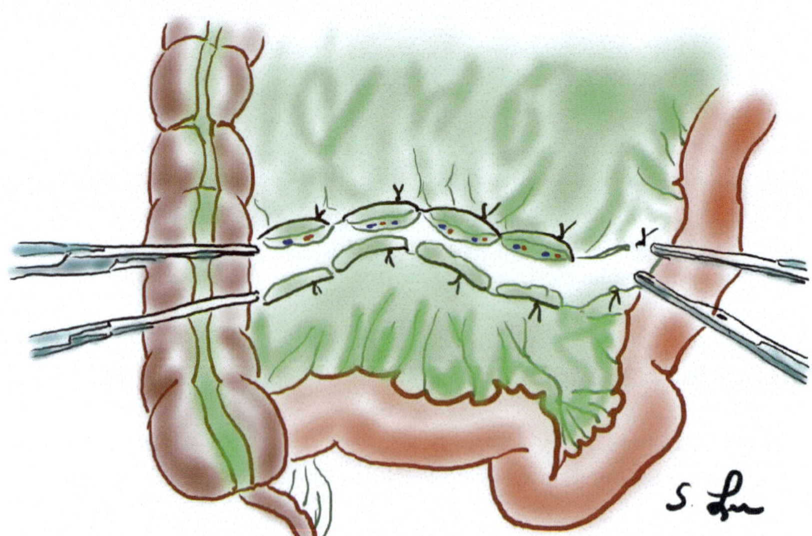

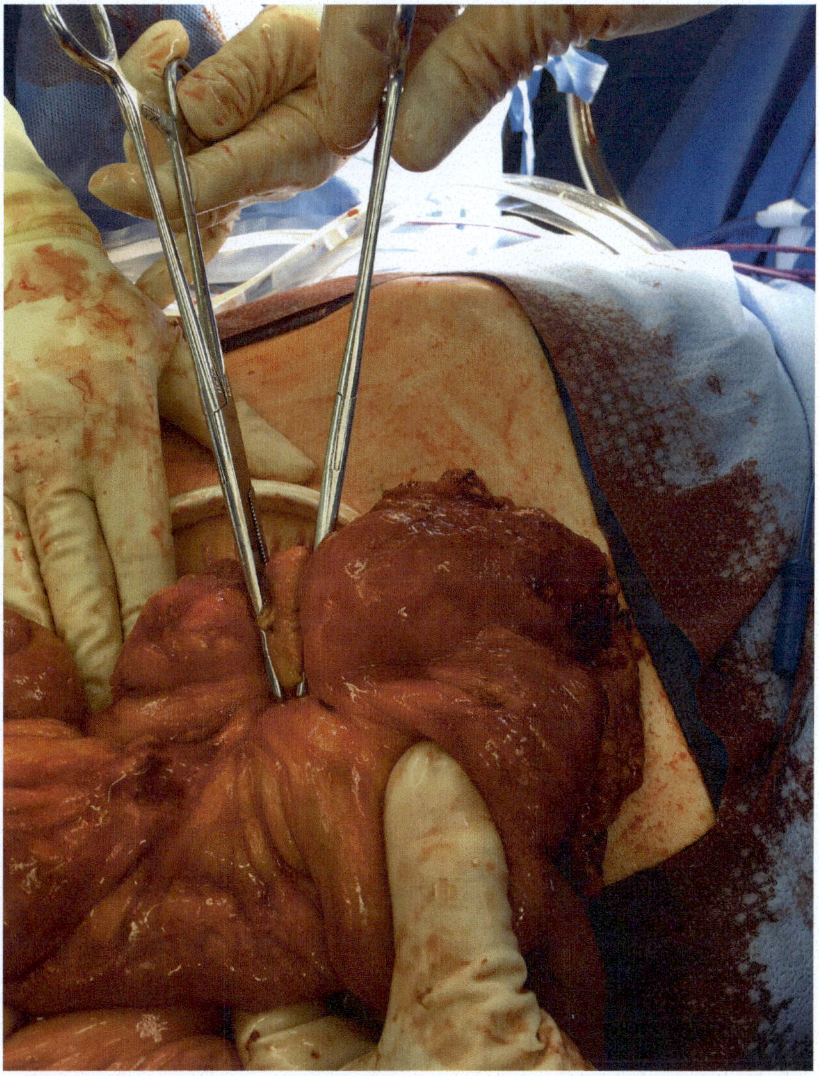

Fig. 28.5 Kocher clamps replaced on the mesentery to divide and suture

prior to firing. A vascular white load ensures the staple height is adequate for hemostasis.

2. When using energy devices. First place the open jaw on the mesentery, then activate the device, and start to close slowly. Close the jaws all the way down, and activate again for a full round prior to cutting. Can also put one of the jaws within the mesentery and seal in two layers.
3. It is helpful to come across the diseased mesentery in mid-mesentery as long as a nodal catch is not required for the resection. By staying closer to the bowel wall rather than at the base of the mesentery, it is easier to control the bleeding cut edge of the mesentery, and there may be less risk to other structures.
4. It may be necessary to use multiple techniques during the same operation as the thickness and friability of the mesentery varies throughout the segment of bowel to be resected.
5. Ensure all bleeding has stopped prior to concluding the procedure, even apparently minor nuisance bleeding may worsen postoperatively and cause significant postoperative hemorrhage.

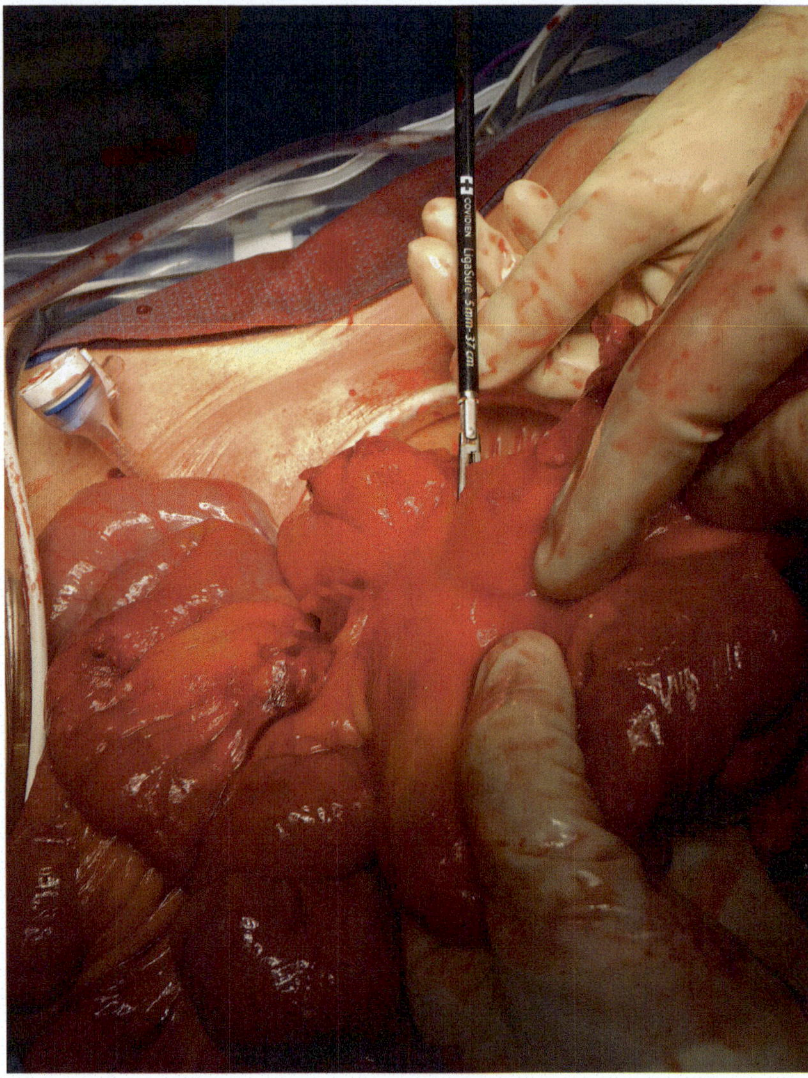

Fig. 28.6 Taking mesentery in two layers using vessel-sealing device

Special Postoperative Care

1. Be cautious with NSAIDs, deep vein thrombosis (DVT) prophylaxis, and therapeutic anticoagulation postoperatively. If there was significant bleeding intraoperatively, check postoperative hemoglobin for baseline.
2. Have a high suspicion for bleeding in patients with tachycardia, hypotension, or a drop in hemoglobin (do not just assume dilution).
3. If bleeding, patient should be taken back to operating room for re-exploration and control of hemorrhage.
4. Otherwise manage per institution-specific enhanced recovery protocol.

Suggested Reading

1. Muldoon R, Herline AJ. Crohn's disease: surgical management. In: Steele SR, Hull TL, et al., editors. ASCRS textbook of colon & rectal surgery. Cham: Springer; 2017.

Ulcerative Colitis with Severe Inflammation and Friable Tissues: How to Avoid Intraoperative Perforation and Manage the Colorectal Stump

29

Sang W. Lee

Clinical Scenario

A 45-year-old woman is undergoing subtotal colectomy for medically refractory acute colitis. The patient's large intestine is extremely inflamed and friable.

Key Points

1. Excessive tugging on the colon may lead to perforation. Gentle manipulation of the tissue is critical.
2. In patients with severe colitis, up to 20–30% of the rectal stumps can dehisce causing pelvic abscesses and peritonitis. Many of these patients are deconditioned and these infections can be difficult to clear.
3. Exteriorization of the rectosigmoid stump is preferred over a Hartmann procedure because it prevents the staple line from leaking intraperitoneally.
4. Venting with a rectal tube can reduce the risk of rectal stump blowout but does not completely prevent this complication. If used, large-caliber tubes such as a 42 French Malecot or a chest tube can adequately decompress the rectum.
5. Mucous fistulas are cumbersome for patients due to their continuous drainage and the need for a second stoma appliance.
6. Securing the rectal stump in the subcutaneous tissues has a lower rate of pelvic sepsis and lower total morbidity than leaving the rectal stump in the abdomen.
7. If the rectosigmoid is severely diseased and friable, a mucous fistula can be created.
8. If the rectosigmoid is too friable to hold sutures, exteriorizing a length of the colon through the mucus fistula site and wrapping it in gauze allows for a seal at the skin level and can be followed by delayed creation of a mucous fistula.

Operative Assessment

1. Patients are often malnourished, on chronic steroids, and immunosuppressed. Possible disruption of a retained rectal stump should be anticipated.
2. In cases where the colon stump is too friable to hold sutures or staples, manipulation of the colon should be kept to a minimum.

Operative Checklist

1. Additional helpful equipment.
   (a) Lighted pelvic retractors (Brite-Tracts)
   (b) Flexible sigmoidoscopy

S. W. Lee (✉)
Department of Surgery – Colon and Rectal Surgery, Keck School of Medicine of University of Southern California, Los Angeles, CA, USA

S. W. Lee et al. (eds.), *Colorectal Surgery Consultation*,
https://doi.org/10.1007/978-3-030-11181-6_29

2. Exposure.
   (a) For laparoscopic access, consider hand-assisted approach to minimize trauma to the tissues causing inadvertent perforation.
   (b) Avoid direct manipulation of the colon using forceps or graspers.
3. Positioning.
   (a) Lithotomy position

Operative Techniques

1. Staple transection and securing the distal sigmoid colon stump in the subcutaneous tissues.
   (a) Retain long enough distal sigmoid colon to reach the lower end of the midline incision or Pfannenstiel incision without tension (~25 cm). Transect the sigmoid stump using a linear stapler. The rectosigmoid stump will protrude beyond the abdominal fascia and into the subcutaneous tissues. The stump is extra-peritonealized by suturing the seromuscular layer of the colon to the peritoneum and anterior fascia. The skin overlying the site can be either closed or left open. Up to 75% of the sigmoid stumps secured in this fashion will stay closed, and, in these patients, the inconvenience of a mucous fistula is prevented (Fig. 29.1). If the stump goes on to disrupt in the subcutaneous tissues, the wound can be managed with routine local wound care and packing, and, in most cases, the perforation heals on its own. Another advantage of this procedure is that at the second operation, mobilizing the colon stump down from the abdominal wall is much easier than mobilizing the rectal stump from the pelvis.
2. Creation of mucous fistula.
   (a) As an alternative to stapling off the distal sigmoid stump, a formal mucous fistula can be formed through the lower end of the midline incision or through a separate incision. If the colon stump can be stapled

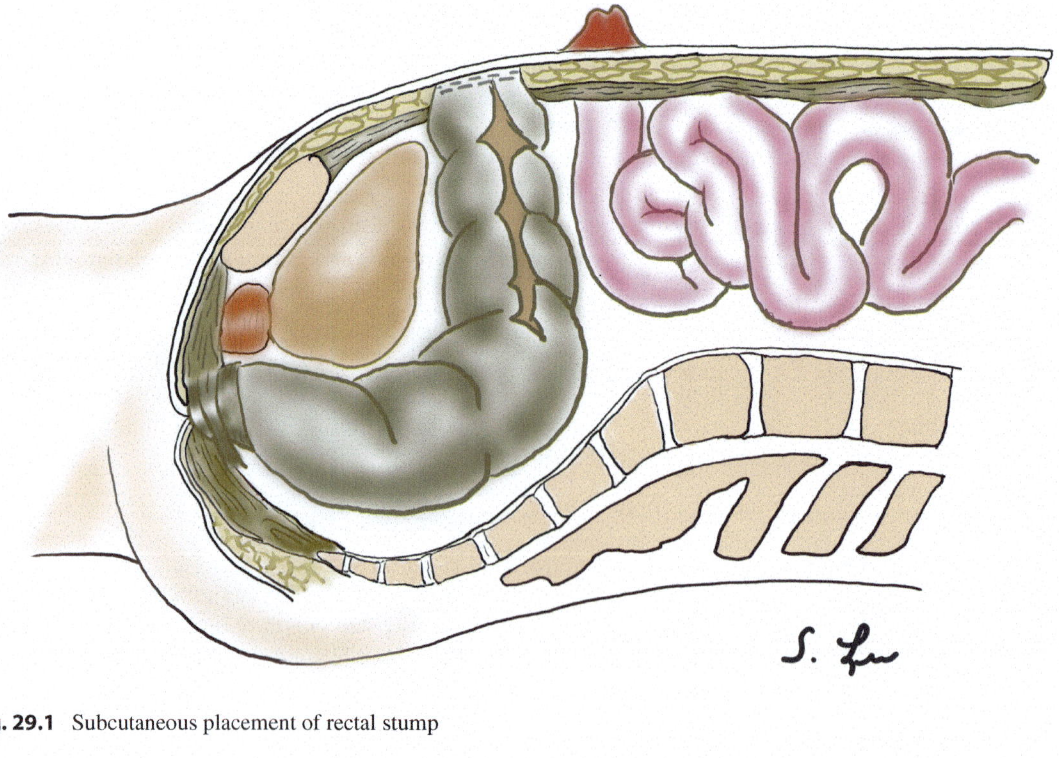

Fig. 29.1 Subcutaneous placement of rectal stump

off safely, our preference is to perform the exteriorization described above.

3. Delayed creation of a mucous fistula.
   (a) If the colon stump is too friable to hold staples or sutures, 5–10 cm of the colon stump can be left protruding beyond the skin wrapped in a Kerlix or lap pad. Silk sutures are tied around the gauze to provide anchorage to the abdominal wall. Over time, the colon wall adheres to the surrounding abdominal wall creating a seal. Five to seven days postoperatively, the stump is transected at the skin level and is secured with several interrupted sutures to mature a mucous fistula.
4. Rectal tube placement.
   (a) A large bore (38 or 42 French) Malecot or a chest tube is inserted into the anus and left in the distal pouch. The tube is secured using drain sutures tied around the tube and anchored to a thick duoderm placed around the perianal area.

Technical Pearls (Tips and Tricks)

1. Before transecting the colon, retain the sigmoid colon long enough to comfortably reach just above the skin level. It is easy to underestimate the length of colon required for this reach.
2. Close the fascia in continuous fashion until it closes snuggly around the colon stump. Place interrupted suture between the fascia and seromuscular layers of the colon to prevent the rectal stump retracting into the peritoneal cavity.
3. Delayed mucous fistula maturation can be performed at the bedside. The Kerlix around the stump is removed and the colon wall transected just above the skin level. The mucous fistula is matured by placing several interrupted sutures between the colon wall and the skin using absorbable sutures, per usual.

Special Postoperative Care

1. Routine postoperative care is recommended
2. If wound infection develops after rectal stump exteriorization, partial opening of the wound with moist saline packing should be continued until drainage tapers off

Suggested Reading

1. Gu J, Stochhi L, Remzi F, Kiran RP. Intraperitoneal or subcutaneous: does location of the (colo)rectal stump influence outcomes after laparoscopic total abdominal colectomy for ulcerative colitis? Dis Colon Rectum. 2013;56(5):615–21.
2. Michelassi F, Milsom JW. Operative strategies in inflammatory bowel disease. New York: Springer; 1999.
3. Trickett JP, Tilney HS, Gudgeon AM, Mellor SG, Edwards DP. Management of the rectal stump after emergency sub-total colectomy: which surgical option is associated with the lower morbidity? Color Dis. 2005;7(5):519–22.

Patient Develops Anastomotic Stricture After Low Anastomosis with Diverting Ileostomy

30

Nivedh V. Paluvoi and Sang W. Lee

Clinical Scenario

A 32-year-old male with medically refractory ulcerative colitis is now 3 months status post total proctocolectomy with ileal pouch anal anastomosis (IPAA) and diverting loop ileostomy. Hypaque enema prior to ileostomy reversal shows anastomotic stricture. Endoscopic evaluation in the operating room reveals a web at the pouch anal anastomosis, and you are unable to identify the proximal lumen.

Key Points

1. Anastomotic stricture to varying degrees occurs in 3–30% of colorectal or pouch anal anastomoses.
2. Diagnosis is made by digital rectal examination or on radiographic or endoscopic evaluation prior to diverting stoma reversal (Fig. 30.1).
3. When unable to clearly identify the lumen, do not blindly force a digit, bougie, or endoscope through the web or stricture.

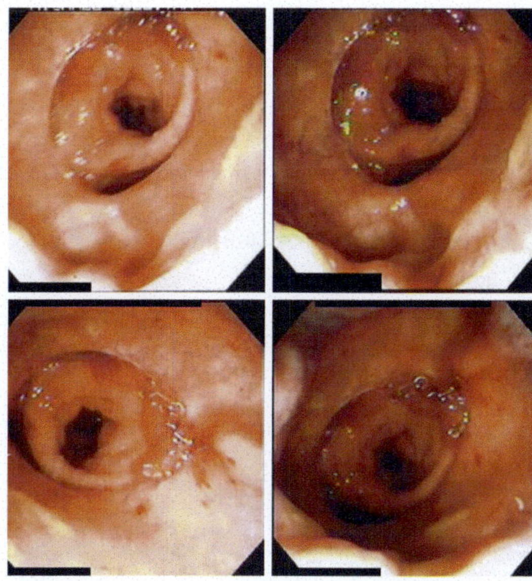

Fig. 30.1 Anastomotic stricture in a proximally diverted patient via flexible sigmoidoscope

4. When endoscopic evaluation of the anastomosis from the distal to proximal approach does not clearly reveal the lumen, a proximal to distal approach from the efferent limb of the diverting stoma may be useful.
   (a) Visualization of transillumination proximal to the anastomosis allows the surgeon to identify the lumen.
5. When the initial operation was performed for malignancy, keep in mind that the stricture may represent recurrence at the anastomosis and the patient should be evaluated appropriately.

N. V. Paluvoi
University of Miami, Department of Surgery, Division of Colorectal Surgery, Pasadena, CA, USA

S. W. Lee (✉)
Department of Surgery – Colon and Rectal Surgery, Keck School of Medicine of University of Southern California, Los Angeles, CA, USA

S. W. Lee et al. (eds.), *Colorectal Surgery Consultation*, https://doi.org/10.1007/978-3-030-11181-6_30

Operative Assessment

1. Where is the anastomosis located in relation to the anal verge?
2. Is there a visible lumen?
   (a) If the lumen is visible, serial dilatation is possible using sequentially larger "through the scope" balloons.
   (b) If the lumen is not visible, a colonoscope can be advanced through the efferent limb of the diverting loop ileostomy to reach the anastomosis.

Operative Checklist

1. Endoscopic tower with a colonoscope
2. Rigid sigmoidoscope with a long metal suction device
3. Endoscopic balloon dilator made available

Operative Techniques

1. Endoscopy through the efferent limb of the diverting stoma.
   (a) With the patient in either the left lateral position or the lithotomy position, the endoscope is gently inserted through the efferent limb of the stoma and passed to the level of the strictured anastomosis. Depending on the level of the anastomosis, either an anoscope or a rigid proctoscope is inserted from below, while transillumination is performed via the endoscope. The light from the endoscope is identified from the distal side of the anastomosis, and a small incision is made into the lumen toward the light using an electrosurgical device. Once the lumen is entered, the lumen can be serially dilated either using a balloon dilator or a bougie (Fig. 30.2).

Technical Pearls (Tips and Tricks)

1. Transillumination of the endoscope must clearly be visualized prior to incising in order to prevent perforation of the bowel wall.
   (a) The operative lights should be moved away from the field during this portion to maximize visibility of transillumination.

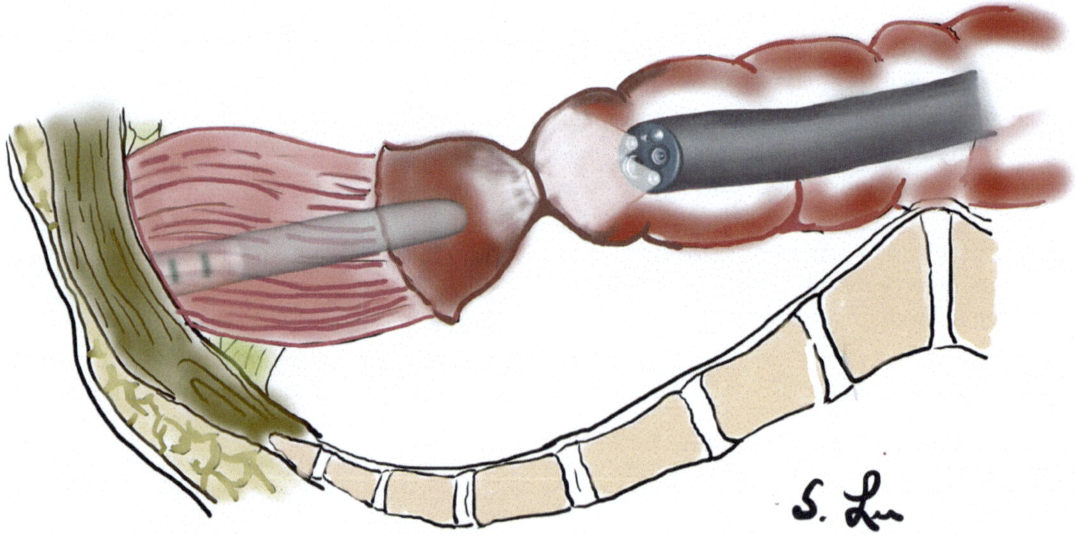

Fig. 30.2 An endoscope is gently inserted through the efferent limb of the stoma and passed to the level of the strictured anastomosis. Depending on the level of the anastomosis, either an anoscope or a rigid proctoscope is inserted from below, while transillumination is performed via the endoscope. The light from the endoscope is identified from the distal side of the anastomosis, and a small incision is made into the lumen toward the light using an electrosurgical device

2. Smaller-caliber endoscopes are preferred to the standard colonoscope when performing endoscopy through the defunctionalized efferent limb.
3. Prior to reversal of the diverting stoma, the anastomosis should once again be evaluated with radiologic imaging and endoscopy to confirm patency.

Special Postoperative Care

1. The patient should be warned that he/she may experience bleeding after this procedure.
2. As is with any endoscopy, a patient presenting with abdominal pain and distention should raise concern for perforation.

Suggested Reading

1. Sinh P, Shen B. Endoscopic evaluation of surgically altered bowel in patients with inflammatory bowel diseases. Inflamm Bowel Dis. 2015;21(6):1459–71.
2. Umanskiy K, Hyman N. Anastomotic complications. In: Steele SR, Hull TL, Read TE, Saclarides TJ, Senagore AJ, Whitlow CB, editors. The ASCRS textbook of colon and rectal surgery. 3rd ed. Heidelberg, New York, Dordrecht, London: Springer Publ; 2016. p. P161–71.

Presacral Bleeding

31

Sarah Koller and Howard M. Ross

Clinical Scenario

You are performing a laparoscopic low anterior resection on a 55-year-old, obese female. She has a mid-rectal T_2 tumor and did not require neoadjuvant chemoradiation. Your dissection is going well, until you encounter some minor venous bleeding in the pelvis. You suction and pack the pelvis and continue with your dissection until the bleeding begins welling up quickly, prohibiting you from continuing the dissection (Fig. 31.1).

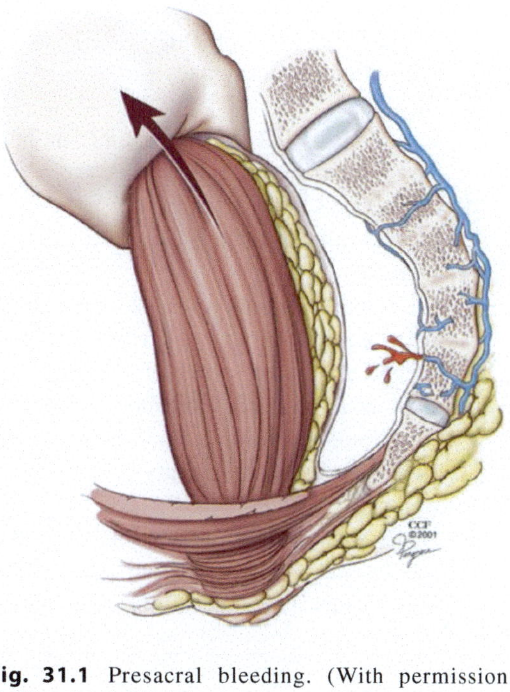

Fig. 31.1 Presacral bleeding. (With permission. © Cleveland Clinic)

Key Points

1. Copious presacral bleeding can occur during rectal dissection and can be a lethal complication.
2. Communication between the surgical and anesthesia teams is critical.
3. Initial management involves packing the pelvis and determining the exact location of bleeding.
4. Know the options and approach bleeding in a systematic fashion.
5. Surgical options to control presacral bleeding include tacking, muscle welding or tamponade, and pelvic packing. Which option to use depends on whether bleeding is focal or diffuse, as well as the rapidity of the bleeding and the stability of the patient.

S. Koller
Department of Surgery, Lewis Katz School of Medicine at Temple University and the Temple University Health System, Philadelphia, PA, USA

H. M. Ross (✉)
Division of Colon and Rectal Surgery, Lewis Katz School of Medicine at Temple University and the Temple University Health System, Philadelphia, PA, USA
e-mail: Howard.Ross@tuhs.temple.edu

S. W. Lee et al. (eds.), *Colorectal Surgery Consultation*,
https://doi.org/10.1007/978-3-030-11181-6_31

Operative Assessment

1. Pack the pelvis and notify anesthesia of potential need for transfusion
2. Remove packs systematically to assess where the bleeding is coming from
3. Review checklist of options with entire operating room team
4. Convert to open surgery, as needed, for better visualization and control

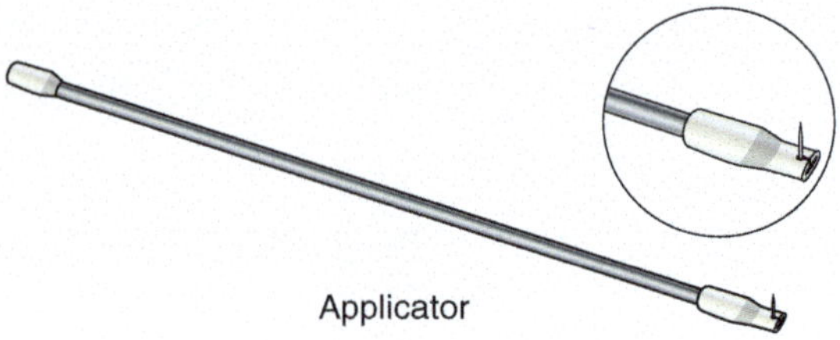

Fig. 31.2 Thumbtack applicator

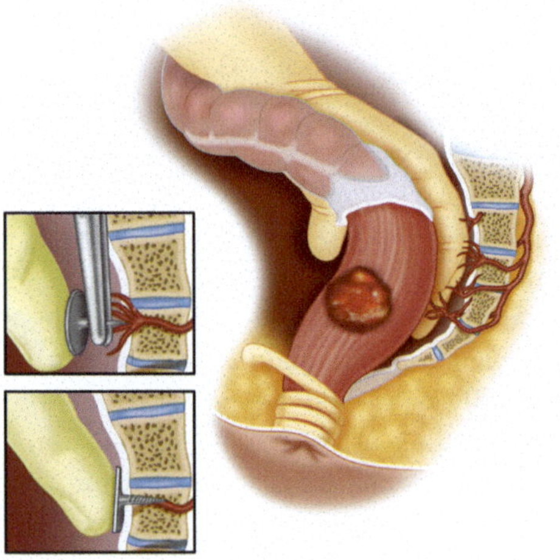

Fig. 31.3 Thumbtack placement

Operative Checklist

1. Additional helpful equipment.
   (a) Multiple laparotomy pads
   (b) Head light
   (c) St. Mark's lighted retractors and a Bookwalter retractor
   (d) Sacral tacks and applicator
   (e) Blood available in the room
2. Exposure.
   (a) All adjacent organs must be retracted in order to adequately visualize the deep pelvis and assess the source of bleeding. All maneuvers to gain exposure should be employed, including converting to an open procedure if necessary.
3. Positioning.
   (a) While attempting to control bleeding, the patient may be placed in either the Trendelenburg or neutral, supine position.

Operative Techniques

1. Tacking. When bleeding is focal, metallic thumbtacks may be applied to these discrete areas. They may be applied by hand (Fig. 31.2) or with a tack applier (Fig. 31.3). First, stop the bleeding by applying direct pressure to the bleeding site with a fingertip or a sponge on a stick. Remove any blood and clot from the surgical field. Using a forceps, remove the tack from its holder and place it directly over the bleeding site. Push the tack into the bone using fingertip pressure. Apply steady pressure until the pin is fully engaged with the head of the tack flush with the bony cortex. A second tack may be placed if bleeding continues and appears to be coming from an additional site, although tack heads should not be overlapped as this will limit the pressure applied to the bleeding site. Alternatively, a tack applicator may be used, again employing fingertip pressure to seat the tack in place. Pressing a tack into the sacral bone requires significant strength.
2. Muscle welding. This technique is best used when bleeding is more diffuse and a discrete area of bleeding is not appreciated. While applying digital pressure to the area of bleeding, resect an approximately 2 × 2 cm

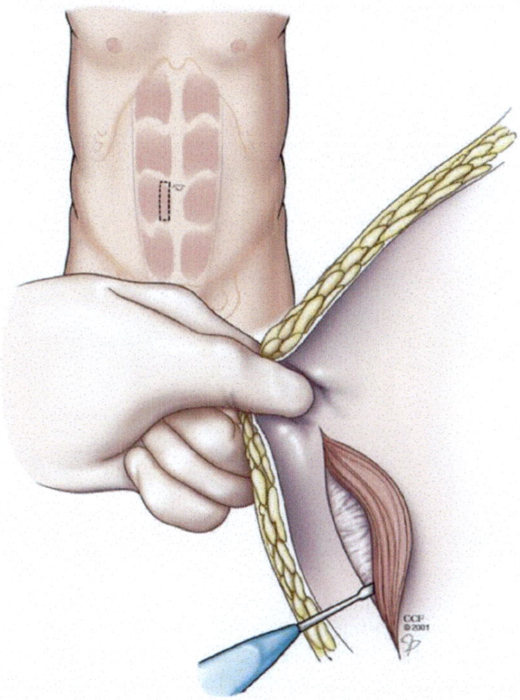

Fig. 31.4 Harvest rectus for welding or tamponade. (With permission. © Cleveland Clinic)

piece of anterior rectus muscle using electrocautery (Fig. 31.4). Place the piece of rectus muscle over the bleeding presacral area, grasp with a dissecting forceps, and apply electrocautery to the muscle via the forceps on full power. The muscle fragment may remain adhered to the bone, or it may fall away, but the source of bleeding will remain welded closed. If the bleeding continues, the same maneuver may be repeated with another fragment of rectus muscle. Ensure that the electrocautery is turned high enough. The muscle may also stick to the forceps but may also help control the bleeding.

3. Muscle tamponade. Resect a 4 × 2 cm fragment of anterior rectus muscle in the same manner. While controlling bleeding with direct pressure with a sponge, apply two 2-0 Vicryl sutures across the bleeding presacral area and leave untied. Apply the rectus muscle over the area of bleeding, and tie down the sutures, causing a tamponade effect (Fig. 31.5).
4. Pelvic packing. If the patient is bleeding very quickly and is becoming unstable or coagulopathic, there may not be time to implement the above techniques. Pelvic packing with multiple laparotomy pads or a 5-yard roll and temporarily closing the abdomen may be lifesaving. The tamponade allows time for resuscitation, warming, and correction of coagulopathy in the ICU. The patient is returned to the OR to remove the packs in 24–48 hours.
5. If these maneuvers fail, consider consultation with interventional radiology for catheter embolization or control of internal iliac artery inflow.

Technical Pearls (Tips and Tricks)

1. Presacral bleeding can be difficult to manage and patients can lose a significant amount of blood when it occurs. It is import to act quickly to get control.
2. Traditional methods to control bleeding such as clips, ligatures, and electrocautery are usually ineffective and are discouraged due to their tendency to worsen presacral bleeding.
3. A combination of all the above operative techniques may be required.
4. Packing should be used if patients become unstable or if all other techniques fail.

Special Postoperative Care

1. Check serial hemoglobins and transfuse as necessary.
2. If bleeding was significant, the patient may benefit from ICU level of care.
3. If packing was employed, the patient will need to return to the OR to remove packs and formally close the abdomen in 24–48 hours.

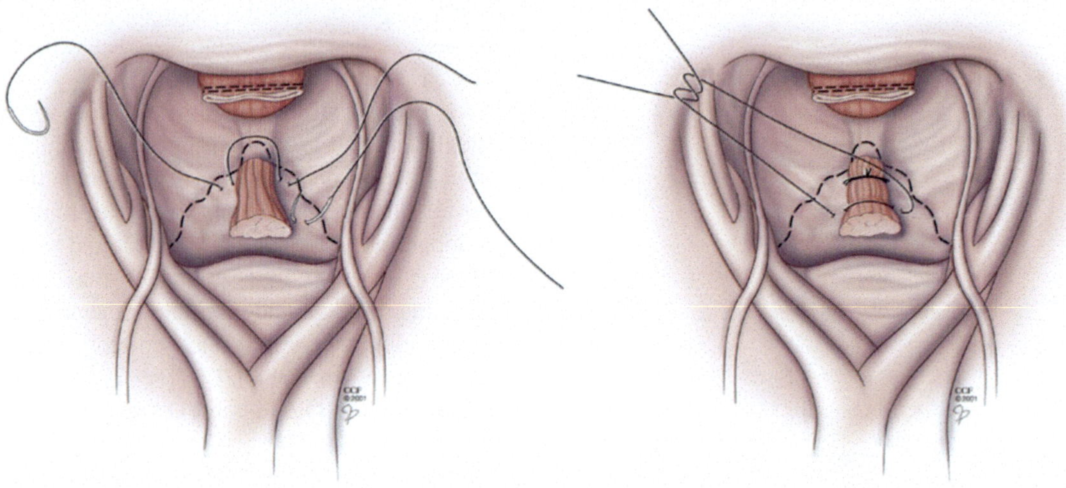

Fig. 31.5 Rectus tamponade. (With permission. © Cleveland Clinic)

Suggested Reading

1. Casal Núñez JE, Pérez Domínguez L, Vigorita V, Ruano Poblador A. Efficacy of rectus muscle fragment welding in the control of presacral venous bleeding. ANZ J Surg. 2018;88(3):182–4.
2. Celentano V, Ausobsky JR, Vowden P. Surgical management of presacral bleeding. Ann R Coll Surg Engl. 2014;96(4):261–5.
3. Harrison JL, Hooks VH, Pearl RK, Cheape JD, Lawrence MA, Orsay CP, Abcarian H. Muscle fragment welding for control of massive presacral bleeding during rectal mobilization: a review of eight cases. Dis Colon Rectum. 2003;46(8):1115–7.
4. Hemorrhage Occluder Pins, Tools for Surgery, www.toolsforsurgery.com/HOP/. Accessed 29 Nov 2017.
5. McPartland KJ, Hyman NH. Damage control: what is its role in colorectal surgery? Dis Colon Rectum. 2003;46(7):981–6.
6. Remzi FH, Oncel M, Fazio VW. Muscle tamponade to control presacral venous bleeding: report of two cases. Dis Colon Rectum. 2002;45(8):1109–11.

32 Cannot Extract the Circular Stapler

Daniel L. Feingold and Ravi P. Kiran

Clinical Scenario

After firing the circular stapler during a sigmoidectomy for diverticulitis, the wing nut is turned counterclockwise as per the manufacturer's recommendations for use, but the stapler will not disengage from the tissues and does not allow extraction.

Key Points

1. Circular staplers, like all mechanical staplers, are prone to misfiring and other technical misadventures. On occasion, when unscrewing the circular stapler wing nut to disengage the stapler from the anastomosis, the anvil of the stapler springs back or otherwise catches a lip of mucosa preventing effortless extraction of the stapler. There are a number of maneuvers to use in this situation to extract the device without traumatizing the fresh anastomosis.

D. L. Feingold (✉) · R. P. Kiran
Division of Colorectal Surgery, Department of Surgery, Columbia University, New York, NY, USA
e-mail: df347@cumc.columbia.edu

S. W. Lee et al. (eds.), *Colorectal Surgery Consultation*,
https://doi.org/10.1007/978-3-030-11181-6_32

Operative Assessment

1. Recognize the stapler has not disengaged by seeing the stapler pulling the colon and the anastomosis deeper into the pelvis, and avoid traumatizing the fresh anastomosis.

Operative Checklist

1. Additional resources and equipment
   (a) A colonoscope to assess the anatomy

Operative Technique

1. Secure the anvil of the stapler and fire the stapler per usual protocol.

Technical Pearls

1. Once the stapler is fired, attempt to extricate the device by rotating the stapler wing nut as instructed by the manufacturer's recommendations counterclockwise, and then gently raise the stapler handle and pull back on the stapler while placing careful countertraction on the colon coming down to the pelvis. The manual pressure fixes the colon from above preventing twisting of the tissues and may help the stapler disengage.

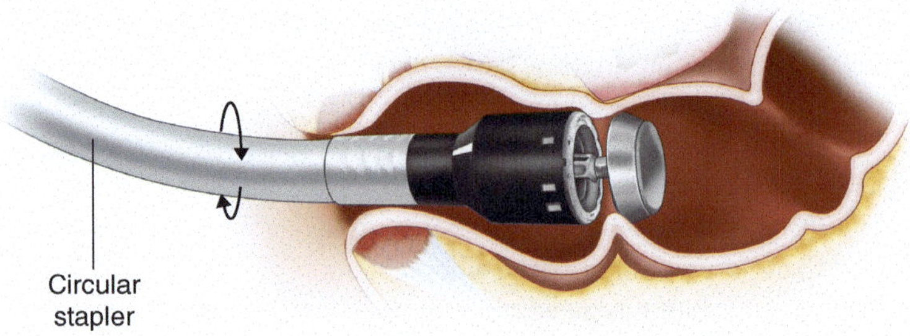

Fig. 32.1 Rotate the stapler along its long axis clockwise or counterclockwise to try to extract the stapler

2. Carefully rotate the stapler along its long axis 90° clockwise and then 90° counterclockwise. If this does not release the stapler, gently and smoothly rotate the stapler 360° in one direction along its long axis taking care to accommodate the curved shaft of the stapler as it bows the rectum. If the stapler does not release, again carefully rotate the stapler 360° the other way (Fig. 32.1).
3. Do not rotate the wing nut counterclockwise much more than the recommended four half turns as the anvil will disconnect from the body of the stapler making retrieval of the anvil more difficult. In the event the anvil does separate from the stapler, an O-ring forceps can be used to grab the shaft of the anvil and manipulate it free of the staple line.
4. If the stapler fails to disengage, the surgeon, using both hands, can take hold of the stapler between patient's legs and of the colon going to the anastomosis in order to control tension across the anastomosis while trying to separate the device from the anastomosis.
5. There is usually enough laxity in the tissues and enough reach of the proximal colon that the stapler can pull and internally prolapse the anastomosis lower into the pelvis so that the anvil is within reach of a digital exam. Using a finger with a sweeping motion, the surgeon can carefully detach the anvil from the mucosa.
6. If these manipulations are unsuccessful, a colonoscope can be passed alongside the shaft of the stapler to evaluate. It is difficult to maintain insufflation as the anus is stented open, but the tip of the scope can help separate the anvil from the mucosa.
7. In cases where the stapler does not disengage despite the above suggestions, the surgeon can purposely disengage the anvil from the stapler by further turning the wing nut counterclockwise and then manipulate the anvil proximally into the colon above the anastomosis. By floating the anvil and then aligning and straightening the two sides of the anastomosis, the anvil can be manually milked into the rectum and then retrieved.
8. Once the hardware is extracted, carefully check the fresh anastomosis with a leak test, per routine. If the leak test is positive, follow the earlier chapter dealing with this situation.

Special Postoperative Care

1. Nothing per anus, per usual, after a low pelvic anastomosis.

Suggested Reading

1. Offodile AC, Feingold DL, Nasar A, Whelan RL, Arnell TD. High incidence of technical errors involving the EEA circular stapler: a single institution experience. J Am Coll Surg. 2010;210:331–5.

Part IV

Technical Tips and Tricks for Difficult Laparoscopic Cases

General Technical Recommendations for Difficult Laparoscopic Cases

33

Andrew Godwin and David E. Rivadeneira

Clinical Scenario

A 65-year-old obese male referred to you by a gastroenterologist after a screening colonoscopy with polypectomy revealed moderately differentiated adenocarcinoma with lymphovascular invasion in the sigmoid colon. The gastroenterologist marked the polypectomy site with a clip. During the operation the clip could not be found.

Key Points

1. For any operation to go smoothly with the least amount of complications, thorough planning before the surgery is of the utmost importance. Not only does the surgeon need to be competent to perform the operation, they also must ensure the operation is made patient-specific. Have an operative plan set into place.
2. Verify room setup is complete, which involves having all supplies and equipment present, accessible, and ready. Make sure that all the equipment is functioning prior to incision.
3. Proper positioning: Supine? Lithotomy? Split leg? Prone? It is most helpful to decide on the ideal positioning when you evaluate the patient in your office well in advance of the operation itself. This is the time the patient is fresh in your mind and you can anticipate how the correct positioning may influence the surgery.
4. Make sure you have good visualization and exposure. Move the scope to a different trocar, and see if looking from a slightly different viewpoint gives a better approach.
   (a) Place additional trocars if needed, but think about what instruments are going to be used through these trocars and anticipate port size. There is very little downside to placing an additional 5 mm port.

Operative Assessment

1. Take time to examine the patient and start planning trocar sites.
   (a) Does the specific disease process that you are treating influence the way you approach the operation?
   (b) Is body habitus going to pose a problem and do you need longer trocars or instruments?

A. Godwin
Northwell Health-Lenox Hill Hospital, New York, NY, USA

D. E. Rivadeneira (✉)
Surgical Strategic Initiatives, Northwell Health, New Hyde Park, NY, USA

Surgical Services and Colorectal Surgery, Huntington Hospital, Huntington, NY, USA

Hofstra University-Northwell School of Medicine, Hempstead, NY, USA
e-mail: DRivadeneira@northwell.edu

S. W. Lee et al. (eds.), *Colorectal Surgery Consultation*,
https://doi.org/10.1007/978-3-030-11181-6_33

   (c) Does the patient have history of prior operations?
   (d) Will you have to modify port placement based on body habitus and or prior incisions?
2. Survey the layout.
   (a) After safe entry into the abdominal cavity, study the operative field.
   (b) Is the operation still possible laparoscopically?
   (c) Are there dense adhesions and can lysis be performed safely without harming surrounding structures?
3. Make sure the area of the colon can be properly identified for surgical excision. Tattoo marking is the most efficient way to localize targets intraoperatively. Having an x-ray demonstrating a clip's location can still result in difficulty localizing a lesion intraoperatively.

(a) Have an operative plan set into place. The operative plan is the way a surgeon can anticipate unique circumstances and address these proactively in advance of surgery rather than reactively during surgery. Does the case require ureteral stenting? Is there a hernia that may interfere with your usual extraction site? Does the uterus need to be removed to gain access to the low pelvis? Should the patient meet with an enterostomal therapist in advance of the surgery date? Should you arrange for one of your partners to assist for part of the case? These kinds of considerations will facilitate a successful operation

Operative Checklist

1. Have the anticipated laparoscopic and standard open equipment and instruments available. Have extra-long laparoscopic trocars and graspers for obese patients.
2. Have all colonoscopy or proctoscopy equipment available. Colonoscopy with CO_2 is invaluable in these situations.

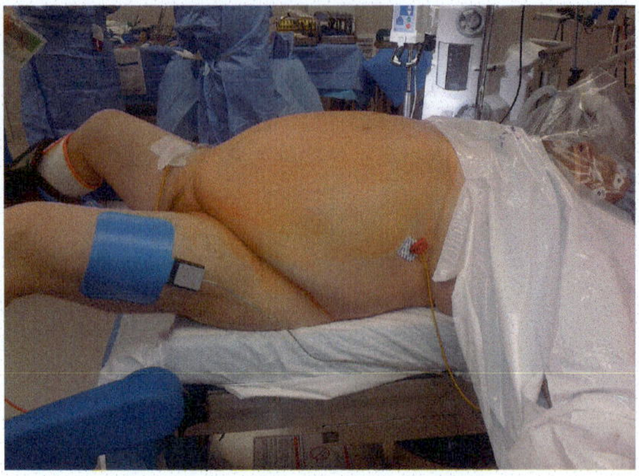

Fig. 33.1 Morbidly obese patient: still able to use gravity for positioning and consider hand-assist

Operative Techniques

1. In this clinical scenario, the surgeon decided to perform an intraoperative colonoscopy with CO_2 prior to starting the case to verify the polypectomy site and was successful in identifying the area.
2. Patient body habitus made laparoscopy difficult, so the decision to convert to hand-assisted technique made operative intervention easier (Fig. 33.1).
3. When dealing with difficult operations where the planes are obscured by the disease process or from prior procedures, taking the time to identify anatomical landmarks and going from "known to the unknown" will help save time and possibly avoids hazardous complications.
4. Advanced laparoscopists understand the need and power of conversion. Certain operations will need to be converted in order to facilitate safe operation. Reasons for conversion may include abnormal anatomy, intraoperative bleeding, difficult disease process (size of tumor, degree of inflammation, etc.), obesity, etc. When an operation is converted, the surgeon has an opportunity to view the operative field from a different perspective, and this can enhance the surgeon's ability to address similar anatomy laparoscopically in the future.

Technical Pearls (Tips and Tricks)

1. If not making significant progress in one area, then try a different approach, medial to lateral or lateral to medial, inferior to superior or vice versa.
2. Proactive conversion to hand-assisted or open procedure is better than reactive conversion. It allows for appropriate planning and the operative team to be more prepared.
3. Never let frustration get the better of you and cloud your judgment. Surgery should never be forced especially in elective cases.
4. If needed for proper retraction, add one or two extra 5 mm trocars.
5. Use gravity as an additional retractor.
6. Do not underestimate the importance of informed consent. Prepare the patient and the family for the operation by discussing risks, benefits, alternatives, and pertinent complications. This detailed discussion sets reasonable expectations to better prepare the patient for undergoing the proposed operation.

Special Postoperative Care

1. Postoperative care will be dictated by the magnitude of the surgery.

Suggested Reading

1. Lee S, Ross H, Rivadeneira DE, Steele S, Feingold D. Advanced colonoscopy and endoluminal surgery. Cham: Springer; 2017.
2. Ross H, Lee S, Mutch M, Rivadeneira D, Steele SR. Minimally invasive approaches to colon and rectal disease: technique and best practices. New York: Springer Publishing; 2015.
3. Ross H, Lee S, Champagne B, Pigazzi A, Rivadeneira DE. Robotic colorectal surgery. New York: Springer Publishing; 2015.

Dislodged Laparoscopic Cannulas

34

Emily Steinhagen and Scott R. Steele

Clinical Scenario

A 45-year-old female with a BMI of 20 is undergoing laparoscopic sigmoid resection for diverticulitis. In addition to a supra-umbilical 10 mm port for the laparoscopic camera, there are two 5 mm ports on the right side of the abdomen and one on the left. During the dissection, one of the trocars keeps slipping out when instruments are pulled back or exchanged.

Key Points

1. When the end of the trocar pulls out and lays in the subcutaneous tissue, it can lead to subcutaneous emphysema and crepitus, and ports that repeatedly fall out can also leak CO_2 from around the skin incision.
2. The skin incision should be made the appropriate size for the cannula to avoid it sliding out each time the instrument is exchanged or manipulated.
3. Though there are several different types of cannulas, there is limited evidence about how cannula features impact trocar dislodgement.
4. It has been suggested that radially expandable sheaths or ribbed/threaded cannulas decrease cannula slippage compared to smooth devices.
5. Blunt tip trocars appear to be more stable compared to those with a bladed tip, likely due to the need for them to be screwed into place.

Operative Assessment

1. Is the cannula in a position that will need to be upsized to accommodate a stapler, or a specimen bag? If so, management may include earlier exchange to a larger cannula.
2. Is the port in a position that can or will be utilized for specimen extraction? In the clinical scenario above, the left-sided port may be in a position ideal for extraction and placement of the stapler anvil, therefore, strategies for trocar placement or extraction may be adjusted accordingly and you could remove that slipping trocar.
3. The expected duration of the case is an important consideration as some solutions are more durable.

E. Steinhagen
University Hospitals Case Medical Center, Department of Surgery, Cleveland, OH, USA

S. R. Steele (✉)
Case Western Reserve University School of Medicine, Cleveland, OH, USA

Department of Colorectal Surgery, Cleveland Clinic, Cleveland, OH, USA

S. W. Lee et al. (eds.), *Colorectal Surgery Consultation*,
https://doi.org/10.1007/978-3-030-11181-6_34

Operative Checklist

1. Create an incision that is sized appropriately for the cannula. When feasible, the trocar should be placed in a single attempt to reduce the size of the tract.
2. Is there a way to address the cannula dislodgement without switching out to another port? This is often the fastest and most cost-effective approach.
3. Is the cannula going to be replaced with a larger one or a wound protector later in the procedure? If so, performing this earlier will solve the problem.

Operative Approaches

1. A stitch can be placed in the fascia. This can be done in either a figure-of-eight or purse-string fashion. Once the cannula is in place, the suture can be placed on tension and clamped to decrease the size of the incision and hold it in place. There are laparoscopic port systems designed to have fixation sutures wrapped around them during the procedure. This is more common in larger-sized cannulas. If a larger than typical incision is needed to visualize the fascia for Hasson technique entry, this type of cannula is a logical choice (Fig. 34.1).
2. Place a "U" stitch in the skin around the port, and tie it down to prevent further CO2 escaping and to secure the port. Pull the ends of the suture around the insufflation valve/arm of the port, and secure the suture with a snap at the appropriate length. This helps reduce the CO_2 leak that commonly happens in this situation and effectively secures the port to stay in place.
3. A penetrating towel clamp on the skin and subcutaneous tissue may be an effective technique for limiting sliding. The towel clamp should be placed in close proximity to the trocar but not around it.
4. Balloon ports may be utilized to maintain cannula position in the abdomen. These cannulas are available in 5 mm size as well as the larger port sizes. Consider whether it makes sense to switch to a different cannula when there is sig-

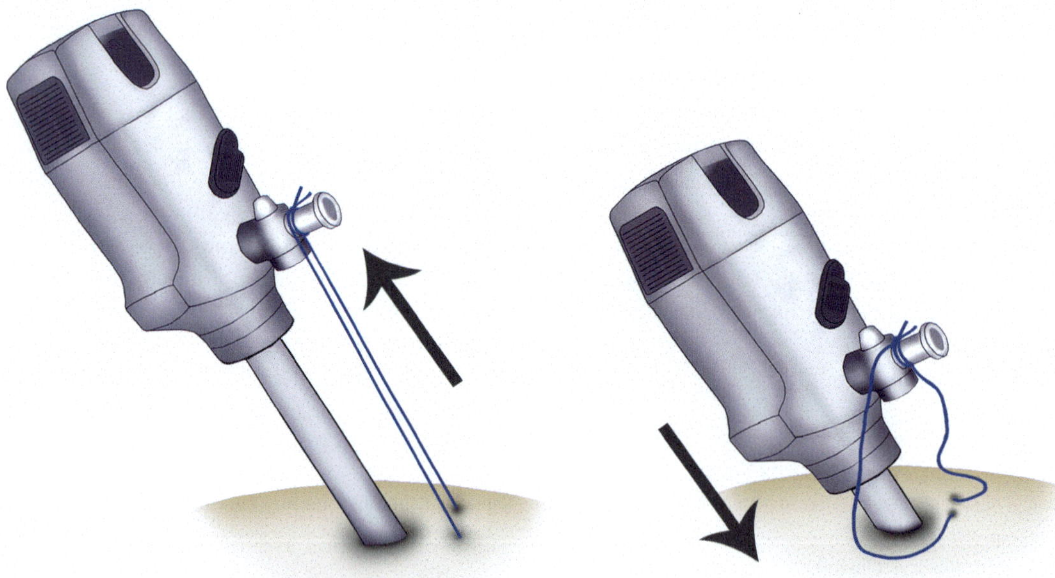

Fig. 34.1 A stitch can be placed in the fascia. (With permission. Nakajima K, Milsom JW, Böhm B. Basic laparoscopic surgical skills. In: Milsom JW, Böhm B, Nakajima K, editors. *Laparoscopic colorectal surgery*. New York: Springer; 2006. p. 66–96)

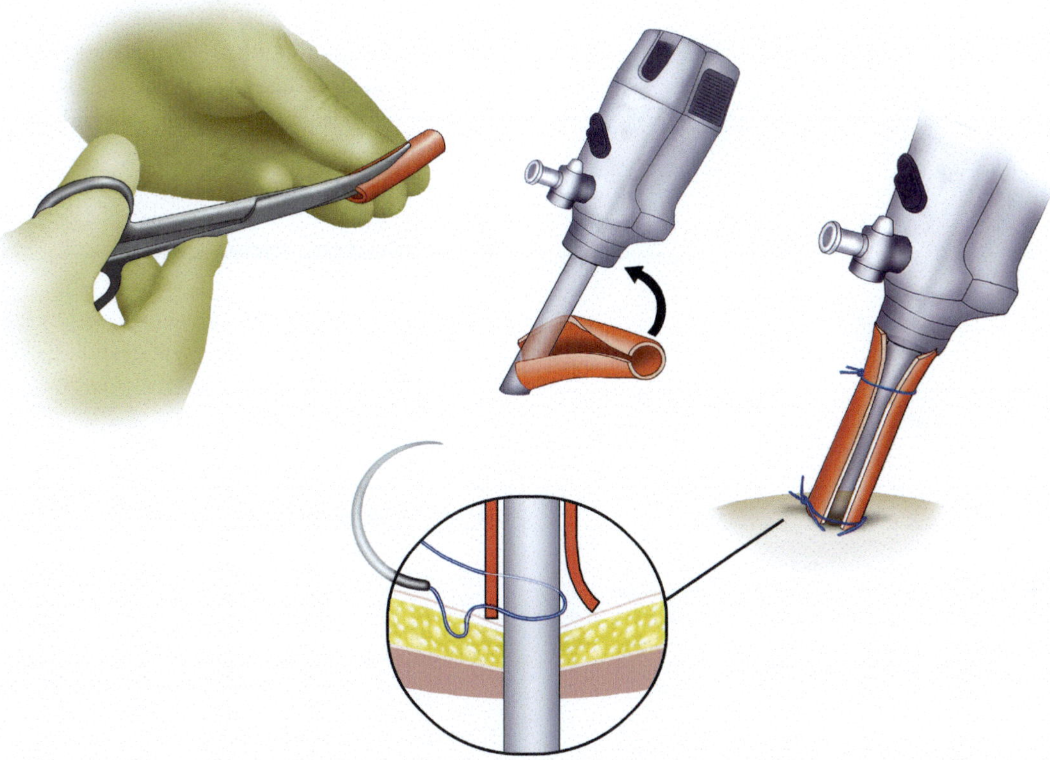

Fig. 34.2 Upsizing of the cannula can be facilitated by wrapping and fixing a red rubber catheter around the port. (With permission. Nakajima K, Milsom JW, Böhm B. Basic laparoscopic surgical skills. In: Milsom JW, Böhm B, Nakajima K, editors. Laparoscopic colorectal surgery. New York: Springer; 2006. p. 66–96)

nificant dislodgement early in the case and there is a compelling reason to avoid upsizing the cannula.

5. The cannula may be upsized to facilitate completion of the case. This is ideal when the port site is going to be upsized anyway either to accommodate a stapler, a specimen bag, or other instrument that requires a larger port later in the case. This can also be facilitated by wrapping and fixing a red rubber catheter around the port (Fig. 34.2).
6. Port "fixators" have been described, which are secured to the skin and are purported to increase trocar stability; in one study they also decreased operative time even when taking into account the amount of time it took to secure the device in place [2]. This can also be done by a Rummel tourniquet maneuver around the port using a red rubber catheter (Fig. 34.3).
7. If the initial incision was relatively larger, for a 10 or 12 mm trocar, inserting an extra small wound protector may be the easiest solution. There are wound protector systems with a cap, through which the cannula can be placed. Alternatively, a glove can be utilized as a cover. One of the glove fingers is removed several centimeters distal to the origin of the finger, and the cannula is placed through it with a suture tied around to hold it in place.

Technical Pearls (Tips and Tricks)

1. Appropriate incision size for the selected trocar is fundamental.
2. If significant torque on the trocar is anticipated, particularly in a patient without significant subcutaneous tissue, a balloon trocar may be selected.

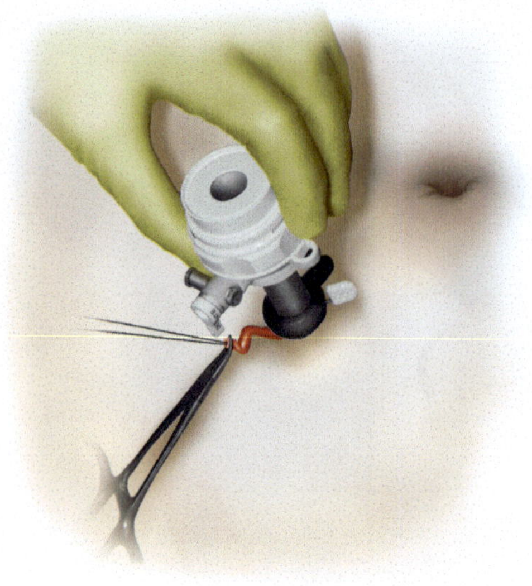

Fig. 34.3 Rummel tourniquet maneuver around the port using a red rubber catheter. (With permission. Lee S. Laparoscopic stoma formation. In: Milsom JW, Böhm B, Nakajima K, editors. *Laparoscopic colorectal surgery*. New York: Springer; 2006. p. 304–13.)

3. The appropriate solution to a slipping trocar depends on the location, the duration of the case, and the availability of different materials or devices for addressing the problem.
4. Ports that fall out and need to be replaced repeatedly may result in larger and irregular fascial defects that can result in port site hernias. In these situations, consider closing the fascia of these port sites at the end of the operation.

Special Postoperative Care

1. Large amount of subcutaneous emphysema will typically pass on its own, despite its concerning appearance.

Suggested Reading

1. Hamade AM, Issa ME, Haylett KR, Ammori BJ. Fixity of ports to the abdominal wall during laparoscopic surgery: a randomized comparison of cutting versus blunt trocars. Surg Endosc. 2007;21(6):965–9. https://doi.org/10.1007/s00464-006-9142-3.
2. Vrentas V, Herrmann A, Cezar C, Tchartchian G, Diesfeld P, De Wilde RL. Reducing trocar movement in operative laparoscopy through use of a fixator. J Minim Invasive Gynecol. 2013;20(6):842–7. https://doi.org/10.1016/j.jmig.2013.05.010.

35 How to Keep the Small Bowel from Getting in the Way of a Laparoscopic Operation

Nivedh V. Paluvoi and Sang W. Lee

Clinical Scenario

A 64-year-old female is undergoing a laparoscopic sigmoid colectomy for recurrent diverticulitis. After port placement, the small bowel is constantly falling into the operative field, causing the surgeon to frequently change instruments to reposition the small bowel out of the field.

Key Points

1. Gravity is extremely useful in managing the position of the small bowel during colorectal surgery.
   (a) Frequent changes in steep positioning may be required to prevent small bowel from falling into the operative field.
   (b) A gel pad should be placed over the operating table prior to the patient being positioned to prevent sliding during steep positioning. Specific foam pads are also available for this purpose. These kinds of positioning devices should be part of your standard OR setup for all colorectal abdominal cases.
2. Placing a radiopaque sponge through a larger trocar during laparoscopic surgery may be necessary to adequately retract the small bowel.
3. A moist laparotomy pad or a radiopaque towel can be placed through the hand access incision prior to placement of the port in hand-assisted laparoscopic surgery.

Operative Assessment

1. Which quadrant is the target structure located in?
2. Is the patient appropriately positioned to prevent the small bowel from disrupting the operative field?
   (a) The working quadrant should be positioned higher than all other quadrants to allow the small bowel to fall out of the field.
   (b) In this scenario, the patient should be placed in Trendelenburg position with right side down to maximize visualization.
3. What is the size of largest trocar?
   (a) A radiopaque sponge can be placed into the abdomen to assist in packing the small bowel away.
4. Is the procedure being performed with a hand-assist port?

N. V. Paluvoi
University of Miami, Department of Surgery, Division of Colorectal Surgery, Pasadena, CA, USA

S. W. Lee (✉)
Department of Surgery – Colon and Rectal Surgery, Keck School of Medicine of University of Southern California, Los Angeles, CA, USA

S. W. Lee et al. (eds.), *Colorectal Surgery Consultation*,
https://doi.org/10.1007/978-3-030-11181-6_35

(a) A laparotomy pad or surgical towel can be placed into the abdomen through this port to assist in packing the small bowel away.

Operative Checklist

1. Positioning.
   (a) As described earlier, the patient should be positioned to maximize the use of gravity in preventing the small bowel from disrupting the operative field (Fig. 35.1).
   (b) If need be, the patient can be placed into a steep position for even further use of gravity if tolerated from a hemodynamic and respiratory standpoint.
      (i) Preoperative placement of a gel pad on the OR table prevents the patient from sliding during steep positioning.

Operative Techniques

1. Stacking of intestines.
   (a) Instead of pushing small intestines out the way, purposeful stacking the intestines away from the operative field can be effective.
   (b) Grab the edges of greater omentum and place them over the liver. This maneuver also retracts the transverse colon out of the way.
   (c) Laparoscopically run the small intestines and stack the loops from proximally to distally.
   (d) For left-sided diseases, empty out the pelvis by retracting the small intestines out of the pelvis.
2. Placement of a radiopaque sponge.
   (a) When positioning alone does not allow for adequate exposure, a surgical sponge can be placed into the abdomen via a laparoscopic port. Generally, the sponge must be placed through at least a 10 mm port. The sponge should be completely unfolded outside of the abdomen and a corner of should be grasped with a locking laparoscopic grasper. The grasper with the sponge is then introduced into the abdomen. The sponge may then be placed over the small bowel and packed away from the operative field using two laparoscopic graspers. Inspection of the abdomen prior to removal of the laparoscope should be done to confirm that no surgical item is retained.
3. Placement of a moist laparotomy pad or a radiologically detectable towel.
   (a) When doing hand-assisted laparoscopic surgery (HALS), a laparotomy pad or surgical towel can easily be placed into the abdomen prior to placement of the access port. The presence of the pad or towel can facilitate rapid packing of the small bowel out of the operative field if gravity alone does not suffice. If this is not done prior to placement of the gel port, a laparotomy pad or towel can still be easily placed into the abdomen through the port device. The pad or towel is similarly used to pack the small bowel away from the operative field. Inspection of the abdomen prior to removal

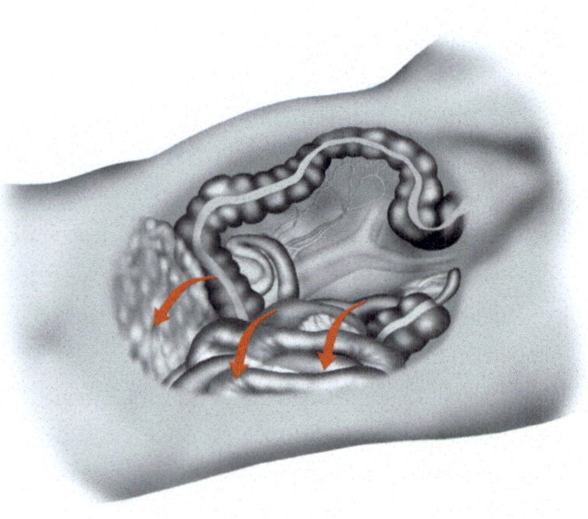

Fig. 35.1 The working quadrant should be positioned higher than all other quadrants to allow the small bowel to fall out of the field. (With permission. Leroy J, Henri M, Rubino F, Marescaux J. Sigmoidectomy. In: Milsom JW, Böhm B, Nakajima K, editors. *Laparoscopic colorectal surgery*. New York: Springer; 2006. p. 145–69)

of the laparoscope should be done to confirm that no surgical item is retained.

Technical Pearls (Tips and Tricks)

1. The working quadrant should be positioned higher than all other quadrants to allow the small bowel to fall out of the field.
2. When placing a sponge, laparotomy pad, or towel into the abdomen, it is of extreme importance that an intra-abdominal count is maintained by the circulating nurse.
   (a) The surgeon must clearly communicate with the OR team when a sponge, laparotomy pad, or towel is placed into or removed from the abdomen.
   (b) It is helpful to have a system in place that is familiar to the OR team that you work with to keep track of any sponges placed in the abdomen. Having a physical marker reminding the team that a laparotomy pad has been placed in the abdomen can help prevent having a retained foreign body. Consider, when you place a pad in the abdomen, clamping a hemostat on the upper, front part of your OR gown to signify there is a pad in the abdomen. When the pad is removed, remove the clamp from your gown. If there is still a clamp on your gown at the end of the operation, there may be a retained foreign body, and the surgical count needs to be reconciled.
3. If the sponge, laparotomy pad, or towel count is incorrect, the abdomen should be inspected for the retained surgical item.
   (a) If no surgical item is identified, an abdominal and pelvic X-ray must be performed in the operating room to confirm that the item is not within the abdominal or pelvic cavity.
4. Prolonged extreme positioning can risk neurovascular complications to the lower extremities. In cases that require steep Trendelenburg, it is helpful to periodically rest the patient in a more neutral position. This can be done by alternating different parts of the operation that require more or less Trendelenburg positioning.
5. Know your table's capabilities. As you learn how best to position patients, you will be able to maximize the table's positioning to facilitate the operation.
6. In cases where the terminal ileum is adherent to the pelvic brim, consider sharply mobilizing the terminal ileum out of the pelvis.

Special Postoperative Care

1. No changes in postoperative care need to be made with the use of positioning

Suggested Reading

1. Nakajima K, Milsom JW, Margolin DA, Szilagy EJ. Use of the surgical towel in colorectal hand-assisted laparoscopic surgery (HALS). Surg Endosc. 2004;18(3):552–3.
2. Shin J, Lee SW. Laparoscopic complications. In: Steele SR, Maykel JA, Champagne BJ, Orangio GR, editors. Complexities in colorectal surgery. New York: Springer Publication; 2014. p. 477–86.
3. Yeh H, Sung NS, Kim SH. Single docking totally robotic low anterior resection or pull through intersphincteric resection. In: Ross H, Lee SW, Champagne BJ, Pigazzi A, Rivadeneira DE, editors. Robotic approaches to colorectal surgery. Cham: Springer Publ.; 2015. p. 203–17.

36 Laparoscopic Suturing

Daniel Fish and Scott R. Steele

Clinical Scenario

Near the end of a laparoscopic completion proctectomy where the specimen has already been extracted through the perineum, you note a small, focal but deep serosal injury on a loop of small bowel. You have a number of abdominal laparoscopic ports in place but no other abdominal incisions.

Key Points

1. Stable view of the tissues, operator comfort, tissue triangulation, and appropriate equipment choice ease the technical challenge of this maneuver.
2. Change of camera or placement of additional ports carries far less risk of morbidity than ignoring the tissue injury or converting to an open incision; consider placing additional ports, as needed, to facilitate this technique.
3. Stable vision – as the operator will require both hands, an assistant must hold the camera in a stable position to facilitate suturing. A zero-degree scope provides the most stable image for an assistant who is not skilled in camera driving, though 30-degree may depend on operator preference. A larger (10 mm) camera or high-definition camera may provide better image detail.

D. Fish
Department of Colorectal Surgery, Cleveland Clinic, Cleveland, OH, USA

S. R. Steele (✉)
Case Western Reserve University School of Medicine, Cleveland, OH, USA

Department of Colorectal Surgery, Cleveland Clinic, Cleveland, OH, USA

Operative Assessment

1. Secure the operative field – position the table and the target tissues in a configuration such that tissues will not shift out of position and bowel loops will not fall into the field. If necessary, consider having an assistant to hold tissues in place or other structures out of the way with grasper(s).
2. Ergonomic tissue positioning – as the surgeon cannot easily reposition his/her body during laparoscopic suturing, the tissue position should be optimized. The planned suture line should, ideally, be parallel to the plane of the camera and the operator's body.
3. Suturing is facilitated by driving a needle perpendicular to the driver in a plane where force and control are greatest. This can include suturing "on the wall" or "on the ceiling" (see below).
4. Attempting to suture in planes that require the needle to be other than perpendicular in the driver can be very difficult laparoscopically

S. W. Lee et al. (eds.), *Colorectal Surgery Consultation*,
https://doi.org/10.1007/978-3-030-11181-6_36

and is prone to causing tissue damage or other complications or failure.

5. Tissue triangulation – to optimize comfort and movement, position the operator, patient, and monitor in a straight line. The left and right working ports for suturing should be on either side of the camera port within a 120-degree arc, sufficiently far away from each other as to prevent extracorporeal clashing of instruments. If the setup does not allow this arrangement or if working through a single-port platform, consider placing an extra port(s).
6. Needle/suture choice and preparation
   (a) Choice of suture material depends on the specific indication and surgeon preference, but colored suture aids considerably in visualization, and braided suture is often preferable for intracorporeal knot tying as this has less memory, allowing easier manipulation with less unravelling. Compared to monofilament, braided suture is also less susceptible to damage or cracking during suturing and tying. Braided suture also has greater surface roughness which decreases the likelihood of knot slippage but also poses greater risk of tissue trauma as it passes through tissue, emphasizing the need for the pulley technique (see below).
   (b) Barbed suture (e.g., V-lock) can be used that can avoid the need for laparoscopic knot tying.
   (c) Suture length.
      (i) For intracorporeal tying, lengths between 8 and 20 cm are often used, depending on the working space and the number of planned uses for each piece of suture. For the novice, 12 cm is a manageable length.
      (ii) For extracorporeal tying, an extra-long suture should be used, at least 75 cm and preferably greater than 100 cm.
   (d) Needle size and shape should be chosen based on the planned use, but consideration must be given to passing the needle through the port. The camera can be temporarily downsized to place a needle through the larger camera port if necessary.
   (e) Blind passage of a needle is not recommended due to concern for inadvertent tissue injury or intraperitoneal misplacement.

Operative Techniques

1. Inserting the needle. The full trocar diameter can be used by locking the grasper on the suture so that the needle hangs freely (like a fishing lure) as it passes through the trocar. The greatest needle control and least likelihood of catching on the trocar or tissues can be achieved by grasping the suture close to its junction with the needle, often a few centimeters away.
2. Loading the needle. Hold the needle slightly loose in the non-dominant grasper close to the needle tip. Use a needle driver in the dominant hand to torque the needle into the correct plane (most commonly perpendicular to the needle driver) by pulling or pushing on the suture near the suture/needle junction. Once the needle is in the desired position, grasp and lock the dominant-hand needle driver on the needle, and release the non-dominant grasper.
3. Driving the needle. Use instruments in both hands that allow secure needle grasping so that the non-dominant hand can complete the needle rotation as it passes out of the tissue (Fig. 36.1). A ratcheted laparoscopic needle driver is usually used in the dominant hand; common choices for the non-dominant hand include a second needle driver, which can be ratcheted very securely but also can cause tissue trauma if closed on tissue. A Maryland grasper, which is not ratcheted, is less traumatic on tissue. You can suture on the "floor," "wall," or even "ceiling" (such as the posterior surface of the abdominal wall) simply by rotating the wrist.

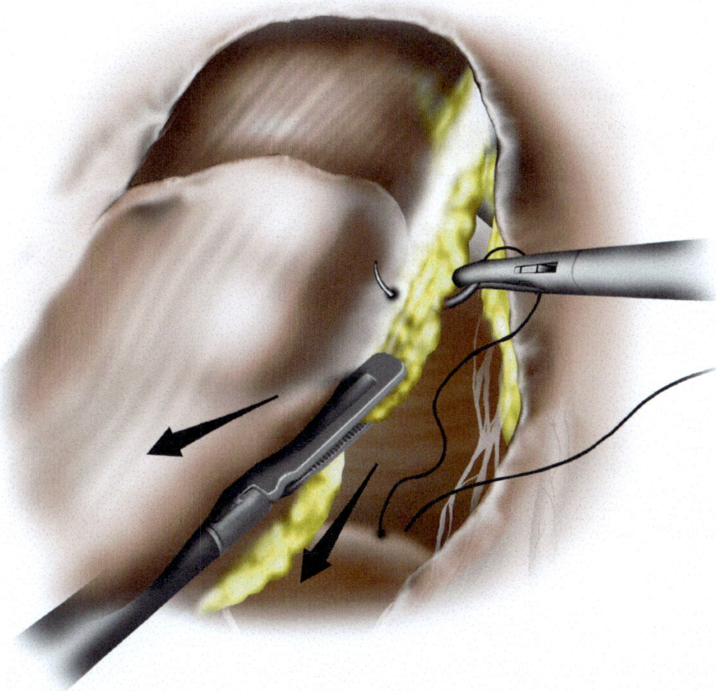

Fig. 36.1 Proper tissue tension (arrows) allows for the natural curve of the needle to pass through the tissue

4. Pulling suture through tissue – the suture can be pulled through the tissue with minimal trauma by pulling it through in the same direction as the needle was driven. Use the non-dominant-hand grasper shaft as a "pulley" such that the suture can be pulled in whichever direction is convenient while maintaining this straight course through the tissue.
5. Tying.
   (a) Intracorporeal knot tying closely resembles conventional instrument tying and can be performed with minimal tissue strain.
      (i) Pull the suture almost completely through the tissue to create a short 1–2 cm tail. While holding the suture or needle with the tail-side instrument, create a "C-loop" in the suture extending from the point of emanation from the tissue, bowing away from the suture line, and ending at the grasping instrument. The other instrument can be used to fashion the curvature of the "C."
      (ii) Wrap the suture around the free instrument twice by pressing the shaft into the suture and moving the tip of the instrument underneath the suture.
      (iii) Grab the tail end with the free instrument tip, and pull it through the created loops to create a surgeon's knot that can be brought down flat, approximating the tissue and moving the tail to the other side of the field, just like in conventional, open knot tying.
      (iv) This process is then repeated in a mirror fashion by exchanging the hands such that the other hand instrument is now opposite the tail and holds the needle or suture, while the hand now closer to the tail fashions the C-loop, wraps around the suture, grabs the tail and pulls it through the loop, and then cinches down another flat knot.

(v) Further throws are placed as appropriate again in alternatingly fashion.
(vi) Once the knot tying is completed, the suture is cut, and a locking grasper is introduced through the port through which the needle will be extracted. The surgeon then withdraws the needle under direct vision (Fig. 36.2).

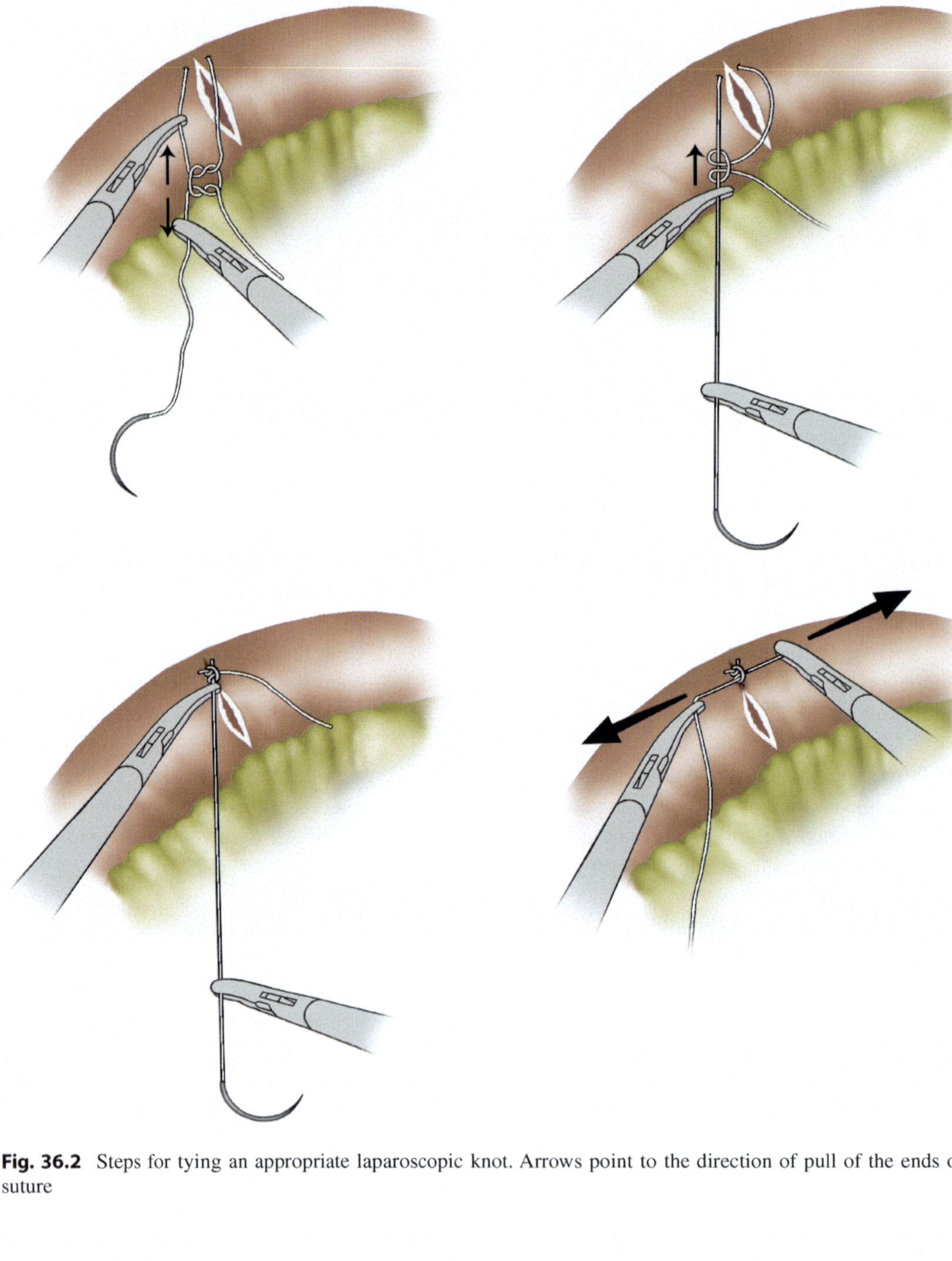

Fig. 36.2 Steps for tying an appropriate laparoscopic knot. Arrows point to the direction of pull of the ends of the suture

(b) Extracorporeal tying may be faster and less technically demanding, although it utilizes a slip knot and has potential to create significant strain on the tissues.
 (i) A very long suture is passed into the body such that one limb remains extracorporeal through the trocar.
 (ii) After driving through the desired tissue, the needle is immediately brought back out through the same trocar, and knots are tied using one of two techniques.
  1. The individual throw technique is more straightforward and includes creating single-handed, single overhand throws and pushing each throw down through the trocar and to the tissue with an open or closed knot pusher.
  2. The Roeder knot technique utilizes a single, complex knot designed to slip in one direction. A single overhand throw is created and held between two fingers in the non-dominant hand. One tail is wrapped three times with the dominant hand around both of the limbs back toward the trocar and then is threaded back between the two limbs, over the top of the lowest wrap. Both tails are then carefully pulled to tighten the knot, and the non-wrapping tail is held tight, and the knot is slipped down into the trocar and to the tissue using a knot pusher.
  3. With either technique, the target tissue should remain under direct vision throughout to monitor suture tension and that the tissue is not traumatized (Figs. 36.3, 36.4, and 36.5).

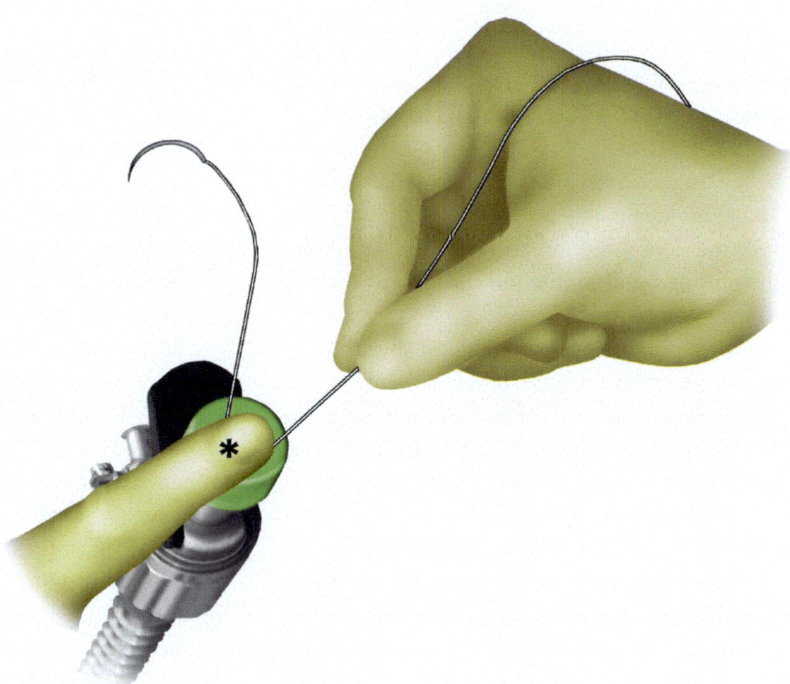

Fig. 36.3 Suture ends are brought through the trocar, and the tip is covered to allow for pneumoperitoneum to not dissipate

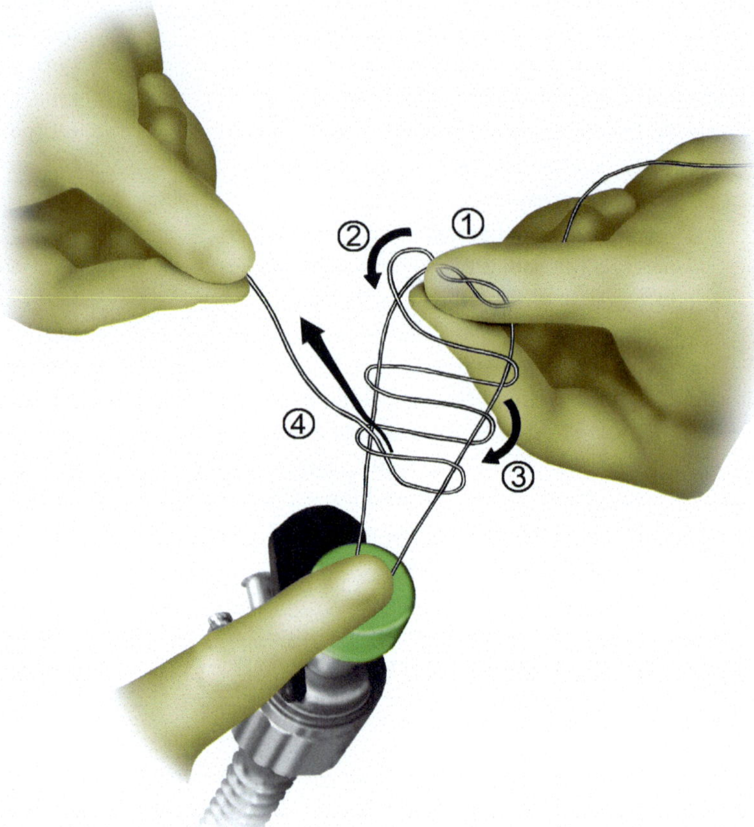

Fig. 36.4 The knot is constructed (numbers indicate the steps and arrows indicate the direction of the suture passing)

Technical Pearls (Tips and Tricks)

1. When intracorporeally tying, grasper choice and technique can aid in easing the process of forming loops around the grasper, grabbing the tail, and pulling the tail through to form a throw.
   (a) Non-curved, taper-tipped graspers (such as a standard needle driver) may allow the loop to slide off of the tip; this can be avoided by opening the jaws after passing behind the suture so as to prevent suture from slipping past.
   (b) A common mistake is to tightly wrap the loops of suture around the grasper. Graspers with side hinges that flex outward may inhibit sliding of tight loops off and over the suture tail. Similarly, graspers with crevices near the tip in which suture can become caught may also inhibit sliding of tight loops, requiring you to redo the throw maneuver. Tight looping can also prevent sufficient opening of the jaws to grab the tail. Striving to keep the suture loops loose until the tail has been pulled through avoids these issues. Moving both instruments together as a unit toward the tail helps reduce tension on the loops, as well.
2. When extracorporeally tying, the closed knot pusher may be technically easier to use as it will not slip off the knot. Both sutures must be held with tension for effective knot pushing.
3. Laparoscopic suturing devices such as Endo Stitch(r) can also facilitate laparoscopic suturing and knot tying.

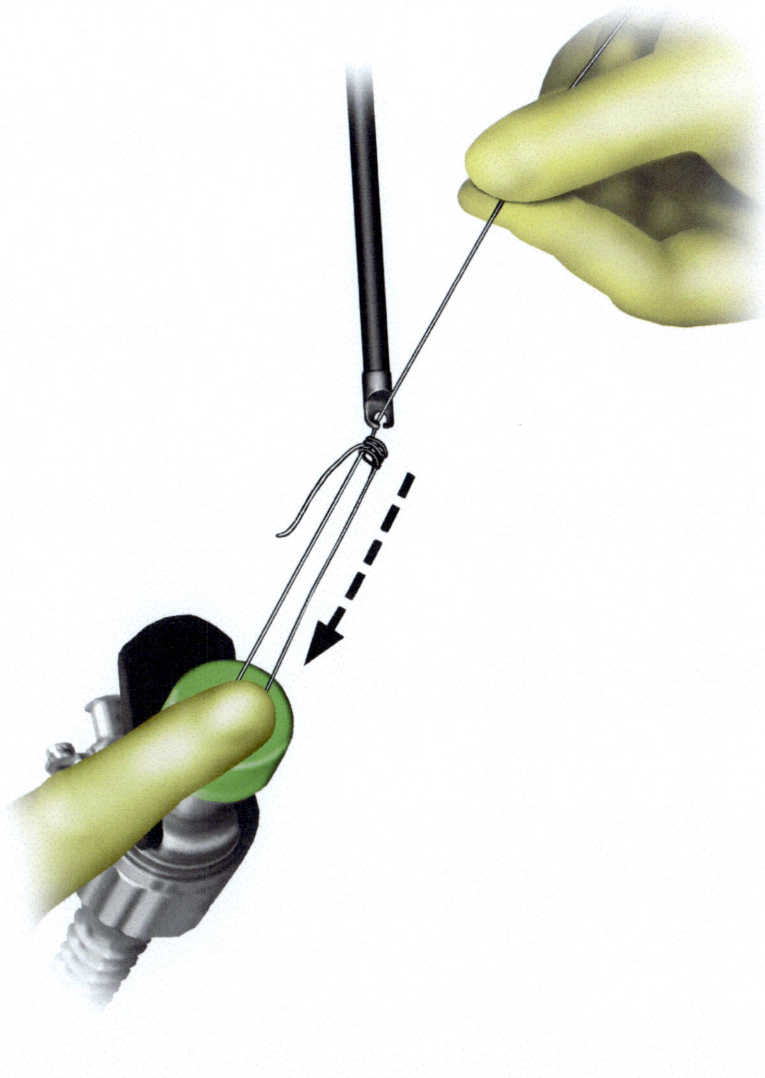

Fig. 36.5 The knot pusher is used to pass the knot through the trocar

Special Postoperative Care

1. None required other than to continue routine enhanced recovery where applicable.

Suggested Reading

1. Soper NJ, et al. Principles of tissue approximation. In: Beck WC, Holzman MD, editors. From The SAGES manual. Springer Publishing, Philadelphia, PA: 2012.

Re-look After Laparoscopic Resection

37

Howard M. Ross

Key Points

Having a strategy to recreate pneumoperitoneum after colon extraction increases the likelihood of completing an operation without increasing incision length or converting to an open operation. The importance of having options minimizes frustration at the end of an operation when surgeons might be tired or the situation may be urgent. Multiple techniques exist to allow rapid restoration of pneumoperitoneum.

Clinical Scenario

You perform a completely laparoscopic left colon resection for a descending colon cancer. Anastomosis was created between the transverse colon and the rectum via end-to-end anastomosis. Mobilization of the splenic flexure seemingly went without incident, and the extraction of the specimen was through a 5 cm Pfannenstiel incision. After the anastomosis was created, you note there is blood in the left upper quadrant. You believe a careful re-inspection of the spleen and left colic artery stump is needed.

H. M. Ross (✉)
Division of Colon and Rectal Surgery,
Lewis Katz School of Medicine at Temple University
and the Temple University Health System,
Philadelphia, PA, USA
e-mail: Howard.Ross@tuhs.temple.edu

Operative Assessment/Operative Checklist

1. Recreating pneumoperitoneum after specimen extraction may require additional equipment which may include:
   (a) A 0 – silk suture to create a purse-string closure of the peritoneum and a short segment of a red rubber catheter to allow the purse string to be cinched closed
   (b) A wound protector with a cap (an example is the Gel Port, Applied Medical, Rancho Santa Margarita, CA) (Fig. 37.1)
   (c) Suture to close fascia
   (d) A wound protector that can be twisted closed

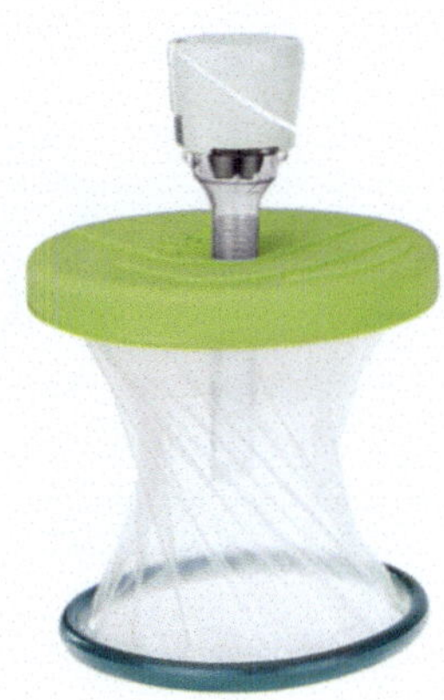

Fig. 37.1 Wound protector with cap

S. W. Lee et al. (eds.), *Colorectal Surgery Consultation*,
https://doi.org/10.1007/978-3-030-11181-6_37

Operative Techniques

1. To recreate pneumoperitoneum after having created a wound for specimen extraction:
   (a) An existing wound protector can be twisted and clamped with an instrument like a Kelly (Fig. 37.2).
   (b) A wound protector with replaceable cap can be inserted.
   (c) A purse-string closure of the peritoneum can be rapidly created (Fig. 37.3). The purse string can be cinched reversibly by threading the suture through a short segment of a red rubber catheter.

Technical Pearls (Tips and Tricks)

1. The operative team should have equipment necessary to recreate pneumoperitoneum in the operating room.
2. Practicing selected techniques to recreate pneumoperitoneum can be helpful for surgeons and surgical teams. Many surgeons perform routine second-look laparoscopy at the end of every laparoscopic colon resection.

Special Postoperative Care

1. None required

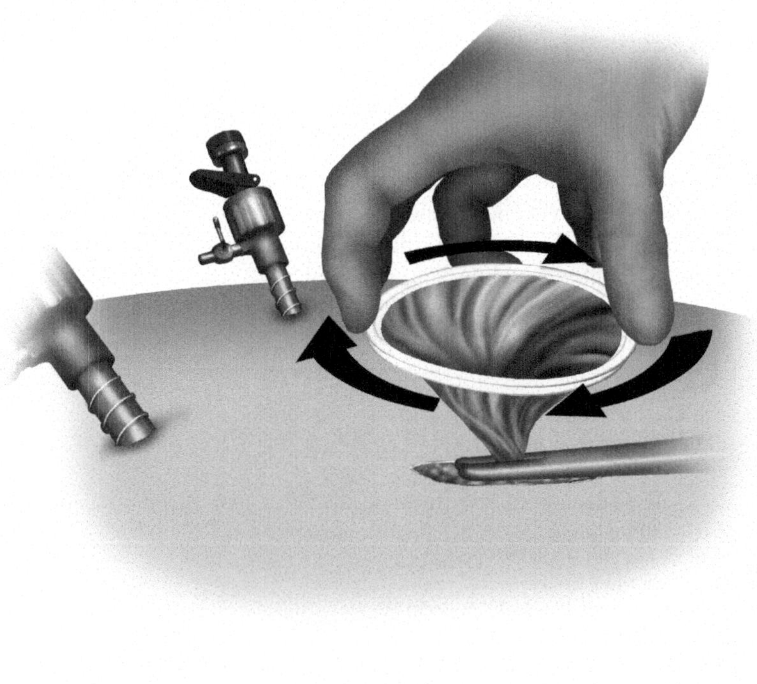

Fig. 37.2 Twisting of a wound protector to recreate pneumoperitoneum

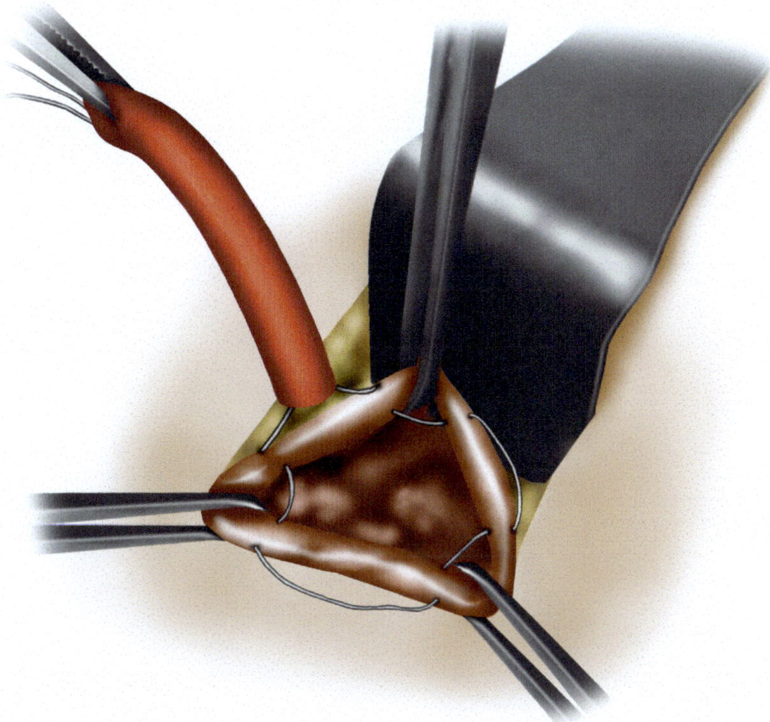

Fig. 37.3 Creation of a purse string for closure of peritoneum

Retraction of a "Floppy Uterus" Encountered During Minimally Invasive Rectal Resection

38

Howard M. Ross and Meredith Gunder

Clinical Scenario

Ms. M, a 31-year-old woman, was found to have a T_1 mid-rectal cancer and presents for laparoscopic LAR. After ports are placed, access to the pelvis is prevented from a uterus that continually falls into the deep pelvis. Simple position changes do not provide relief, and the operation cannot progress given the uterus position. Ms. M. definitely wants to preserve her uterus and desires children.

Key Points

1. The ability to have an unobstructed view of the pelvis is mandatory when performing operations on the mid and distal rectum.
2. Retraction of a "floppy uterus" is simple and effective when surgeons are familiar with the available technical options.
3. Suspension of the uterus can be readily achieved via a Keith needle placed through the uterine fundus, suture looped around the broad ligament, or the use of a retractable fan retractor.

H. M. Ross (✉)
Division of Colon and Rectal Surgery,
Lewis Katz School of Medicine at Temple University and the Temple University Health System,
Philadelphia, PA, USA
e-mail: Howard.Ross@tuhs.temple.edu

M. Gunder
Department of Surgery, Temple University Hospital,
Lewis Katz School of Medicine at Temple University,
Philadelphia, PA, USA

Operative Assessment

1. If the pelvis cannot be visualized adequately due to the uterus obstructing exposure, uterine suspension should be performed.

Operative Checklist

1. Additional helpful equipment includes a Keith needle and an expandable fan retractor.

Operative Techniques

1. Suspension of the uterus via Keith needle is performed with the patient in Trendelenburg position. Direct visualization of the needle at all times is critical. The needle is placed through the skin, through the anterior portion of the uterus where suspension will be maximal, and then placed back through the skin (Fig. 38.1). If the entry and exit points in the skin are close in distance, a single clamp may be used to anchor the suture.
2. Suspension of the broad ligament is performed by looping the suture around the broad

S. W. Lee et al. (eds.), *Colorectal Surgery Consultation*,
https://doi.org/10.1007/978-3-030-11181-6_38

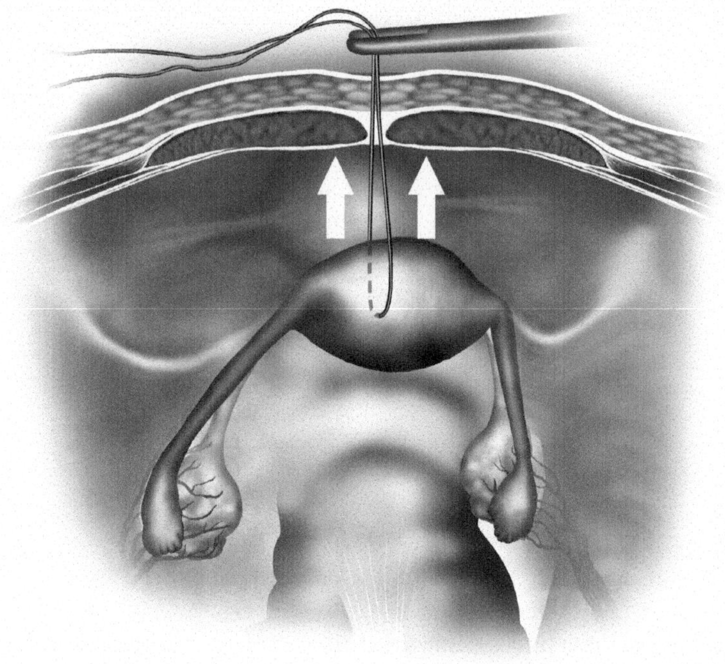

Fig. 38.1 Suture retraction of the uterus. (With permission. Leroy J, Henri M, Rubino F, Marescaux J. Sigmoidectomy. In: Milsom JW, Böhm B, Nakajima K, editors. *Laparoscopic colorectal surgery*. Springer, New York; 2006. p. 145–69)

ligament with same precaution of needle visualization mentioned above.

3. A fan retractor can provide effective uterine retraction. It is inserted underneath the uterus and expanded to give the desired effect. The upward force of retraction on the uterus can be maintained by an assistant or by use of an instrument clamping system.
4. An additional port can always be placed to facilitate additional approaches to retraction.
5. A uterine manipulator used in gynecology can be helpful, if personnel are familiar with its use.

Technical Pearls (Tips and Tricks)

1. Create uterine retraction early in the operation. Suspension techniques are simple and effective. Delaying their utilization is unnecessary.

Special Postoperative Care

1. After removal of the uterine suture, monitor effectively for bleeding.

Suggested Reading

1. Ashley SW. Left hemicolectomy and sigmoid colon. In: Matteotti R, editor. Minimally invasive surgical oncology state-of- the-art cancer management. Springer; New York, NY: 2016. p. 224.
2. Lichliter WE. Techniques in total mesorectal excision surgery. Clin Colon Rectal Surg. 2015;28(1):21–7. https://doi.org/10.1055/s-0035-1545066.
3. Puntambekar SP, Patil AM, Rayate NV, Puntambekar SS, Sathe RM, Kulkarni MA. A novel technique of uterine manipulation in laparoscopic pelvic onco-surgical procedures: "the uterine hitch technique". Minim Invasive Surg. 2010;2010:836027. https://doi.org/10.1155/2010/836027.

Bleeding During Colectomy 39

Shirley Shih and David E. Rivadeneira

Clinical Scenario

You are performing a low anterior resection for a rectosigmoid cancer in a 68-year-old male, smoker, diabetic with significantly calcified vessels. You identified the inferior mesenteric vascular pedicle and proceed to apply the energy-based vessel sealing device when suddenly extensive bleeding occurs from the pedicle and a pulsatile stream of blood covers the tip of your laparoscope and obscures your entire screen with red. Now what?

Key Points

1. Methods to approach major vascular pedicle bleeding during a laparoscopic colectomy:
   (a) Maintain a calm composure and think clearly without panicking.
      (i) Although easier said than done, it is imperative that the surgeon maintains composure and a clear head during this critical time. The surgeon must maintain "equanimity under duress" and stay in control, exude confidence, and communicate clearly with the staff. The chance of having a good outcome will depend on everyone in the operating room; however, the tone will be set by the surgeon. This approach allows the operating theater to remain drama free and for the nurses and technicians to provide you with the assistance and equipment you need efficiently and expeditiously.
2. Be prepared for the worst when dealing with ligation of major vascular pedicles.
   (a) Always prepare before coming across a major vascular pedicle. Expect failure of any blood vessel sealing device, such as bipolar or ultrasonic energy devices, clips, and staplers as they can all fail. Have a game plan ready to deal with a major failure of one of these devices, if and when this happens.
   (b) Make sure to communicate with your assistant to maintain the exposure if there is bleeding from a major vascular pedicle. Often the first response from the assistant

S. Shih
Northwell Health, Department of Colorectal Surgery, Woodbury, NY, USA

D. E. Rivadeneira (✉)
Surgical Strategic Initiatives, Northwell Health, New Hyde Park, NY, USA

Surgical Services and Colorectal Surgery, Huntington Hospital, Huntington, NY, USA

Hofstra University-Northwell School of Medicine, Hempstead, NY, USA
e-mail: DRivadeneira@northwell.edu

S. W. Lee et al. (eds.), *Colorectal Surgery Consultation*,
https://doi.org/10.1007/978-3-030-11181-6_39

is to drop the tissues being held and attempt to suction the area or grasp the bleeding pedicle indiscriminately. That should not be done. Instruct the assistant to maintain the exposure while the surgeon guides the efforts. Before coming across a pedicle, it is helpful to remind your assistant that in the event of bleeding, do not let go of the tissue, etc.

(c) Have a clear visualization of the vascular pedicle and a grasper nearby in order to grasp the bleeding vessel. Do not reapply vessel sealing devices, clips, or staplers in a pool of blood without a clear view of the bleeding vessels, as this may lead to inadvertent injury to other structures, such as the ureter or bowel. You often have more time than you think. Take time to clearly get the area clear of blood and secure the pedicle.

(d) Pre-knotted endoloop ligature. Before coming across a pedicle, it is good practice to confirm that there is a pre-knotted endoloop available in the room and that the suction irrigator has been primed and is working. You don't need to open the endoloop at this point; just have it available for this type of scenario. An endoloop will often allow you to secure and ligate a large bleeding pedicle with relative ease.

(e) As demonstrated by the clinical scenario, patients with calcified vessels require special attention, as the calcified vessels may not seal properly with energy-based devices. Calcified vessels will often cause annoying oozing from a vascular staple line. If an energy device or stapler is used across a significantly calcified vessel, it may be best to reinforce the stump closure with an endoloop ligature.

Operative Assessment

1. Identify and plan for rapid control of a bleeding pedicle, should this occur. Remember that the vascular pedicle will often contain both arterial and venous vessels.
2. Communicate with the anesthesia team regarding significant hemorrhage so supportive measures can be initiated, including:
   (a) Type and cross.
   (b) Transfusions of not only PRBC but also FFP and other blood products, as needed.
   (c) Pressure bags for resuscitation and for administration of blood products.
   (d) Insertion of central lines, additional large bore IV lines, or arterial lines, as needed.
   (e) Notify the staff that the patient may need close monitoring in the postoperative setting.
   (f) Gain exposure via suctioning/irrigating, adding a 5 mm port for further assistance, introducing a 4×4 gauze, converting to hand-assisted approach, and isolating and controlling the bleeding pedicle manually.
   (g) Electrocautery can be applied to smaller-caliber vessels or friable oozing tissue
3. Topical coagulants such as surgical are best used for small-caliber vessel bleeding and usually will have minimal role in large bleeding vessels.
4. Medium- to large-caliber vessels.
5. Suture ligation of medium to large vessels can be used once proximal and distal control has been obtained.
6. Topical coagulants such as Floseal (thrombin with gelatin) are more appropriate for moderate arterial bleeding. When placed in contact with blood, it serves as source of fibrinogen for reasonable bleeding control. Has the bleeding been adequately controlled to the point where hemodynamic instability is not contributing to coagulopathy?
   (a) Has anesthesia caught up in terms of IV resuscitation and transfusion of blood products?
   (b) Have all available OR methods been utilized in obtaining hemostasis?
   (c) Is there additional assistance required in the OR? Vascular consult? Another experienced surgical attending?

Operative Checklist

1. Laparoscopic endoloop available in the room.

2. Suction/irrigation setup: suction the field and make the area as dry as possible. Remember not to cauterize or use energy-based devices, clips, or staplers without having a clear view of the bleeding pedicle.
3. Raytec (radiopaque 4×4) gauze readily available to put down the trocar and use for tamponade propose.
4. Laparoscopic Maryland or fine-tip graspers will allow you to precisely hold blood vessels.
5. Energy-based blood vessel sealing device of surgeon's choice.
6. Clips or Hem-o-lok® polymer clips (Teleflex, Morrisville, NC, USA).

Operative Technique

1. Maintain the exposure, and grasp the bleeding pedicle with a laparoscopic Maryland or bowel grasper.
2. Once you have controlled the bleeding pedicle with a grasper, use suction or gauze to clean up the area. You can use the gauze and pressure to help tamponade the bleeding pedicle. Ensure that no other inadvertent tissue is being caught up and potentially injured. If you can, reapply the vessel sealing device to the bleeding pedicle; it may require several applications to achieve hemostasis. If a stapler has failed, there is usually very little space to apply another stapler line. Regular laparoscopic clips and synthetic Hem-o-lok can be applied (Fig. 39.1).
3. Application of an endoloop is essential when dealing with bleeding from a major pedicle, usually can be placed safely through a 5 mm assistant port. The suture is formed in a ligature loop with a knot. Once the ligature is in place, simply snap the scored end, and pull upward to tighten the loop and secure the knot (Fig. 39.2).
4. Conversion to a hand-assisted laparoscopic technique may be necessary if you are unable to control the bleeding using the discussed methods. Hand-assisted approach will allow for rapid manual compression of the pedicle and, usually, immediate cessation of bleeding. During this time your anesthesia team should be prepared to transfuse, as necessary. While you maintain manual compression of the pedicle, you should clean up and dry the surgical bed and again identify essential structure so they are not inadvertently injured as you achieve hemostasis.
5. If all maneuvers fail to achieve hemostasis, convert to an open approach, and address the pedicle.

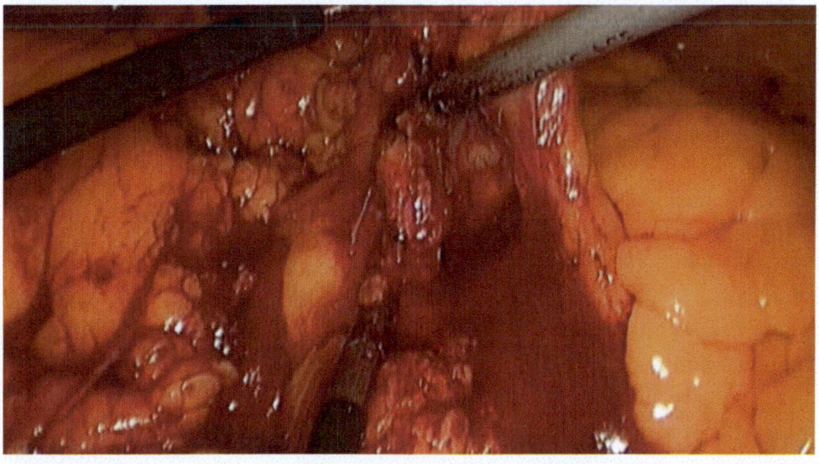

Fig. 39.1 Laparoscopic grasper and energy device controlling the mesenteric root bleeding

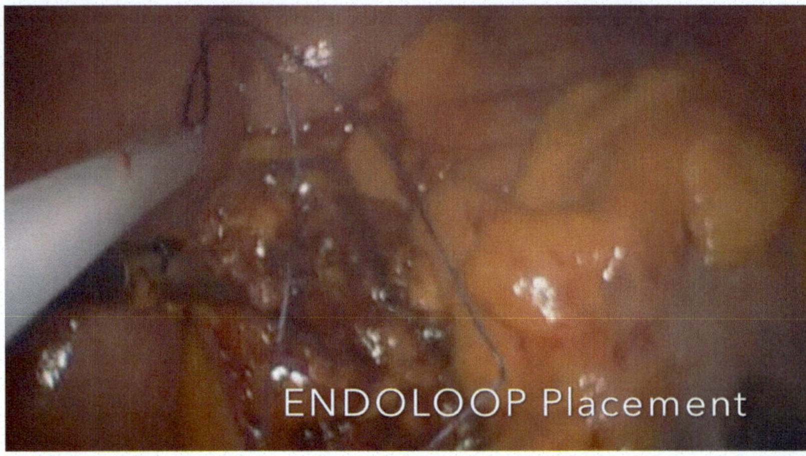

Fig. 39.2 Placement of the endoloop around a bleeding pedicle

Technical Pearls (Tips and Tricks)

1. Be prepared! Always assume that any device you use to come across a major vascular pedicle will fail and you will have massive bleeding.
2. Alert your assistant to keep the exposure and not to drop the retracted tissues in an attempt to assist.
3. Keep a laparoscopic grasping instrument near the pedicle that you are coming across. Often, when reviewing videos of vascular pedicle bleeding, one of the first things that is apparent is that there is no grasper near the pedicle as it starts to bleed.
4. Have an endoloop available in the operating room. You don't have to open this unless it is needed, and therefore you don't have to waste the expense in most cases. In the authors' experience, this has come in handy in many cases.
5. Be especially careful and cautious with patients with calcified vessels, as these vessels may not seal properly with energy-based devices. In these patients a laparoscopic stapler with a vascular cartridge may be preferred.
6. Do not clip, seal, burn, or staple a pedicle without clearly identifying critical structures. You often have more time than you think. Use suction to get clear, blood-free visualization. Remember that the bleeding always seems worse with a laparoscopic view. When dealing with a bleeding ileocolic pedicle, make sure to see the duodenum, right ureter, and gonadal vessels clearly. When dealing with the middle colic pedicles, make sure to clearly see the duodenum, pancreas, and superior mesenteric pedicle, as an injury to any of these could be devastating. When dealing with left colic or inferior mesenteric pedicle, you should clearly see the left ureter, gonadal vessels, and hypogastric nerves.

Postoperative Care

1. If bleeding is minimal to moderate, then nothing special is needed.
2. If bleeding is significant, then postoperative hemoglobin and hematocrit is ordered and blood transfusion given if clinically indicated.

Suggested Reading

1. Lee S, Ross H, Rivadeneira DE, Steele S, Feingold D, editors. Advanced colonoscopy and endoluminal surgery. Cham: Springer; 2017.

2. Merchea A, Wolff BG. Pelvic bleeding. In: Steele SR, Maykel JA, Champagne BJ, Orangio GR, editors. Complexities in colorectal surgery: Decision making and management. Seiten: Springer; 2014. p. 305–9.
3. Ross H, Lee S, Mutch M, Rivadeneira D, Steele SR, editors. Minimally invasive approaches to colon and rectal disease: technique and best practices. New York: Springer Publishing; 2015.
4. Ross H, Lee S, Champagne B, Pigazzi A. In: Rivadeneira DE, editor. Robotic colorectal surgery. New York: Springer Publishing; 2015.

Cannot Find the Ureter

40

Scott R. Steele and Andrew T. Schlussel

Clinical Scenario

A 55-year-old morbidly obese female is undergoing a laparoscopic sigmoid colectomy for recurrent diverticulitis. Eight weeks ago, she presented with a complicated episode of diverticulitis where she developed a 5 cm pericolonic abscess requiring percutaneous drainage. She recovered from this acute episode but continued to have left lower quadrant abdominal pain. The colon was being mobilized in a lateral to medial fashion, and the left ureter could not be identified during the dissection.

Key Points

1. How is the ureter injured?
   (a) Failure to recognize surrounding structures and understand anatomic relationships.
   (b) Disease severity and/or location.
   (c) Poor dissection technique.
2. Consider which patients may have complicated anatomy that may interfere with the identification of the ureter, and consider ureteral stenting.
   (a) Reoperative surgery.
   (b) Severe recurrent and/or complicated diverticulitis.
   (c) History of radiation.
   (d) Large malignancies.
   (e) Morbidly obese patients undergoing pelvic surgery.
   (f) Inflammatory bowel disease.
      (i) Crohn's disease.
      (ii) Ulcerative colitis with fulminant colitis.
   (g) Any anatomic variations like a double ureter.
3. Identify the iliac artery where the ureter will cross over.
4. The ureter should always be identified on the left side.
   (a) This should be performed prior to division of any vascular pedicle.
5. Identification of the right ureter during right colectomy is not typically needed but may be required depending on the dissection.

Operative Assessment

1. The ureter is a retroperitoneal structure that measures 25–30 cm in length and lies on the anterior surface of the psoas muscle (Fig. 40.1).

S. R. Steele (✉)
Case Western Reserve University School of Medicine, Cleveland, OH, USA

Department of Colorectal Surgery, Cleveland Clinic, Cleveland, OH, USA

A. T. Schlussel
Madigan Army Medical Center, Department of Surgery, Tacoma, WA, USA

S. W. Lee et al. (eds.), *Colorectal Surgery Consultation*,
https://doi.org/10.1007/978-3-030-11181-6_40

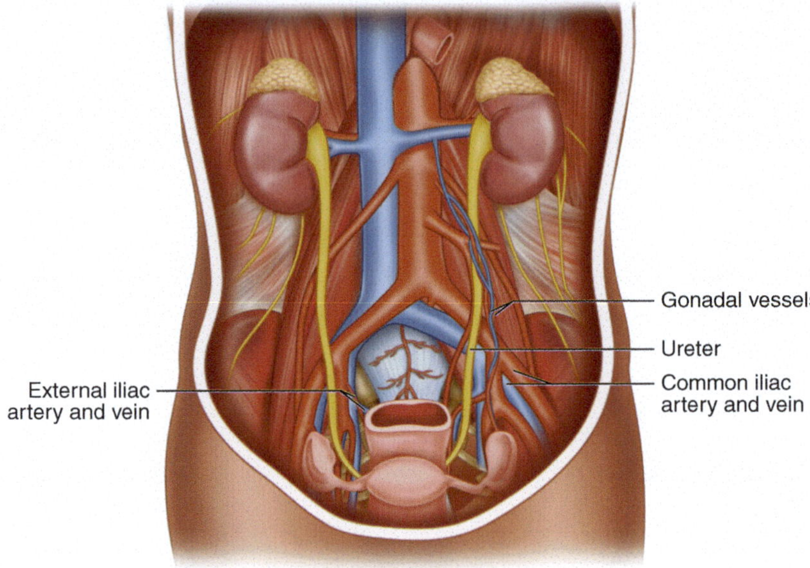

Fig. 40.1 Ureter anatomy

2. The ureter courses over the pelvic brim and then crosses the bifurcation of the common iliac artery on the left and the external iliac on the right.
3. The gonadal vessels will cross the ureter anteriorly as it enters the pelvis.
4. The proximal ureter on the right is located posterior to the duodenum.
5. The proximal ureter on the left is lateral to the inferior mesenteric vessels.
6. The distal ureters are located medial to the gonadal vessels
7. Observe for Kelly's sign (vermiculation of the ureter when it is pressed) as this will assist in differentiating the ureter from other structures.

Operative Checklist

1. Ensure the patient is in proper position on the table, and use table positioning/gravity to move the bowel out of the way.
2. Ureter stents can be used as indicated and should be planned ahead for placement.
3. Methylene blue given intravenously may help identify the ureter or injury site.
4. Emerging experience in ICG fluorescence can help identify the ureter, where available.

Operative Techniques

1. Operative exposure and medialization of the left colon
   (a) Lateral-to-medial approach (Fig. 40.2)
      (i) Requires tension and counter tension.
      (ii) Can utilize the hook monopolar cautery to allow for controlled and focused cauterization along the white line of Toldt and gentle tissue pushing with the heel of the hook. Dissecting the filmy attachments in the avascular plane will medialize the colon (Fig. 40.3).
      (iii) Do not work in a hole. Continue the dissection proximally and then back down distally to widen the dissection field and identify the ureter.
      (iv) Controlled and focused cauterization using the hook device in this region can limit thermal spread. Alternatively and to avoid using monopolar energy

Fig. 40.2 Left-side ureter anatomy from a lateral approach

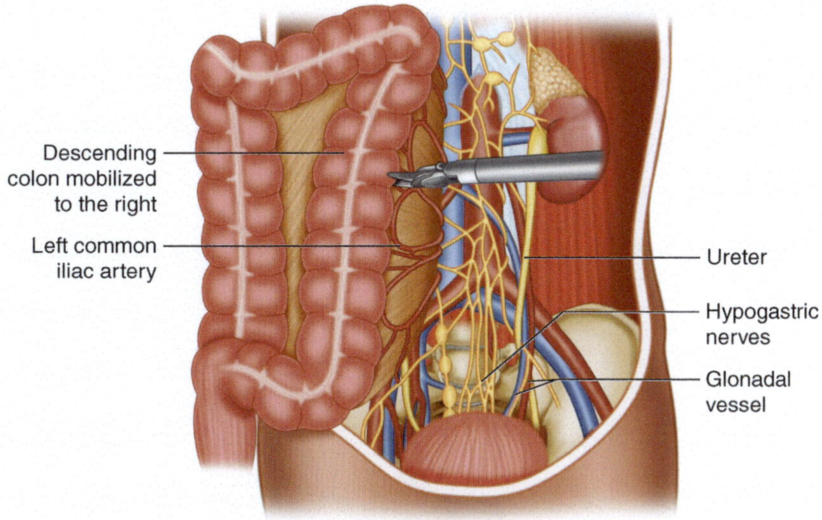

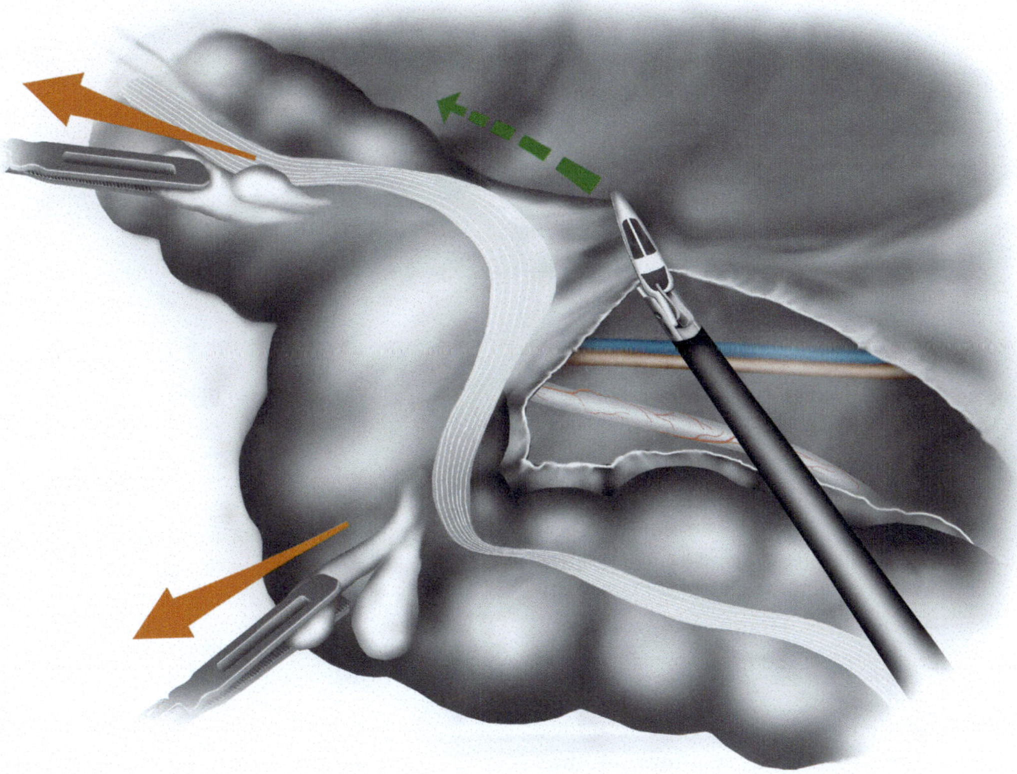

Fig. 40.3 Takedown of the lateral attachments of the left side of the colon to identify the ureter. (With permission. Leroy J, Henri M, Rubino F, Marescaux J. Sigmoidectomy. In: Milsom JW, Böhm B, Nakajima K, editors. *Laparoscopic colorectal surgery*. New York: Springer; 2006. p. 145–69)

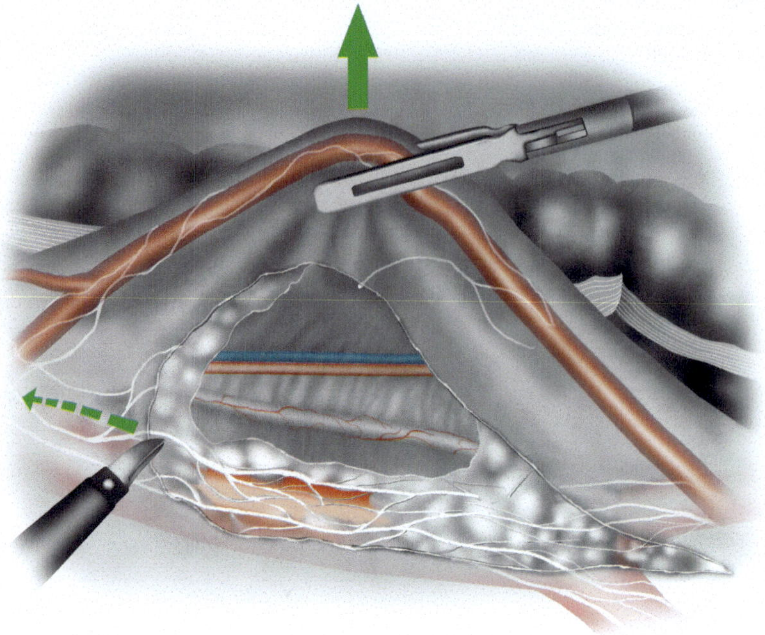

Fig. 40.4 Retroperitoneal window posterior to the inferior mesenteric vascular pedicle from a medial approach (arrows indicate the direction of the instrumentation). (With permission. Leroy J, Henri M, Rubino F, Marescaux J. Sigmoidectomy. In: Milsom JW, Böhm B, Nakajima K, editors. *Laparoscopic colorectal surgery*. New York: Springer; 2006. p. 145–69)

in the abdomen, a bipolar energy device is commonly used for this dissection.

(b) Medial-to-lateral dissection.
  (i) Elevate the inferior mesenteric vascular pedicle to place the mesentery under tension.
  (ii) Score the mesentery distal to the inferior mesentery vascular pedicle (Fig. 40.4).
  (iii) A laparoscopic blunt grasper is inserted into the plane between the mesentery and the retroperitoneum. The mesentery is then elevated toward the anterior abdominal wall.
  (iv) This plane should be bluntly dissected laterally toward the abdominal wall; the ureter will be identified and should be bluntly dissected posteriorly off of the mesentery.
  (v) Ensure the dissection is not too deep and the ureter is not adherent to the mesentery on the "ceiling" of the dissection (Figs. 40.5 and 40.6).
  (vi) The inferior mesenteric artery and vein should be circumferentially isolated to ensure it is completely mobilized off of the left ureter as to not inadvertently transect the ureter or cause thermal injury.

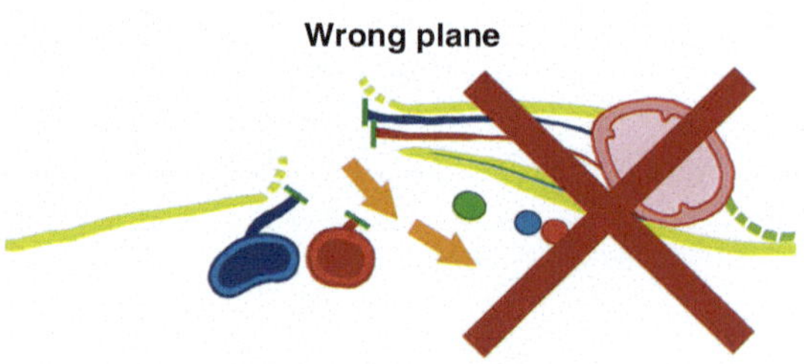

Fig. 40.5 Wrong plane of dissection will lead behind the ureter and expose it to increased risk of injury

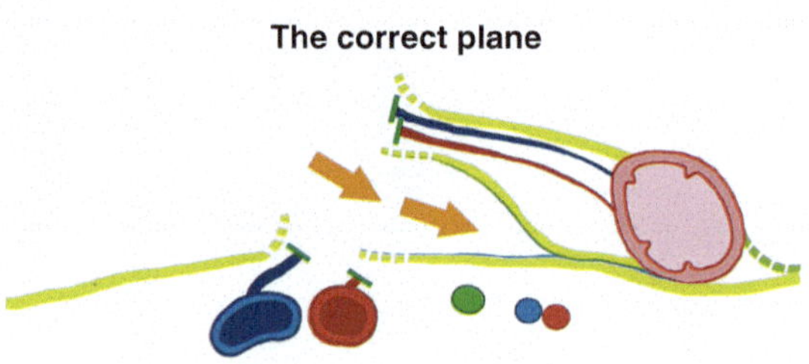

Fig. 40.6 The correct plane of dissection to keep the ureter in the retroperitoneum

Technical Pearls (Tips and Tricks)

1. Consider a medial-to-lateral approach when the colon is adherent to the abdominal wall due to a chronic or active inflammatory process. This technique will allow the surgeon to develop a plane under the area of concern and identify the ureter prior to dissection through fibrotic tissue.
2. If the ureter is not identified in the retromesenteric space caudal to the inferior mesenteric artery (IMA), consider making a window in the mesentery cephalad to the main sigmoidal artery, and look for the ureter under the mesentery between the main sigmoidal and the left colic artery. The mesentery here is usually a thin, avascular bare area and can be opened up without using energy. When the mesosigmoid is post-inflammatory, the mesentery above this level is healthier and easier to dissect. Once the ureter is found at the level above the IMA, it can be traced back to the retromesenteric dissection that started below the IMA.
3. Utilize the suction irrigator as a blunt dissector to further develop the plane between the retroperitoneum and mesentery. The blunt tip will help prevent inadvertent damage to the ureter.
4. Be mindful of misidentifying the psoas tendon (appropriately called "the fool's ureter").
5. Recognize the anatomy. If you identify the gonadals at the level of the IMA pedicle, then you know the ureter is medial. If you observe the red fibers of the psoas muscle, you are too deep in the retroperitoneum and need to adjust your dissection.
6. Be careful of extra-thin patients with minimal mesenteric fat. In these cases, the embryonic fusion planes that are dissected during colectomy may not be as easy to follow as in patients with somewhat greater adiposity, and the ureter may be closer to your dissection than you would otherwise appreciate.
7. Change to a hand-assisted approach or convert to laparotomy to improve exposure.
8. Intraoperative ureteral stent placement.
9. Call for assistance during the operation.
10. In hostile cases, though not ideal, it may be reasonable to dissect the mesosigmoid mid-mesentery rather than its base at the level of the retroperitoneum. In this approach, the ureter is usually well below the level of dissection, and dissecting the base of the mesentery is obviated.
11. Prophylactic ureteral stent placement:
    (a) Ureteral injury has a reported incidence of 1.1/1000 cases following laparoscopic colorectal resections; this risk is greater in pelvic operations and in rectal cancer or diverticular case. This is a rare but dreaded complication, and the repair of an iatrogenic ureteral injury may be complex. While there are benefits to stenting, routine use of stents is not recommended. Stents may assist in the recognition of a ureteral injury, yet they have not been demonstrated to result in prevention of this complication.
    (b) The placement of ureteral stents is performed using cystoscopy, and these procedures have inherent complications. There is a risk of iatrogenic ureteral perforation, transient hematuria, urinary tract infections, and possible hydronephrosis due to ureteral edema from trauma. In addition, stent placement incurs an additional cost to the patient as well as time under general anesthesia.
    (c) Lighted ureteral stents may be beneficial during laparoscopic procedures as these catheters have demonstrated an 83% success rate in ureteral identification with transillumination through the retroperitoneum alone with no required dissection. These devices may be useful given the loss of tactile feedback in laparoscopic operations.
    (d) Ureteral stents should be placed selectively.

Special Postoperative Care

1. If stents are placed, they are typically removed the following day.
2. If a Jackson-Pratt drain was placed, consider sending the drain fluid for creatinine if there is suspected ureter injury.

Suggested Reading

1. Beahrs JR, et al. Urinary tract complications with rectal surgery. Ann Surg. 1978;187(5):542–8.
2. Beraldo S, et al. The prophylactic use of a ureteral stent in laparoscopic colorectal surgery. Scand J Surg. 2013;102(2):87–9.
3. da Silva G, Boutros M, Wexner SD. Role of prophylactic ureteric stents in colorectal surgery. Asian J Endosc Surg. 2012;5(3):105–10.
4. Delacroix SE Jr, Winters JC. Urinary tract injures: recognition and management. Clin Colon Rectal Surg. 2010;23(2):104–12.
5. Halabi WJ, et al. Ureteral injuries in colorectal surgery: an analysis of trends, outcomes, and risk factors over a 10-year period in the United States. Dis Colon Rectum. 2014;57(2):179–86.
6. Leanza V, Di Prima AF, Leanza G, Cristina M, Carbonar OA, D'Agatli A, Pafum C. How to prevent ureteral injuries during pelvic gynecological procedures. J Appl Med Sci. 2013;2(3):1–8.
7. Pokala N, et al. A randomized controlled trial comparing simultaneous intra-operative vs sequential prophylactic ureteric catheter insertion in re-operative and complicated colorectal surgery. Int J Color Dis. 2007;22(6):683–7.
8. Senagore AJ, Luchtefeld M. An initial experience with lighted ureteral catheters during laparoscopic colectomy. J Laparoendosc Surg. 1994;4(6):399–403.
9. Tsujinaka S, et al. Prophylactic ureteric catheters in laparoscopic colorectal surgery. Tech Coloproctol. 2008;12(1):45–50.

Ileum Becomes Ischemic Due to Torsion During J-Pouch Creation

41

Sang W. Lee

Clinical Scenario

A 38-year-old woman is undergoing total proctocolectomy with ileal pouch-anal anastomosis (IPAA) for ulcerative colitis refractory to medical management. The colorectal specimen was removed and J pouch was created. When attempting to perform double-stapled IPAA, the cut edge of the small bowel mesentery was noticed to be twisted. While trying to correctly orient the pouch mesentery, the pouch along with the distal small bowel starts to become ischemic (Fig. 41.1).

Key Points

1. As soon as the terminal ileum and ileal mesentery are transected, place a series of markings along the anterior surface near the cut edge of the small bowel mesentery by using either a marker or sutures. The markings can help reorient the mesentery without causing further torsion.
2. Always confirm small bowel orientation before creating the IPAA.
3. To confirm orientation, follow the cut edge of the terminal ileal mesentery from the superior mesenteric artery (SMA) at the level of the duodenum to the ileocolic pedicle to the stapled end of the ileum. It helps to have the patient tilted right side up for this maneuver. If this cut edge is observed without any small bowel crossing over it, then the orientation of the bowel is correct. If the orientation of the small bowel mesentery cannot be verified, the small bowel has to be untwisted starting at the ligament of Treitz. This is the only way to ascertain the correct orientation.

S. W. Lee (✉)
Department of Surgery – Colon and Rectal Surgery, Keck School of Medicine of University of Southern California, Los Angeles, CA, USA

Operative Assessment

1. Always confirm small bowel orientation before creating the pouch-anal anastomosis.
   (a) The cut edge of the small bowel mesentery has to be straight along the right side of the pelvis. Under no circumstances should the anastomosis performed without ascertaining the correct orientation.
2. What type of exposure is needed to reorient the small bowel?
   (a) For laparoscopic cases, re-establish pneumoperitoneum, and run the small bowel starting at the ligament of Treitz.
   (b) For a low midline incision, a hand or single access device could be placed through the incision, and the small bowel could be run laparoscopically. Additional laparoscopic ports can be placed, as needed.

S. W. Lee et al. (eds.), *Colorectal Surgery Consultation*,
https://doi.org/10.1007/978-3-030-11181-6_41

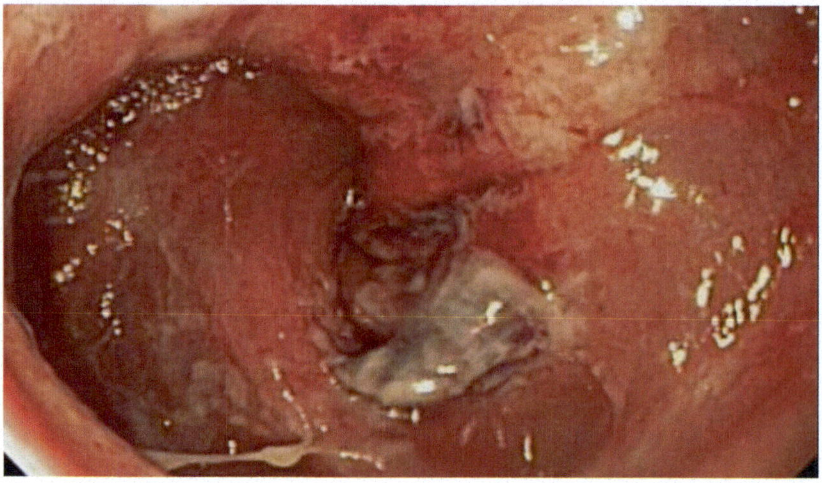

Fig. 41.1 Pouch ischemia from torsion (via endoscopy)

(c) Do not hesitate to extend the incision in order to accomplish what is needed.

Operative Checklist

1. Lighted retractors or headlights for improved visualization in the pelvis are necessary.
2. Hand access device or single incision laparoscopic access device.
3. Laparoscopic setup.
4. Open laparotomy tray with pelvic retractors (lighted retractors, if available) and long pelvic instrument tray if performing open; if performing laparoscopically, have these trays available in case of conversion.

Operative Techniques

1. The best way to prevent torsion is to orient the small bowel as soon as the terminal ileum and its mesentery are transected. A series of horizontal markings can be created along the anterior surface of small bowel using a surgical marker (Fig. 41.2). Alternatively, sutures or surgical clips can be used for marking. The markers can help reorient the small bowel in case of torsion.

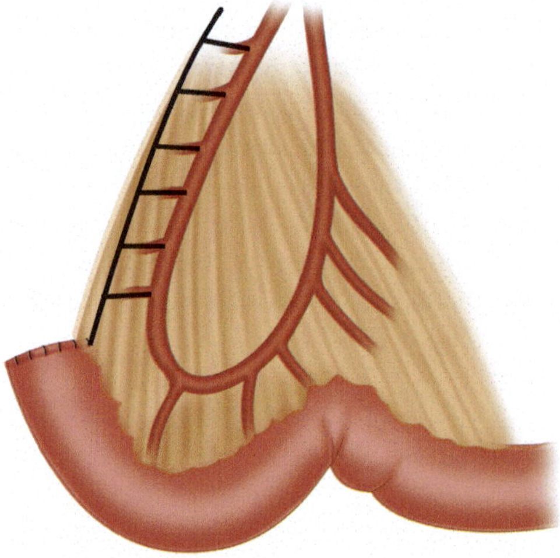

Fig. 41.2 The best way to prevent torsion is to orient the small bowel as soon as the terminal ileum and the mesentery are transected. A series of horizontal markings can be created along the anterior surface of small bowel using a surgical marker

2. To run the bowel in a laparoscopic case, place the patient in Trendelenburg and left side up. Place the loops of the small bowel in the right upper quadrant of the abdomen. Identify to the ligament of Treitz, and run the small bowel

proximally to distally. Placement of additional trocars may be necessary.

Technical Pearls (Tips and Tricks)

1. Mark the anterior small bowel as soon as the ileum and ileal mesentery are transected.
2. Use the markings as a guide when detorsing.
3. If needed, untwist the mesentery by running the small bowel starting at the ligament of Treitz.
4. If torsion is encountered during the second-stage operation through a low midline or Pfannenstiel incision, either a hand or a single incision access device can be placed through the incision to reorient the small bowel.

Postoperative Care

1. Routine postoperative care along an enhanced recovery protocol is recommended

Suggested Reading

1. Kirat HT, Remzi FH. Technical aspects of ileoanal pouch surgery in patients with ulcerative colitis. Clin Colon Rectal Surg. 2010;23(4):239–47.
2. Nivatvongs S. Ulcerative colitis. In: Gordon PH, Nivatvongs S, editors. Principles and practice of surgery for the colon, rectum, and anus. 3rd ed. Boca Raton: Taylor and Francis Group; 2007.

Difficult Laparoscopic Rectal Dissection

42

Deborah S. Keller, Scott R. Steele, and Daniel P. Geisler

Clinical Scenario

An obese, 70-year-old male with rectal cancer 8 cm from the anal verge is undergoing a low anterior resection. There are poor visualization, difficulties exposing the rectum in the narrow pelvis, and issues with keeping the small bowel out of the pelvis. The dissection fails to progress.

Key Points

1. Laparoscopy provides better visualization of the deep pelvis than the open approach. While proper oncologic dissection may be difficult laparoscopically, use changes in position, additional laparoscopic ports, or a hand port to aid exposure before converting to an open approach.
2. Complete, circumferential dissection is needed to safely staple across the rectum without injuring nearby structures such as the ureter, pelvic nerves, vagina, bladder, etc.
3. Begin the dissection posteriorly, and then proceed laterally, alternating sides to continue progressing the dissection distal to the tumor and toward the pelvic floor. Complete the anterior resection last to free the rectal tube for transection.
4. If unable to complete the dissection of the distal third of the rectum from the abdominal approach, consider an additional suprapubic port, hand assistance, or a transanal approach.

Operative Assessment

1. Is keeping the small bowel out of the pelvis an issue?
   (a) Mobilize the small bowel out of the pelvis using gravity – place the patient in steep Trendelenburg position with the right side tilted down so the small bowel falls out of the pelvis and toward the patient's right

D. S. Keller
Department of Surgery, New York-Presbyterian, Columbia University Medical Center, New York, NY, USA

S. R. Steele (✉)
Case Western Reserve University School of Medicine, Cleveland, OH, USA

Department of Colorectal Surgery, Cleveland Clinic, Cleveland, OH, USA

D. P. Geisler
NewYork-Presbyterian/Columbia, Department of Colorectal Surgery, New York, NY, USA

S. W. Lee et al. (eds.), *Colorectal Surgery Consultation*, https://doi.org/10.1007/978-3-030-11181-6_42

side. Some electric operating room tables will allow steeper Trendelenburg positioning if the table is kept left/right neutral.
   (b) In order to effectively retract the small bowel out of the pelvis, it may be helpful to release the attachments of the base of the terminal ileal mesentery to the pelvic inlet. Postoperative or post-inflammatory pelvic adhesions would need to be addressed, as well.
   (c) Pack the small bowel away, if needed, using a sponge introduced through a wound protector or hand-assisted port at the extraction site. Assure any sponges introduced into the abdomen are removed at the end of the case.
2. Is the pelvis obscured by the uterus or adnexa?
   (a) Suture a large uterus to the anterior abdominal wall using a Keith needle or a weighted vaginal speculum.
   (b) Pexy the ovaries to the lateral abdominal wall.
3. Can the proper total mesorectal excision (TME) dissection plane be identified?
   (a) Proper retraction of the rectum will help demonstrate the TME plane posteriorly which is the ideal starting point for this dissection. This can be done with a straight laparoscopic or a hand-assisted fashion. Entering the rectorectal plane allows the CO_2 pneumoperitoneum to auto-dissect the tissues.
   (b) A finger can also be inserted into the rectum to pull it forward to facilitate posterior dissection.
4. Can the anterior rectal plane be clearly distinguished from the vagina/prostate?
   (a) The anterior dissection is 1 or 2 mm anterior to the apex of the pouch of Douglas. Entering here assures the correct anatomical plane, keeping the anterior mesorectal fascia intact.
   (b) Using dilators in the rectum and/or vagina can separate the organs (distracting the rectum posteriorly and the vagina anteriorly) and will help open the plane.
5. Has the dissection been performed far enough distal to the tumor to transect with appropriate margins?
   (a) Reassess with digital examination and/or endoscopy before stapling.

Operative Checklist

1. Abdominal approach
   (a) Basic laparoscopic tray with atraumatic graspers
   (b) Thirty-degree or flexible-tip 110-degree laparoscope
   (c) Rectal dilator set
   (d) Hand-assisted platform (in the room, but not opened)
   (e) Pelvic retractors (lighted retractors if available), a headlight, and long pelvic instrument tray, in case of conversion
   (f) Keith needle to retract the uterus, if needed
2. Transanal approach
   (a) Lone Star retractor
   (b) Second electrocautery and suction setup
   (c) Extra-long instruments
   (d) Lithotomy stirrups

Operative Techniques

1. Perform the abdominal portion of the procedure before proceeding to the pelvic portion. The authors, using a medial-to-lateral approach, identify the inferior mesenteric artery, incise the peritoneum, circumferentially dissect, identify and preserve the left ureter, and then ligate the vessel (Fig. 42.1). Once the artery is ligated, the plane under the mesocolon can be developed laterally and into the pelvis.
2. Commence the mesorectal dissection posteriorly. The rectosigmoid is elevated away

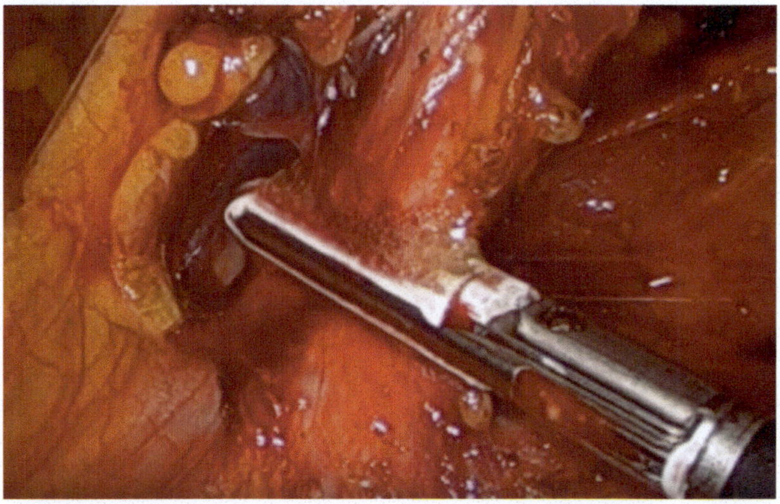

Fig. 42.1 Division of the inferior mesenteric artery (IMA)

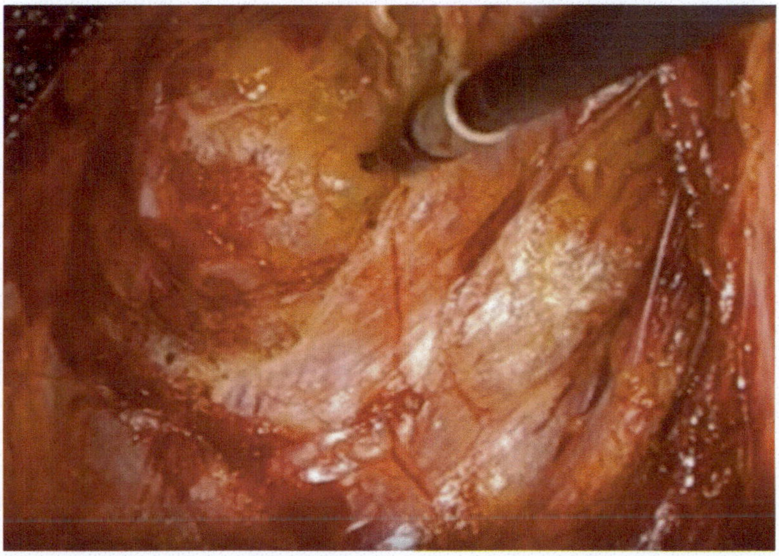

Fig. 42.2 Posterior dissection in the avascular presacral plane

from the sacral promontory using anterior and superior retraction putting the loose areolar tissue under tension and facilitating entry into the presacral space (Fig. 42.2). The posterior aspect of the mesorectum is identified exposing the mesorectal tissue and allowing pneumodissection to open the proper plane. Proceed distally and laterally, opening the fine "angel hair" areolar tissue in a semicircular fashion, taking care to preserve the hypogastric nerves as they pass down into the pelvis anterior to the sacrum. Keep in mind the concavity of the sacrum, and assure the dissection proceeds down the presacral space in this avascular plane toward the pelvic floor and not straight posterior into the bony pelvis.

3. For low, bulky rectal tumors in the anterior position, morbidly obese men, or tumors adherent to the posterior vaginal wall, hand assistance via laparotomy or a hand port may be needed. Manual retraction can help

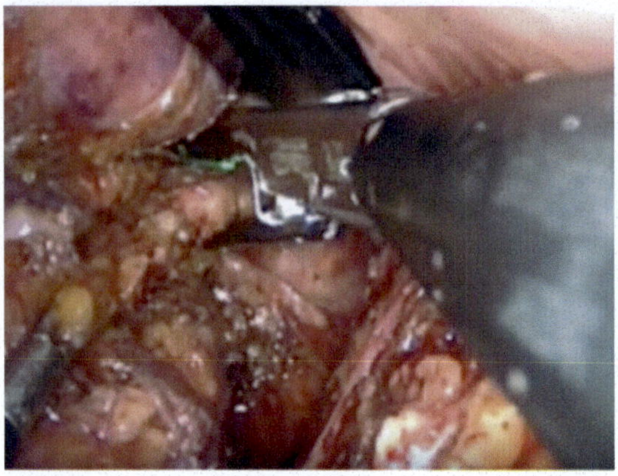

Fig. 42.3 Placement of the stapler in the pelvis for distal resection

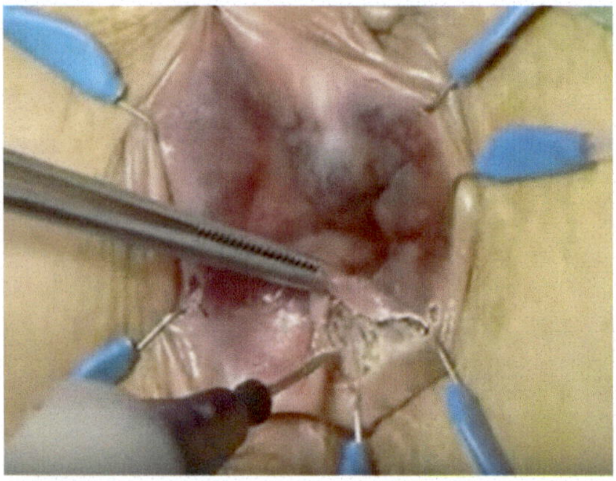

Fig. 42.4 A Lone Star retractor will aid in the intersphincteric dissection

straighten and pull the rectum out of the pelvis, allowing the dissection to be completed. This access also allows placement of the stapler to divide the rectum and extract the specimen (Fig. 42.3).

4. If, despite these maneuvers, the stapler still cannot be passed low enough from the abdominal approach, dissection and division from a transanal approach can be performed (TATA – transabdominal, transanal). A Lone Star retractor is used to efface the anus, then an intersphincteric dissection is performed, the specimen is removed transanally, and a hand-sewn coloanal anastomosis can be performed (Fig. 42.4). In certain situations, an APR will be required.

Technical Pearls (Tips and Tricks)

1. Confirm tumor location using endoscopy and/or digital exam.
2. Place the right-sided ports closer to the midline to facilitate access to the lower pelvis.
3. Placing an additional 5 mm port in the left upper quadrant can help retract the anterior reflection/uterus.
4. If it is difficult to enter the presacral space on the right side, consider using a lateral mobilization.
5. Commence the mesorectal dissection posteriorly, using anterior and superior retraction of the rectosigmoid to place the loose areolar tissue under tension and facilitate dissection.
6. Stapling across the proximal margin can permit better retraction of the rectum for further pelvic dissection.
7. Leave the attachments of the rectum to the lateral sidewall until performing the final lateral mobilization, as this offers helpful countertraction for right-sided and posterior dissections.
8. When performing the lateral mobilization, draw the rectosigmoid medially and anterior to display the space behind the sigmoid and its mesentery. Retracting the mesentery superiorly and medially away from the lateral pelvic sidewall facilitates the lateral dissection.
9. If having difficulty placing the stapler, consider having an assistant manually push up on the perineum to lift the pelvic floor before inserting additional ports; this may lift the rectum enough to allow the first cartridge of the stapler to be fired.
10. Pull up on the rectum through the hand-assisted device (after transecting proximally) to facilitate posterior dissection (Fig. 42.5).

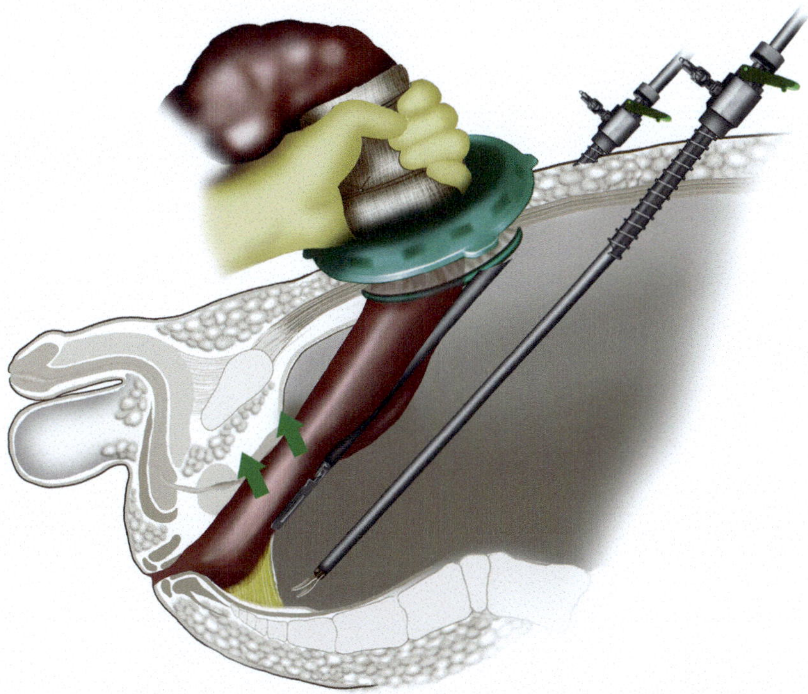

Fig. 42.5 Using the hand-assisted device to facilitate posterior dissection

Special Postoperative Care

1. A standard enhanced recovery pathway is recommended.
2. A drain can be left in the pelvis or transanally if dissection is performed below the mid-rectum; this can be removed as indicated by surgeon preference.

Suggested Reading

1. Champagne BJ, Delaney CP. Laparoscopic approaches to rectal cancer. Clin Colon Rectal Surg. 2007;20:237–48.
2. Cima RR, Pattana-arun J, Larson DW, Dozois EJ, Wolff BG, Pemberton JH. Experience with 969 minimal access colectomies: the role of hand-assisted laparoscopy in expanding minimally invasive surgery for complex colectomies. J Am Coll Surg. 2008;206:946–50; discussion 950.
3. Lindsetmo RO, Champagne B, Delaney CP. Laparoscopic rectal resections and fast-track surgery: what can be expected? Am J Surg. 2009;197:408–12.
4. Rullier E, Sa Cunha A, Couderc P, Rullier A, Gontier R, Saric J. Laparoscopic intersphincteric resection with coloplasty and coloanal anastomosis for mid and low rectal cancer. Br J Surg. 2003;90:445–51.

Techniques for Laparoscopic Distal Rectal Stapled Transection

43

Howard M. Ross

Clinical Scenario

Mr. Rogers completed chemoradiotherapy 10 weeks ago to address his mid-rectal cancer. You are performing a laparoscopic low anterior resection and it is going extremely well. It comes time to transect the distal rectum. Your preferred technique to transect is to place a laparoscopic linear stapler across the rectum in transverse orientation. Mr. Rogers' pelvis is narrow, and the fully adjustable linear stapler cannot enter the deep pelvis. No amount of retraction on the rectum will allow the use of the linear stapler.

Key Points

1. Surgeons operating on the rectum in a minimally invasive manner need to be skilled in a number of techniques to divide the distal rectum.
2. The anatomy of the pelvis combined with a patient's adipose stores can significantly complicate rectal division.
3. Forcing a particular technique in any given operation can result in a rectal perforation, a need to convert to open laparotomy, or an anastomotic leak.
4. Transverse stapled distal division of the rectum with a single stapler firing is the ultimate goal but at times cannot be performed.
5. Pelvic pressure by an assistant or placement of a T™ (Medtronic), PI™ (Medtronic), or Contour stapler (Ethicon) through a Pfannenstiel incision may be helpful.

Operative Assessment

1. Before distal rectal transaction, the rectum must be completely mobilized.
2. Optimizing mobilization and exposure increases the likelihood of successful transection.
3. Stapling should only be attempted once all modifiable factors have been addressed and optimized.

Operative Checklist

1. Additional helpful equipment
   (a) Linear laparoscopic stapler.
   (b) Trans-anastomotic stapler choices including the PI30, TA™ 30 (Medtronic), and/or the Contour curvilinear stapler (Ethicon).
   (c) Wound protector for the Pfannenstiel.

H. M. Ross (✉)
Division of Colon and Rectal Surgery, Lewis Katz School of Medicine at Temple University and the Temple University Health System, Philadelphia, PA, USA
e-mail: Howard.Ross@tuhs.temple.edu

S. W. Lee et al. (eds.), *Colorectal Surgery Consultation*,
https://doi.org/10.1007/978-3-030-11181-6_43

    (d) Fiber-optic endoscope.
2. Exposure
    (a) The pelvis must be completely visualized with the small bowel completely in the upper abdomen.
3. Positioning
    (a) Standard position for laparoscopic rectal dissection that entails arms tucked, head down, and legs in stirrups with thighs parallel to the patient's torso or split-leg positioning.
    (b) Access to the perineum and anus to facilitate placing upward manual pelvic pressure, endoscopy, and stapling.

Operative Techniques

1. Only after bilateral, posterior, and anterior mobilization is complete should distal rectal transection be contemplated.
2. The linear endoscopic stapler works well but can be difficult to place across the rectum in a narrow or adipose-filled pelvis.
3. Effort should be made to divide the rectum perpendicular to the rectum and with as few staple loads as possible (Fig. 43.1).
4. An alternate method of stapling is to create a Pfannenstiel or low midline incision and place a TA, PI, or Contour stapler through the incision and across the distal rectum (Fig. 43.2).
5. A surgical stapler at times can divide the rectum in an anterior to posterior direction.

Technical Pearls (Tips and Tricks)

1. Manual pressure upward on the anus and peritoneum can elevate pelvic floor and facilitate stapling.
2. If there is a question about transection line integrity, flexible endoscopy can be performed prior to creating the end-to-end anastomosis.
3. Do not get frustrated.
4. Have all your options in mind and necessary instruments ready.
5. Conversion is always an option to ensure safety.

Fig. 43.1 Vertical staple

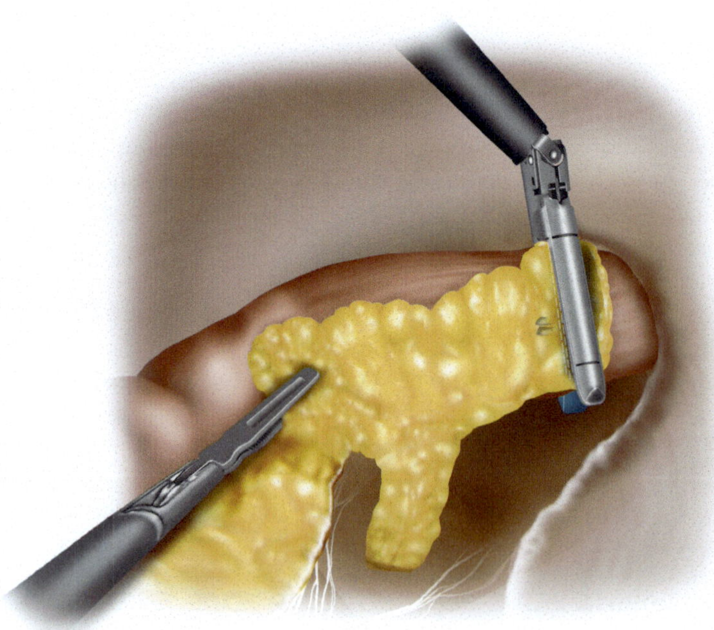

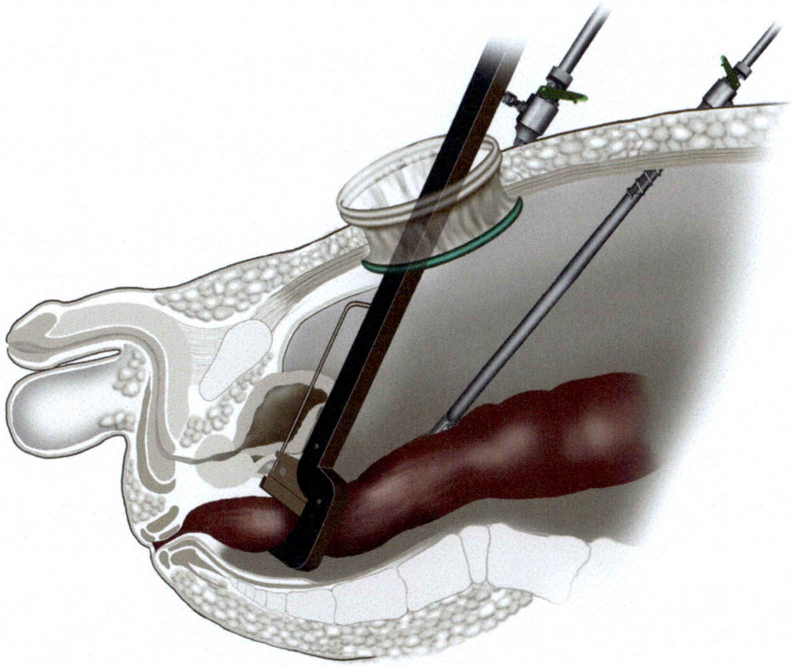

Fig. 43.2 PI™ stapler placed through Pfannenstiel incision

6. Try to avoid "zigzag" staple lines or greater than two stapling passes to divide the distal rectum.
7. Use of additional ports, or a Pfannenstiel wound, to optimize stapler positioning can be helpful.

Special Postoperative Care

1. Pelvic drain placement as per surgeon custom

Suggested Reading

1. Ito M, et al. Relationship between multiple numbers of stapler firings during rectal division and anastomotic leakage after laparoscopic rectal resection. Int J Color Dis. 2008;23(7):703–7.
2. Kim IS, et al. Risk factors for anastomotic leakage after laparoscopic intracorporeal colorectal anastomosis with a double stapling technique. J Am Coll Surg. 2009;209:694–701.
3. Lee S, et al. The relationship between the number of intersections of staple lines and anastomotic leakage after the use of a double stapling technique in laparoscopic colorectal surgery. Surg Laparosc Endosc Percutan Tech. 2017;27(4):273–81.

How to Avoid "Twisting" an Ileocolic or Ileorectal Anastomosis

44

Scott R. Steele and Andrew T. Schlussel

Clinical Scenario

A 36-year-old man with a history of fibrostenotic Crohn's disease is undergoing a laparoscopic-assisted ileocecectomy. The distal terminal ileum is fibrotic with a foreshortened mesentery and creeping fat. The procedure is progressing well laparoscopically; however, due to chronic inflammation surrounding the bowel wall, there is concern that it will be difficult to maintain the correct orientation of the bowel once it is exteriorized for the anastomosis.

Key Points

1. Always adequately mobilize the colon and small bowel prior to exteriorization and creation of the anastomosis.
   (a) This requires full mobilization off of the duodenum.
2. Consider laparoscopic vascular pedicle ligation and mesenteric division when feasible rather than performing these steps in open fashion through the extraction site.
3. When performing a hand-sewn intestinal anastomosis, place a non-crushing bowel clamp on the antimesenteric side of the bowel toward the mesentery to maintain correct orientation.
4. Consider a double-stapled or "Barcelona"-style anastomosis as this eliminates the risk of twisting at the anastomosis.
5. During creation of an ileorectal anastomosis, ensure the small bowel is oriented on the left side of the abdomen with the cut edge of the mesentery facing the right side of the patient.
6. In the morbidly obese patient, consider an intracorporeal anastomosis.
7. Follow the cut edge of mesentery to the root to ensure it is oriented straight the entire length.

Operative Assessment

1. The cut edge of the mesentery to the distal small bowel should go to the second portion of the duodenum.
2. The mesenteric defect can be closed after the ileocolic anastomosis to ensure proper orientation.
3. The cut edge of the mesentery should lie directly against the retroperitoneum for an ileorectal anastomosis.

S. R. Steele (✉)
Case Western Reserve University School of Medicine, Cleveland, OH, USA

Department of Colorectal Surgery, Cleveland Clinic, Cleveland, OH, USA

A. T. Schlussel
Madigan Army Medical Center, Department of Surgery, Tacoma, WA, USA

S. W. Lee et al. (eds.), *Colorectal Surgery Consultation*,
https://doi.org/10.1007/978-3-030-11181-6_44

4. No bowel should be doing through the mesenteric defect if there is proper orientation.

Operative Checklist

1. Ensure the patient is in proper position on the table, and use table positioning/gravity to move the bowel out of the way.
2. Atraumatic bowel graspers to "run" the small bowel and help determine orientation.
3. Laparoscopic needle drivers and suture to mark orientation or close the mesenteric defect.

Operative Techniques

1. Ileocolectomy and anastomosis
   (a) Intracorporeal
      (i) An intracorporeal anastomosis has been described as a means to reduce certain postoperative complications and may mitigate the risk of incorrectly aligning the small bowel and colon prior to creating an anastomosis.
      (ii) This is a technically complex anastomosis and requires an experienced laparoscopic surgeon.
      (iii) Current data has demonstrated no significant difference in rate of "twisting" of the anastomosis when comparing intra- versus extracorporeal methods; however, laparoscopy provides the ability to directly visualize the anatomy in an effort to prevent twisting of the mesentery prior to creation of the anastomosis.
      (iv) An intracorporeal anastomosis is associated with a shorter incision length and a potential decrease in wound complications.
   (b) Extracorporeal
      (i) The surgeon must ensure that adequate mobilization is performed to allow the colon and small bowel to be exteriorized with ease. Whether the dissection is performed in a medial to lateral or lateral to medial fashion, the second portion of the duodenum must be fully visualized, and the ileal mesentery should be mobilized to enable safe and adequate exteriorization.
      (ii) When technically feasible, the authors recommend laparoscopic ligation of the ileocolic pedicle and division of the mesentery to the points of resection. This will allow for increased mobility outside the abdominal cavity and will minimize the risk of tearing the mesentery, which will result in bleeding and impairment of adequate visualization of the anatomy.
      (iii) If a hand-sewn anastomosis is performed, non-crushing bowel clamps should be placed from an antimesenteric to mesenteric direction. This will maintain the correct orientation of the small bowel and colon, ensuring the ends will be lined up appropriately for the anastomosis (Fig. 44.1).

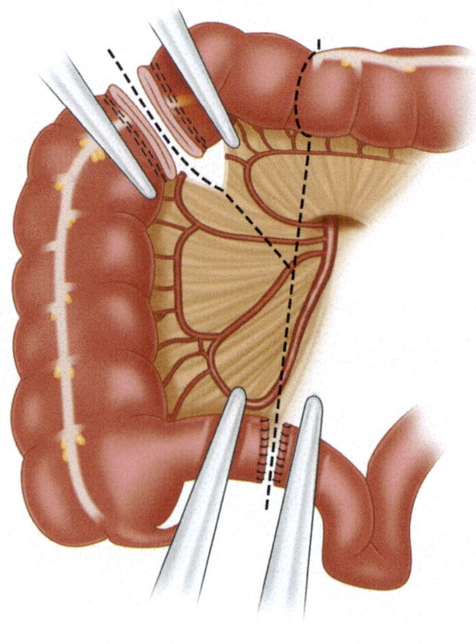

Fig. 44.1 Non-crushing clamps placed across the antimesenteric surface of the bowel prior to anastomosis

(iv) A standard ileocolic anastomosis typically involves transecting the small bowel and colon with a linear cutting stapler, followed by a side-to-side (functional end-to-end) anastomosis along the antimesenteric borders of the bowel. The common enterocolostomy is closed with either a stapler or suture technique. It is critical when performing this anastomosis that the surgeon maintains the correct orientation of the bowel. The mesentery should be facing toward the patient's left side with the anastomosis on the right.

(c) If there is ongoing concern that the anastomosis is twisted, the surgeon should reenter the abdominal cavity to laparoscopically visualize the anastomosis. If this inspection is not adequate, conversion should be performed.

2. Ileorectal anastomosis
   (a) A stapled ileorectal anastomosis should be created under direct visualization either laparoscopically or through a mini-laparotomy.
   (b) Once the anvil and circular stapler are married, the small bowel should be guided down to avoid twisting around the stapler. To ensure appropriate alignment, the small bowel mesentery should be aligned toward the patient's right side while the bowel wall faces the left (Fig. 44.2). To confirm this anatomic orientation, it is helpful to have the patient in Trendelenburg with the table tilted right side up.
3. Isoperistaltic anastomosis
   (a) An isoperistaltic anastomosis involves joining the small bowel and colon with their stapled ends facing opposite directions. A longitudinal stapled enterocolostomy is then created along the antimesenteric surface (Fig. 44.3). This anastomotic configuration may be beneficial when there is a lack of intestinal mobility.
   (b) This technique is utilized more often during a laparoscopic intracorporeal anastomosis.

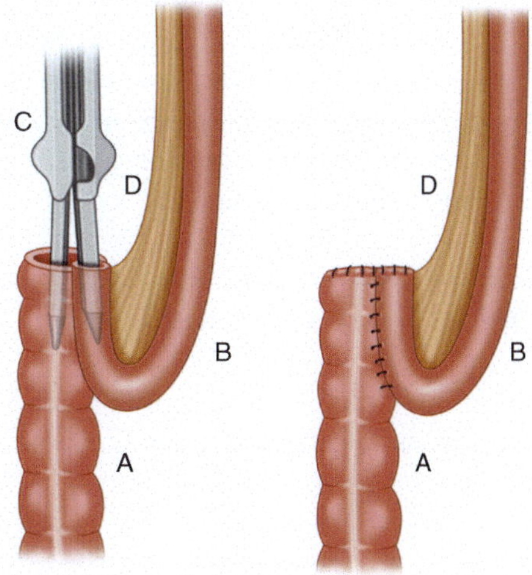

Fig. 44.2 Ileorectal anastomosis

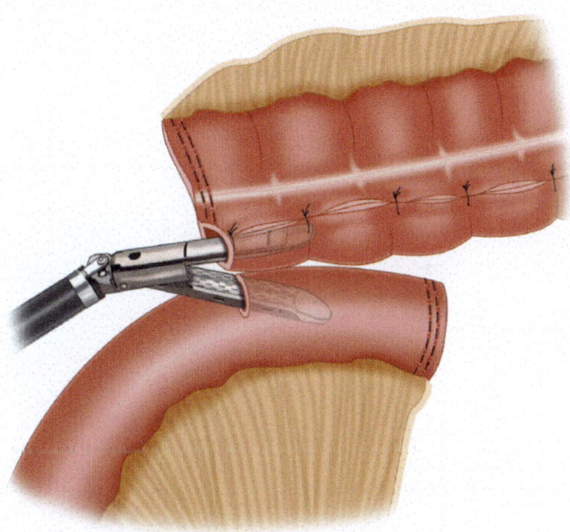

Fig. 44.3 Isoperistaltic anastomosis

   (c) Although aligning the anastomosis in this configuration may ensure appropriate orientation, there is an inherent requirement to rotate the ileal mesentery to complete this successfully. This is more prominent in an ileotransverse colon anastomosis, where a 180-degree rotation of the mesentery is performed, compared to an ileoascending colon anastomosis, which requires only a 90-degree rotation.

(d) No significant difference has been identified when comparing an antiperistaltic to an isoperistaltic configuration; however, the surgeon should be aware of the necessary mesenteric rotation to ensure correct orientation of the anastomosis prior to completing the operation.

Technical Pearls (Tips and Tricks)

1. A double-stapled technique (the "Barcelona" anastomosis) is another option to ensure correct orientation of the anastomosis. This technique avoids twisting of the mesentery, utilizes fewer staplers and stapler loads, and results in fewer transecting staple lines. In this approach, the mesentery of the small bowel and colon is first divided up to the level of transection. An enterotomy and colotomy are made, and a linear anastomosis along the antimesenteric borders is fashioned with a GIA stapler. Using four Alice clamps the common enterocolostomy is closed, slightly offsetting the anterior and posterior staple lines. The anastomosis is then completed while simultaneously transecting the specimen with a second firing of the linear stapler. Using a longer linear stapler to create the common channel is advised as a part of this staple line will be removed with the second firing of the stapler. The benefit of this anastomosis is that the small bowel and colon are transected simultaneously rather than sequentially; therefore, the anastomosis is created with both ends in correct anatomic position (Fig. 44.4).

Special Postoperative Care

1. Routine postoperative care with enhanced recovery protocol as indicated may be utilized.
2. If a twist is suspected, a gastrografin enema will aid in determining the orientation of the bowel.

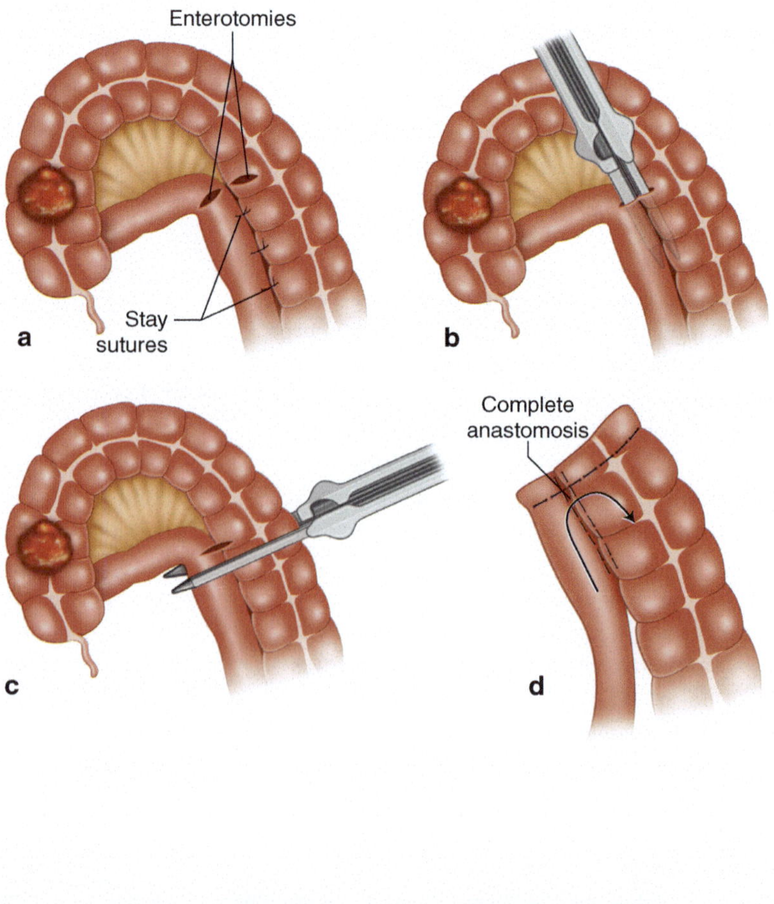

Fig. 44.4 Double-stapled or "Barcelona" anastomosis

Suggested Reading

1. Hellan M, Anderson C, Pigazzi A. Extracorporeal versus intracorporeal anastomosis for laparoscopic right hemicolectomy. JSLS. 2009;13(3):312–7.
2. Matsuda A, et al. Isoperistaltic versus antiperistaltic stapled side-to-side anastomosis for colon cancer surgery: a randomized controlled trial. J Surg Res. 2015;196(1):107–12.
3. Tarta C, Bishawi M, Bergamaschi R. Intracorporeal ileocolic anastomosis: a review. Tech Coloproctol. 2013;17(5):479–85.
4. Tewari M, Shukla HS. Right colectomy with isoperistaltic side-to-side stapled ileocolic anastomosis. J Surg Oncol. 2005;89(2):99–101.

How to Deal with Splenic Injury During Laparoscopic Flexure Mobilization

45

Daniel L. Feingold and Mehraneh D. Jafari

Clinical Scenario

During release of a difficult splenic flexure high in the left upper quadrant, brisk bleeding is noted from a capsular tear at the inferior pole of the spleen (Fig. 45.1).

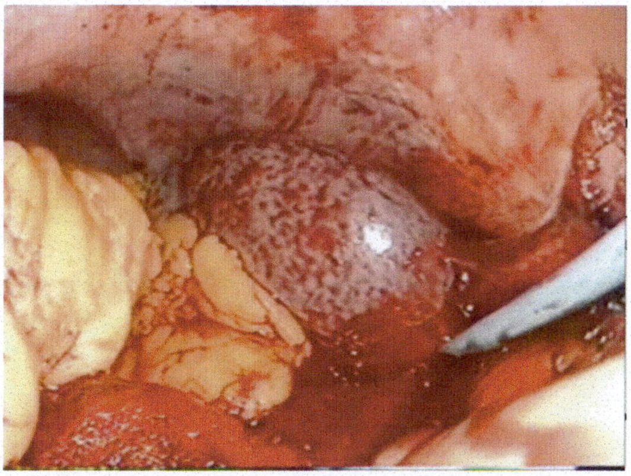

Fig. 45.1 Bleeding from the spleen from a capsular tear

Key Points

1. Bleeding from a splenic injury during flexure takedown is rare but can be challenging to control especially in the setting of urgent colectomy or large bowel obstruction.
2. Splenic injuries during flexure release can usually be managed with monopolar electrocautery and topical hemostatic agents.

Operative Assessment

1. What is the source of the bleeding?
   (a) Capsular bleeding due to traction on the splenocolic ligament or another splenic attachment is the most common mechanism of iatrogenic splenic injury.
   (b) Another possible bleeding source is injury to a splenic vessel, possibly from aberrant hilar anatomy. While controlling this bleeding, avoid further injury to the splenic vessels, and recognize that the pancreas is at risk for injury at this level. While splenic hilum vessels are end arteries and ligation in this setting can cause a readily apparent distribution of splenic infarction, collateral flow via the short gastric arteries may preserve flow in this situation.
2. Be mindful of the blood loss up to this point and the patient's starting hemoglobin, clinical status, and unique threshold for volume

D. L. Feingold (✉)
Division of Colorectal Surgery, Department of Surgery, Columbia University, New York, NY, USA
e-mail: df347@cumc.columbia.edu

M. D. Jafari
UC Irvine Health, Department of Surgery, Division of Colorectal Surgery, Orange, CA, USA

S. W. Lee et al. (eds.), *Colorectal Surgery Consultation*,
https://doi.org/10.1007/978-3-030-11181-6_45

expanders and/or blood transfusion as you control the bleeding.

either splenic salvage or splenectomy may be required.

Operative Checklist

1. Additional resources and equipment.
   (a) Access to a variety of absorbable hemostatic agents.
   (b) In open cases involving an extreme splenic flexure or splenic bleeding, having a dedicated assistant retracting the left upper quadrant with a large body wall retractor can be invaluable.
2. During advanced laparoscopic cases, instrument trays for conversion with body wall retractors should be readily available in the event that rapid conversion to laparotomy is required.

Operative Techniques

1. In order to reduce the risk of morbidity, the decision to takedown the splenic flexure should be individualized based on the patient's anatomy and the extent of colon reach required.
2. The operative platform of the operation underway can limit the options available for control of the bleeding in terms of delivering sponges and hemostatic agents to the left upper quadrant. The specifics of the injury and the requirements of the repair may necessitate a change in the operative approach. Depending on the circumstances, upsizing a laparoscopic port or adding a port may be required. A hand-assisted approach can facilitate hemostasis and can help complete a difficult splenic flexure release.
3. Depending on the degree of bleeding and blood loss, the circumstances of the patient, and the maneuvers that have been tried but failed, conversion to an open approach with

Technical Pearls (Tips and Tricks)

1. Most splenic injuries during flexure mobilization are due to capsular avulsion due to traction on the omentum or any of the connective tissue ligaments in the area. Relying on as little traction as possible to obtain exposure for the dissection can help avoid splenic injury. Placing the patient in steeper reverse Trendelenburg can deliver the field toward the surgeon and uses gravity to facilitate the dissection rather than physical manipulation and traction.
2. When bleeding is encountered, holding direct pressure with a sponge can temporize while needed products are brought into the operating room and a decision is made regarding how best to access the left upper quadrant in this situation.
3. High setting monopolar electrocauterization can usually control capsular bleeding. The "spray" mode may be more useful than "fulgurate" to achieve hemostasis. Light irrigation onto the bleeding site when delivering the energy can keep the cautery instrument from adhering to the char of the tissues.
4. Directly applying pressure with absorbable topical hemostatic agents (made from oxidized cellulose, collagen, gelatin, thrombin, plasma, etc.) held in place with a sponge can also control the bleeding.
5. In cases of a deeper laceration and failure of topical therapy, suturing the spleen may be required. This is typically done using absorbable monofilament sutures with pledgets in simple interrupted fashion using a large tapered needle. It is helpful to combine suture splenorrhaphy with absorbable hemostats by using the sutures to hold the hemostatic agent in place. If the case is still laparoscopic, use the largest needle that fits through a 10 mm port.

6. In situations of profuse bleeding with hemodynamic instability and a blood transfusion requirement, splenectomy may be required.
7. A 10 mm laparoscopic suction does a better job of evacuating blood and clot than a typical 5 mm suction device.
8. Patients undergoing advanced laparoscopic cases typically should have access with two peripheral IVs, and communicating with the anesthesia team when bleeding is encountered improves care.
9. In cases of otherwise uneventful splenic flexure takedown, it is important to survey the left upper quadrant prior to completing the operation and closing to verify there is no bleeding that needs to be addressed.

Special Postoperative Care

1. Given the raw surface of the spleen and depending on the blood loss, consider possibly modifying your postoperative care protocol in terms of deep venous thrombosis chemoprophylaxis as well as Ketorolac use.

Suggested Reading

1. Isik O, Aytac E, Ashburn J, et al. Does laparoscopy reduce splenic injuries during colorectal resections? An assessment from the ACS-NSQIP database. Surg Endosc. 2015;29:1039–44.

Entering the Reoperative Hostile Abdomen Laparoscopically

46

Laura Greco and Howard M. Ross

Clinical Scenario

Mrs. O presents with a newly diagnosed cecal cancer. She is a morbidly obese 72-year-old diabetic who had an appendectomy via long right paramedian incision when she was 7 years old. Mrs. O's surgeon and the patient both favor a laparoscopic approach to optimize postoperative recovery and minimize the risk of wound complications. Mrs. O's surgeon utilizes a left upper quadrant incision 2 cm below the midclavicular line and places the first port in open fashion. Additional two ports are placed in the left lower quadrant. Careful, sharp dissection allows complete adhesiolysis and a laparoscopic right colon resection (Figs. 46.1 and 46.2).

Key Points

1. Risk of anterior wall adhesions increases with increasing number of prior abdominal surgeries. In patients with prior abdominal surgery, risk of adhesions is 60–90%. Visceral injury from trocar placement accounts for 40% of visceral injuries from laparoscopic surgery.
2. Presence of dense adhesions is associated with increased risk of conversion (odds ratio of 2.3).
3. According to one review, 69% of visceral injuries during laparoscopic surgery occurred in patients with adhesions or history of prior abdominal surgery.
4. The decision to place the initial port in open fashion or via Veress needle technique is up to surgeon and their experience.
5. Maintaining a low threshold for conversion as a missed bowel injury can be a devastating injury.
6. Reoperation in the setting of adhesions requires patience. It is important to schedule enough time for these kinds of operations and to arrange for adequate assistance.
7. Sharp adhesiolysis helps prevent thermal injury.
8. Structures that cannot be completely visualized should not be divided.

Operative Assessment

Goal: Safe initial entry of the first port and rapid assessment if the operation can ultimately be completed laparoscopically.

L. Greco
Department of Surgery,
Temple University Hospital, Philadelphia, PA, USA

H. M. Ross (✉)
Division of Colon and Rectal Surgery,
Lewis Katz School of Medicine at Temple University and the Temple University Health System,
Philadelphia, PA, USA
e-mail: Howard.Ross@tuhs.temple.edu

S. W. Lee et al. (eds.), *Colorectal Surgery Consultation*,
https://doi.org/10.1007/978-3-030-11181-6_46

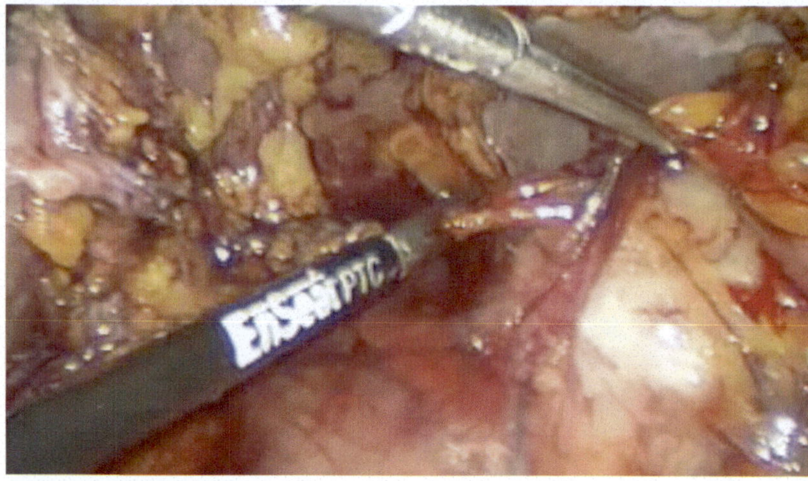

Fig. 46.1 Bowel wall adhesions to the anterior abdominal wall

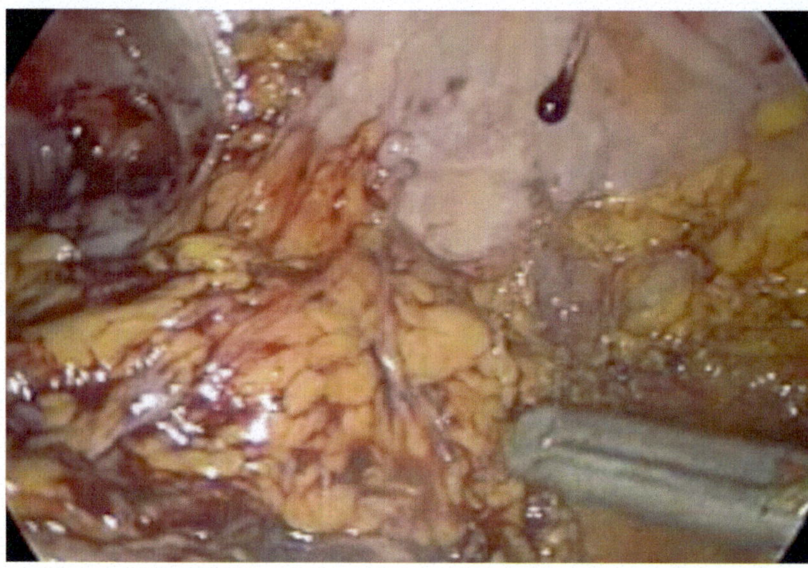

Fig. 46.2 Dense omental adhesions and intra-loop adhesions seen laparoscopically

1. Initial port placement
   (a) Location
      (i) Left upper quadrant
         1. Left upper quadrant entry with Veress needle has been shown to be effective in patients at risk for periumbilical anterior abdominal wall adhesions. The Veress needle can be placed at Palmer's point about 2 cm below the costal margin in the midclavicular line or in the ninth intercostal space lateral to the midclavicular line. In a series of 918 patients who underwent access in the left upper quadrant for laparoscopic lysis of adhesions, 54% of patients had adhesions in the periumbilical region that would have increased their risk for bowel injury upon entrance to the abdomen. In various studies evaluating left upper quadrant placement of first ports for laparoscopy, the incidence of enterotomy is low.

2. Both Palmer's point and the ninth intercostal space lateral to the midclavicular line have been shown to be safe and effective locations for placement of Veress needle for establishment of pneumoperitoneum.

(ii) Placement of ports away from prior surgical sites

1. Presence of adhesions to the prior surgical incision sites is common. In animal models, it has been demonstrated that adhesions directly to prior operative wound occur in 33% of cases, suggesting that laparoscopic access through sites of prior surgery would be associated with increased risk of enterotomy.

(b) Ultrasound evaluation for location of adhesions

(i) Various studies have assessed the efficacy of preoperative transabdominal ultrasound to identify peritoneal adhesions for the purpose of placement of laparoscopic ports away from adhesions. To evaluate for the presence of adhesions, the degree of visceral sliding with respiration was assessed. Patients with adhesions at the area being examined had little to no sliding. In one study, transabdominal ultrasound identified the location of bowel adhesions to the anterior abdominal wall with a sensitivity of 77.8% and specificity of 97.9% but a positive predictive value of only 49%.

2. Open vs. closed laparoscopic entry

(a) There have been many studies and reviews published comparing open (Hasson) versus closed laparoscopic entry into the abdomen with many concluding there was no difference in the rate of visceral injury between the methods. One review article found that open entry was associated with lower rate of failed entry and there was no difference in rate of injury with either method. Another review article that focused specifically on patients with prior abdominal surgery and adhesions also found that there was no difference in visceral injury between entry methods and that open entry was associated with longer time to entry. Based on these findings, the method of laparoscopic entry should be at the discretion of the surgeon as neither method has been associated with an increased risk of injury.

Operative Checklist

1. Additional helpful equipment
   (a) Laparoscopic scissors
   (b) 5-mm laparoscopic Babcock graspers
   (c) Blunt graspers
   (d) 30-degree 5-mm laparoscope
   (e) 30-degree 10-mm laparoscope

Operative Techniques

1. Place the first port safely relying on your judgement and experience.
2. Rapidly assess feasibility and avoid the frustration of converting after an extensive laparoscopy.
3. Lyse adhesions carefully and sharply.
4. Do not divide tissues you can't completely visualize.
5. Go slow.
6. Be patient.
7. Balance desire for laparoscopic procedure with risk of creating missed enterotomy and the realities of what a laparoscopic procedure actually delivers when compared to open procedure (2 days length of stay and smaller incision in a patient who already has a large scar from prior operation).

Technical Pearls (Tips and Tricks)

1. Patience is a virtue.
2. Lyse adhesions carefully and sharply.
3. Traction is your friend.

4. An extra 5 mm port is often helpful.
5. Disposable tip cold scissors are extremely sharp and enable delicate, fine adhesiolysis.
6. Leaving peritoneum and even layers of the abdominal wall on the serosa of adherent small bowel is preferable to dissecting the small bowel off of the peritoneum and injuring the bowel.

Special Postoperative Care

1. Appreciate that an enterotomy can occur. Understand that a missed enterotomy is a dangerous entity.

Suggested Reading

1. Ahmad G, Gent D, Henderson D, O'Flynn H, Phillips K, Watson A. Laparoscopic entry techniques. Cochrane Database Syst Rev. 2015;(8):CD006583. https://doi.org/10.1002/14651858.CD006583.pub4.
2. Argarwala N. Safe entry techniques during laparoscopy: left upper quadrant entry using the ninth intercostal space—a review of 918 procedures. J Minim Invasive Gynecol. 2005;12(1):55–61.
3. Bhoyrul S, Vierra MA, Nezhat CR, Krummel TM, Way LW. Trocar injuries in laparoscopic surgery. J Am Coll Surg. 2001;192(6):677–83.
4. Chang FH, Chou HH, Lee CL, Cheng PJ, Wang CW, Soong YK. Extraumbilical insertion of the operative laparoscope in patients with extensive intraabdominal adhesions. J Am Assoc Gynecol Laparosc. 1995;2(3):335–7.
5. Childers J, Brzechffa P, Surwit E. Laparoscopy using the left upper quadrant as the primary trocar site. Gynecol Oncol. 1993;50(2):221–5.
6. Englum BR, Hopkins MB, Migaly J. Overcoming technical challenges: reoperative surgery. In: Ross H, Lee S, Mutch M, Rivadeneira D, Steele S, editors. Minimally invasive approaches to colon and rectal disease. New York: Springer; 2015.
7. Kothari SN, Fundell LJ, Lambert PJ, Mathiason MA. Use of transabdominal ultrasound to identify intraabdominal adhesions prior to laparoscopy: a prospective blinded study. Am J Surg. 2006;192(6):843–7, ISSN 0002-96101.
8. Kumar S. Veress needle insertion through left lower intercostal space for creating pneumoperitoneum: experience with 75 cases. J Minim Access Surg. 2012;8(3):85–9. https://doi.org/10.4103/0972-9941.97590.
9. Parker J, Reid G, Wong F. Microlaparoscopic left upper quadrant entry in patients at high risk of periumbilical adhesions. Aust N Z J Obstet Gynaecol. 1999;39:88–92. https://doi.org/10.1111/j.1479-828X.1999.tb03452.x.
10. Read TE, Salgado J, Ferraro D, et al. "Peek port": a novel approach for avoiding conversion in laparoscopic colectomy. Surg Endosc. 2009;23:477. https://doi.org/10.1007/s00464-008-0047-1.
11. Tinelli A, Malvasi A, Guido M, Tsin DA, Hudelist G, Stark M, Mettler L. Laparoscopy entry in patients with previous abdominal and pelvic surgery. Surg Innov. 2011;18(3):201–5. https://doi.org/10.1177/1553350610393989. Epub 2011 Jan 18.
12. Tittel A, Treutner KH, Titkova S, et al. New adhesion formation after laparoscopic and conventional adhesiolysis. Surg Endosc. 2001;15:44. https://doi.org/10.1007/s004640000256.
13. van der Voort M, Heijnsdijk EA, Gouma DJ. Bowel injury as a complication of laparoscopy. Br J Surg. 2004;91(10):1253–8.
14. Van Goor H. Consequences and complications of peritoneal adhesions. Color Dis. 2007;9(S2):25–34.

Manage Inferior Epigastric Bleeding

47

Titilayo Adegboyega and David E. Rivadeneira

Clinical Scenario

A 73-year-old male is undergoing a laparoscopic low anterior resection for cancer. He has been on Plavix and aspirin for recent cardiac stent placement. An expanding hematoma is noted in the right lower quadrant with blood trickling down the trocar. The anesthesiologist communicates concerns about transient hypotension, which may be from CO_2 insufflation.

Key Points

1. Injury to the inferior epigastric artery (IEA) can occur during a variety of colorectal procedures. Awareness of the variety of ways the IEA can be injured is important.
   (a) Primarily, the IEA is at risk during trocar placement for laparoscopic surgery.
   (b) The location of colostomy and ileostomy within the rectus sheath increases the risk of IEA injury.
   (c) Specimen extraction sites as well as drains can also injure this vessel.
2. The management of injury to IEA begins first with a good understanding of anatomy.
   (a) The IEA arises from the external iliac artery immediately above the inguinal ligament and ascends obliquely along the medial margin of the deep inguinal ring.
   (b) It pierces the transversalis fascia, passes in front of the arcuate line, and runs between the rectus abdominis and posterior rectus sheath.
   (c) It is located about 5 cm lateral to the umbilicus.
   (d) Above the umbilicus, it divides into numerous branches and collateralizes with descending branches of the superior epigastric artery
3. Various strategies can be employed to avoiding injury to the IEA.
   (a) Trocars should be placed more laterally (lateral to the rectus muscle), when possible (Fig. 47.1).
   (b) Transillumination of thinner abdominal walls can help avoid injury when placing trocars.
   (c) If the IEA is not readily apparent, the vessel can be identified lateral to the internal

T. Adegboyega
Huntington Hospital-Northwell Health, Department of Colorectal Surgery, Huntington, NY, USA

D. E. Rivadeneira (✉)
Surgical Strategic Initiatives, Northwell Health, New Hyde Park, NY, USA

Surgical Services and Colorectal Surgery, Huntington Hospital, Huntington, NY, USA

Hofstra University-Northwell School of Medicine, Hempstead, NY, USA
e-mail: DRivadeneira@northwell.edu

S. W. Lee et al. (eds.), *Colorectal Surgery Consultation*,
https://doi.org/10.1007/978-3-030-11181-6_47

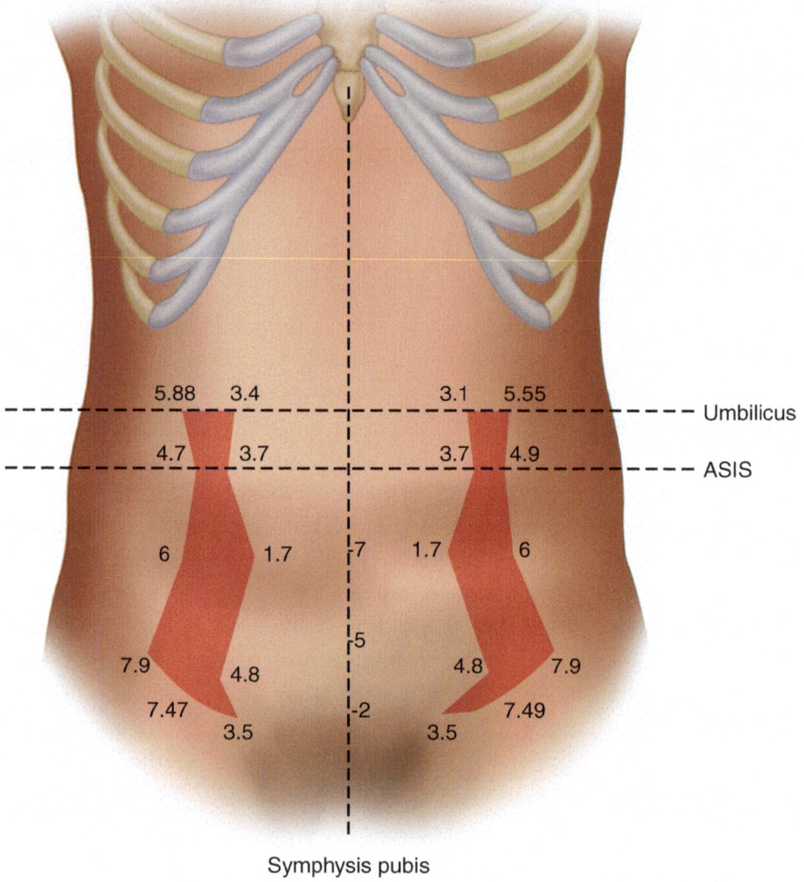

Fig. 47.1 Red areas represent the location of the inferior epigastric artery. *ASIS* anterior superior iliac spine. Numbers indicate distance away from the midline. Trocars should be placed outside of the highlighted area. This can be easily accomplished by placing trocars lateral to the rectum sheath

opening of the inguinal ring and then followed cephalad along its course.

4. When injury occurs, early recognition of injury is paramount to minimizing morbidity and mortality and allows for rapid control of the vessel and avoidance of further blood loss.

Operative Assessment

1. Is the patient stable?
   (a) Communication with the OR team is important.
   (b) The hemodynamic status of the patient determines the next steps which may include tamponading the bleeding by applying manual pressure or balloon-tipped devices, giving fluids, obtaining blood products, and, in some cases, use of vasopressors. Concurrently, the surgeon needs to evaluate the injury and the available options for definitive control of the bleeding.
2. Identify injury.
   (a) In this case, the site of injury is obvious as the expanding hematoma and bleeding are visible in relation to the trocar.
3. Remain laparoscopic or convert to open?
   (a) The initial goal is to control the bleeding from the IEA first before proceeding with the remainder of the surgery. The injury may be controlled laparoscopically or through a cutdown incision at the trocar site.
   (b) Regardless of the means utilized to control the bleeding, the surgeon still needs to decide how to proceed with the remainder of the surgery depending on the overall

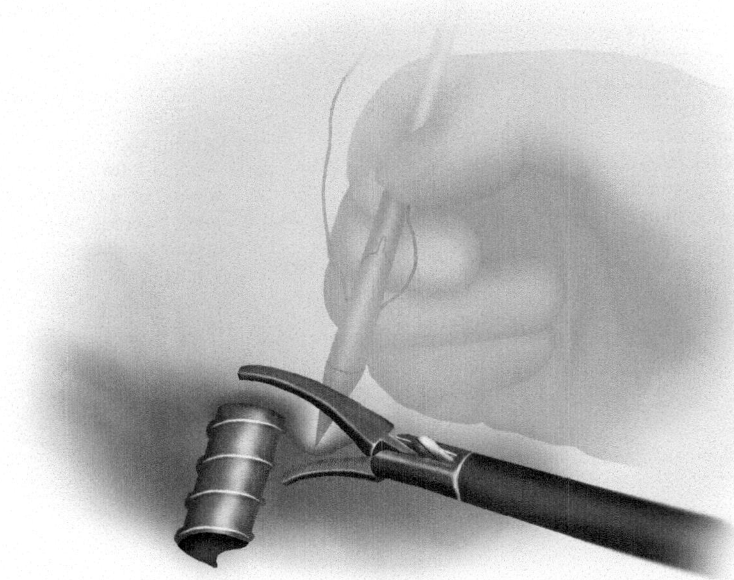

Fig. 47.2 Cannula wound closure. Introducing the suture passer into the abdomen. Countertraction is applied by a laparoscopic instrument at the puncture site. (With permission. Nakajima K, Milsom JW, Böhm B. Basic laparoscopic surgical skills. In: Milsom JW, Bohm B, Nakajima K, editors. *Laparoscopic colorectal surgery*. New York: Springer; 2006. p. 66–96.)

status of the patient, comorbidities, and time spent controlling the bleeding.

Operative Checklist

1. Preoperative preparation
   (a) Ensure a type and screen is performed and that blood products are available in high-risk patients.
   (b) Review patient history such as prior surgeries which may influence or limit trocar placement.
2. Equipment
   (a) Have suture passer (Figs. 47.2, 47.3, 47.4, and 47.5) and long sutures available.
   (b) Have an open instrument tray available when performing laparoscopic surgery should it be needed for rapid conversion to arise.

Operative Techniques

1. Laparoscopic approach
   (a) If there is minimal bleeding from a small branch of the IEA, monopolar electrocautery can be utilized to control bleeding. It is important to note that this has the potential of worsening the bleeding, and laparoscopic devices such as the Ligasure or Harmonic are better suited as they allow for a purchase across a vessel to create a hemostatic seal.
   (b) Place laparoscopic clips via a trocar from the contralateral side of the injured epigastric vessel. The vessel may need to be circumferentially isolated to adequately secure clips and minimize risk of dislodgement.
   (c) Suture ligation of the inferior epigastric vessel can control bleeding and can be performed via a variety of options like using a Keith needle, suture passer, or trocar closure device such as the Carter-Thomason. It is important to ligate the vessel proximal and distal to injury. After achieving hemostasis laparoscopically, regardless of the specific method used, it is important to release or aspirate the pneumoperitoneum and to confirm hemostasis with minimal insufflation pressure
   (d) Placing a Foley catheter or a balloon-tipped trocar into the trocar site and inflat-

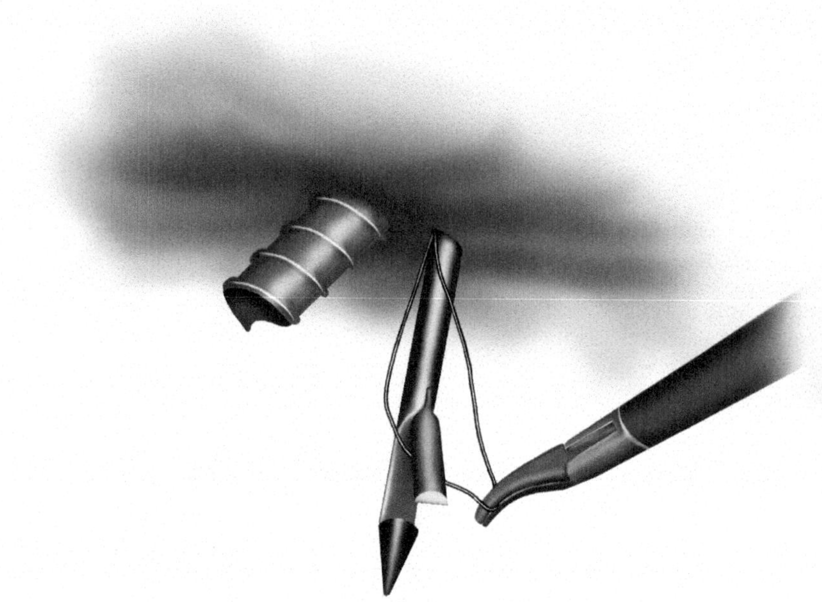

Fig. 47.3 Cannula wound closure. The suture is freed up from the suture passer so it may be removed. (With permission. Nakajima K, Milsom JW, Böhm B. Basic laparoscopic surgical skills. In: Milsom JW, Bohm B, Nakajima K, editors. *Laparoscopic colorectal surgery*. New York: Springer; 2006. p. 66–96)

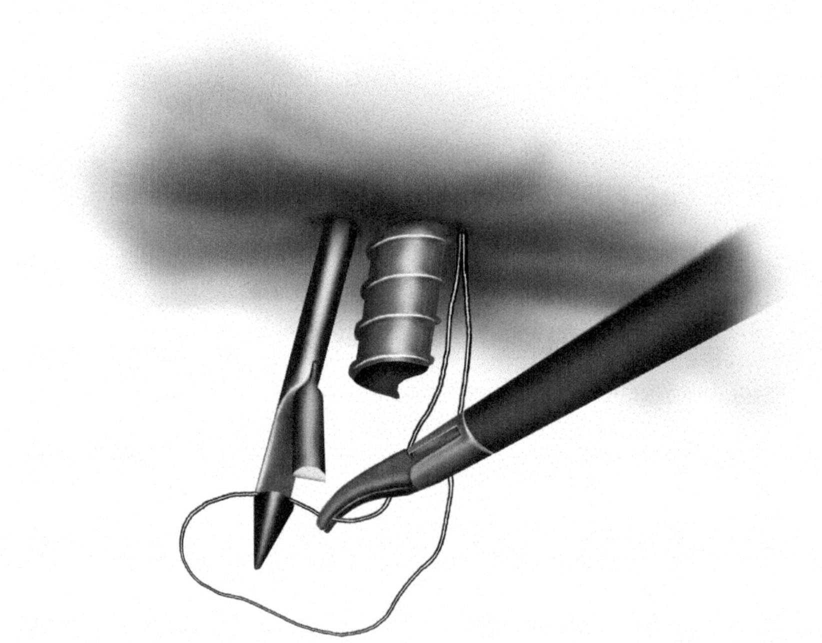

Fig. 47.4 Cannula wound closure. The second puncture by the suture passer permits extraction of the suture and fascial closure. (With permission. Nakajima K, Milsom JW, Böhm B. Basic laparoscopic surgical skills. In: Milsom JW, Bohm B, Nakajima K, editors. *Laparoscopic colorectal surgery*. New York: Springer; 2006. p. 66–96)

ing the balloon intraperitoneally can tamponade the bleeding vessel. This provides temporary compression, minimizes blood loss, and allows time to obtain supplies and trocars needed to perform any of the aforementioned techniques.

2. Open approach
   (a) Injury to the IEA is often more readily identified during open abdominal surgery. All the methods employed for control of the vessel laparoscopically can be employed during open abdominal surgery

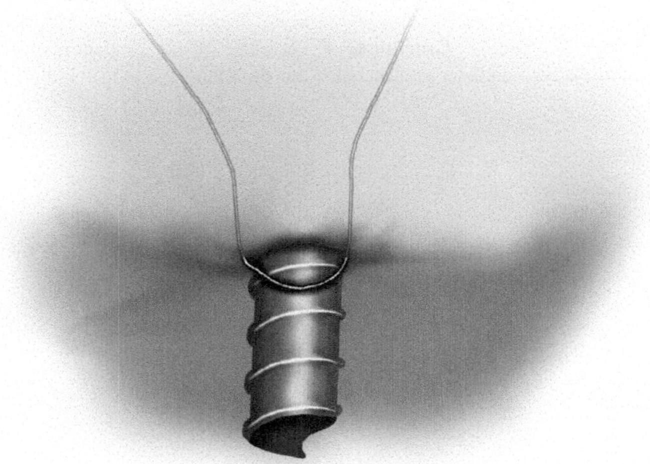

Fig. 47.5 Cannula wound closure. Position of the suture should be checked before cannula removal. (With permission. Nakajima K, Milsom JW, Böhm B. Basic laparoscopic surgical skills. In: Milsom JW, Bohm B, Nakajima K, editors. *Laparoscopic colorectal surgery*. New York: Springer; 2006. p. 66–96)

including use of an energy device, clips, and suture ligation.

   (b) Extending the incision is sometimes needed especially if the injured vessel retracts under the muscle.

3. Interventional radiology
   (a) This is used to manage bleeding that presents in a delayed fashion, results from pulling a drain, or perhaps occurs following the resumption of anticoagulation in the postoperative period. In addition to avoiding reoperation, it serves as a diagnostic and therapeutic option if the exact location of the IEA injury is not clear.
   (b) Transcatheter embolization of IEA bleeding has a 90% success rate.
   (c) Coil or injection embolization and covered stents have also been described.

Technical Pearls (Tips and Tricks)

1. Prevent bleeding based on knowledge of anatomy and direct visualization, when possible.
2. Trocar placement should aim to avoid injury to the vessels.
3. In case of bleeding, quickly control it using the various tamponade techniques described above.
4. Proximal and distal ligation is essential for adequate control.
5. Once the bleeding is addressed, reduce the insufflation pressure, and confirm adequate hemostasis.

Special Postoperative Care

1. Most patients can be managed on the regular surgical floor if the injury to the inferior epigastric artery has been identified and properly managed.
2. In patients who still require resuscitation, a higher level of care may be necessary for fluid management, blood transfusions, and serial hemoglobin.
3. Injuries treated with interventional radiology may require bed rest for a period of time based on the access site.
4. Routine VTE prophylaxis should be initiated when appropriate from a clinical standpoint.

Suggested Reading

1. Ross H, Lee S, Mutch M, Rivadeneira D, Steele SR, editors. Minimally invasive approaches to colon and rectal disease: technique and best practices. New York: Springer Publishing; 2015.

2. Ross H, Lee S, Champagne B, Pigazzi A, Rivadeneira DE, editors. Robotic colorectal surgery. New York: Springer Publishing; 2015.
3. Wick MC, Klocker J, Grundtman C, Jaschke W, Chemelli A. Transcatheter embolization for the management of acute active inferior epigastric artery hemorrhages. J Endovasc Ther. 2013;20:561–7.
4. Wong C, Merkur H. Inferior epigastric artery: surface anatomy, prevention and management of injury. Aust N Z J Obstet Gynaecol. 2016;56:137–41.

Part V

Technical Tips and Tricks for Difficult Colostomy/Ileostomy

Hard to Reach Colostomy/ Ileostomy

48

Christine Hsieh and Sang W. Lee

Clinical Scenario

After performing an emergent Hartmann procedure on a morbidly obese 65-year-old man with feculent peritonitis due to sigmoid diverticulitis, the descending colon is mobilized along the white line of Toldt and the transected end brought up to the abdominal wall toward an infraumbilical site selected preoperatively. Unfortunately, the mesentery is severely foreshortened, and the thickness of the patient's abdominal wall in this location spans over 8 cm.

Key Points

1. Preparation is key. Preoperative stoma site marking by an enterostomal therapy (EST) nurse not only improves ostomates' quality of life and ability to care for their stoma, but their assistance lowers the rate of postoperative complications.
   (a) In emergency situations or when an EST is not available, bear in mind the "ostomy triangle." The stoma should be placed within the rectus muscle inside the borders of a triangle marked by the anterior superior iliac spine, pubic tubercle, and umbilicus, ideally far enough away from the bony prominences, skinfolds, and belt line to facilitate pouching (Fig. 48.1).
      (i) Morbidly obese, chronically bed-bound, or wheelchair-dependent patients may benefit from stomas located superior to the umbilicus for ease of access and care.
      (ii) Think ahead to how the patient will manage their stoma. It is far easier to manage a difficult stoma in a good location than it is to care for a technically perfect stoma in a bad location.
2. The same principles apply to stoma creation as they do to bowel anastomosis: make every effort to minimize tension, preserve blood supply, and ensure adequate perfusion.
   (a) Plan to fully mobilize the intestine selected for stoma creation.
   (b) Be mindful of stoma aperture size at both the fascia and skin level; these must be of adequate size to accommodate the bowel and its mesentery in its current state.

Operative Assessment

1. Is this stoma the best option for the patient?

C. Hsieh
Keck School of Medicine – University of Southern California, Los Angeles, CA, USA

S. W. Lee (✉)
Department of Surgery – Colon and Rectal Surgery, Keck School of Medicine of University of Southern California, Los Angeles, CA, USA

S. W. Lee et al. (eds.), *Colorectal Surgery Consultation*,
https://doi.org/10.1007/978-3-030-11181-6_48

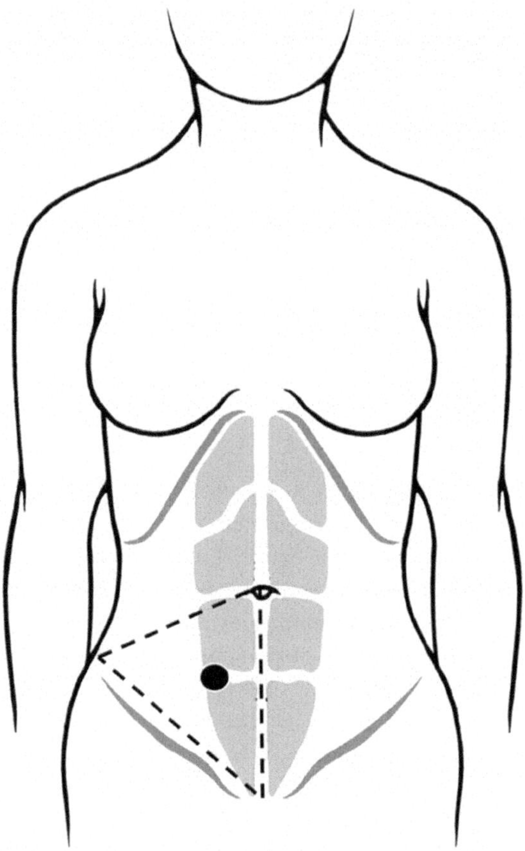

Fig. 48.1 "Ostomy triangle." The stoma should be placed within the rectus muscle inside the borders of a triangle marked by the anterior superior iliac spine, pubic tubercle, and umbilicus

(a) In some cases, creation of an end stoma may be more technically difficult and have potentially higher morbidity than primary anastomosis and proximal diversion with a loop ileostomy.

2. Is the stoma site appropriate for the patient's body habitus and/or lifestyle?
   (a) Obese patients are more likely to suffer from stoma complications than nonobese patients; therefore proper site selection and attention to stoma creation technique are critically important.
      (i) A supraumbilical stoma site is preferable for a number of reasons:
         1. The abdominal wall is typically thinner here compared to the infraumbilical region.
         2. The patient's pannus may artificially bring the umbilicus caudal, and selecting an infraumbilical site in this situation may require several more centimeters of length in order to create a tension-free stoma.
         3. An infraumbilical stoma may be out of the site line of an obese patient, making it difficult to visualize (though some patients are facile with self-care using a mirror) or even to reach the stoma.
   (b) Make note of any physical attributes that may distort landmarks, such as severe scoliosis or a narrow, scaphoid abdomen that may complicate pouching (this may not be readily apparent if a laparoscopic technique is employed).
      (i) Wheelchair-bound patients and their caregivers may find an upper abdomen stoma easier to manage while maintaining the patient in a seated position.
3. Is the bowel adequately mobilized?
   (a) End colostomy: start by mobilizing embryologic fusion planes. The white line of Toldt, splenic flexure, and omentum can all be freed to gain necessary length.
      (i) Further length can be attained by selective vessel ligation.
         1. High ligation of the inferior mesenteric artery proximal to the takeoff of the left colic artery
         2. Ligation of inferior mesenteric vein at the inferior border of the pancreas
   (b) Ileostomy: the small bowel mesentery may be tethered to the retroperitoneum. Releasing the small bowel mesentery up

to the base of the duodenum could yield several more centimeters of reach.
   (i) Ligation of the ileocolic artery will increase mobility of the terminal ileal mesentery and typically does not cause ischemia.
4. Can the bowel pass through the abdominal wall without restricting blood supply or perfusion?
   (a) Consider using a lubricated wound protector within the aperture to facilitate passage.
   (b) The mesentery adjacent to the descending colon can be trimmed, so long as the marginal artery remains intact (typically found within 1 cm of the colon wall).
   (c) Although an oversized aperture predisposes to formation of parastomal hernia, this may be necessary to allow passage of the mesentery and to prevent venous congestion and subsequent ischemia of the stoma.
   (d) Several stoma maturation techniques have been developed for difficult situations (see below).

Operative Checklist

1. Additional helpful equipment
2. Penrose drain
3. Extra-small wound protector
4. Various devices to assess perfusion

Operative Techniques

1. Make the profile of the end of the colon smaller.
   (a) Remove epiploic appendages.
   (b) Trim the mesentery without devascularizing the colon.
   (c) If the colon is distended, decompress the colon by evacuating the content without spillage.
2. Make a bigger opening. Abdominal wall modification.
   (a) When a thick abdominal wall impedes blood supply to the stoma or limits reach, it may be necessary to adjust the aperture itself, knowing that this may contribute to parastomal hernia development in the future.
   (b) Remove a column of subcutaneous fat from the skin opening down to the fascia to facilitate passage and decrease extrinsic compression of the bowel (Fig. 48.2).
   (c) Widen the aperture in the peritoneum, fascia, and/or skin opening.

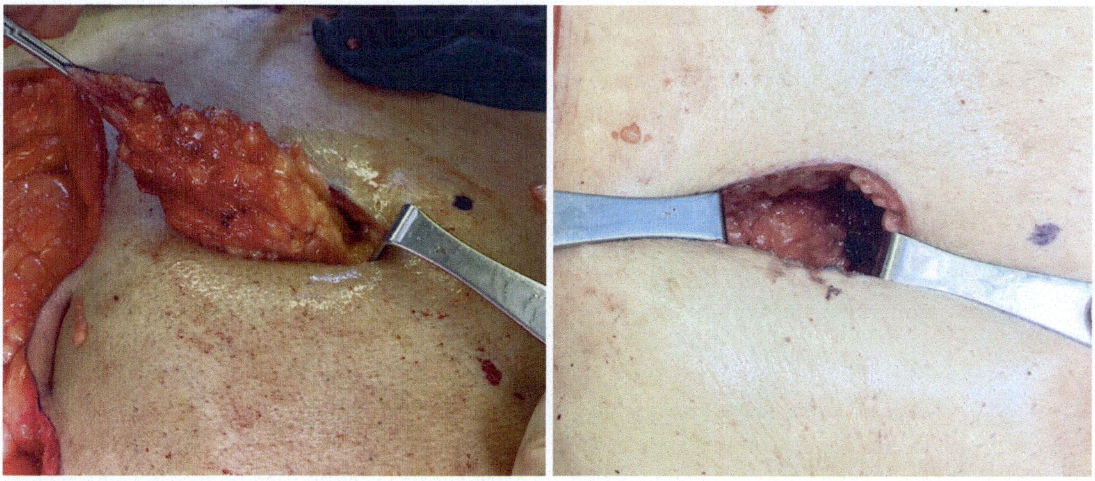

Fig. 48.2 Abdominal wall modification. Remove a column of subcutaneous fat from the skin opening down to the fascia to facilitate passage and decrease extrinsic compression of the bowel

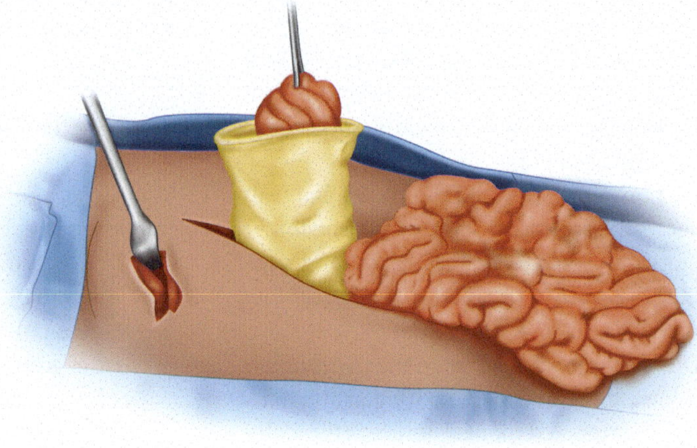

Fig. 48.3 Glove cuff technique: stuff the end of the colon through a 5 or 5 ½ size surgical glove cuff, and deliver the ensheathed colon through the abdominal aperture. Once delivered, cut away the glove

(d) Site the stoma above the umbilicus where, typically, less subcutaneous fat is present in obese patients.

3. Decrease the friction for easier exteriorization.
   (a) Penrose pass technique
      (i) Stuff the end of the colon through a 1 Penrose drain.
      (ii) Deliver the ensheathed colon through the abdominal aperture.
      (iii) Once delivered, cut away the Penrose drain.
   (b) Glove cuff technique (Fig. 48.3)
      (i) Similar technique as above.
      (ii) Instead of a Penrose drain, use a size 5 or 5 ½ glove cuff.
   (c) Wound protector technique (Fig. 48.4)
      (i) Small wound retractor is inserted through the aperture.
      (ii) Once the colon is passed, the inner ring is divided, and the plastic sheath is cut off and removed.
      (iii) There are several benefits to using a wound protector within the stoma aperture.
         1. The circumferential retraction of skin and subcutaneous tissues helps to ease passage of a bulky intestine and mesentery while minimizing trauma. Lubricating the inside of the retractor helps with this, as well.
         2. The wound protector compresses the skin, subcutaneous tissues, and fascia preventing stretching of the tunnel through which the intestine must pass and decreases friction and the force needed to pass the colon through a thick abdominal wall.
4. Loop-end stoma technique (Fig. 48.5).
   (a) This is a useful technique for the patient with a thickened, foreshortened mesentery which tethers the end of the conduit. Rather than unfurl the end of the bowel and potentially risk compromising its blood supply, bring up a more proximal portion of the bowel using a Penrose to help distribute the tension and mature this in the same fashion as a loop ileostomy.

Technical Pearls (Tips and Tricks)

1. Mesenteric "pie-crusting": score the peritoneum in 1 cm increments overlying the vascular arcade to the segment of bowel intended for stoma creation to gain an addition 2–3 cm

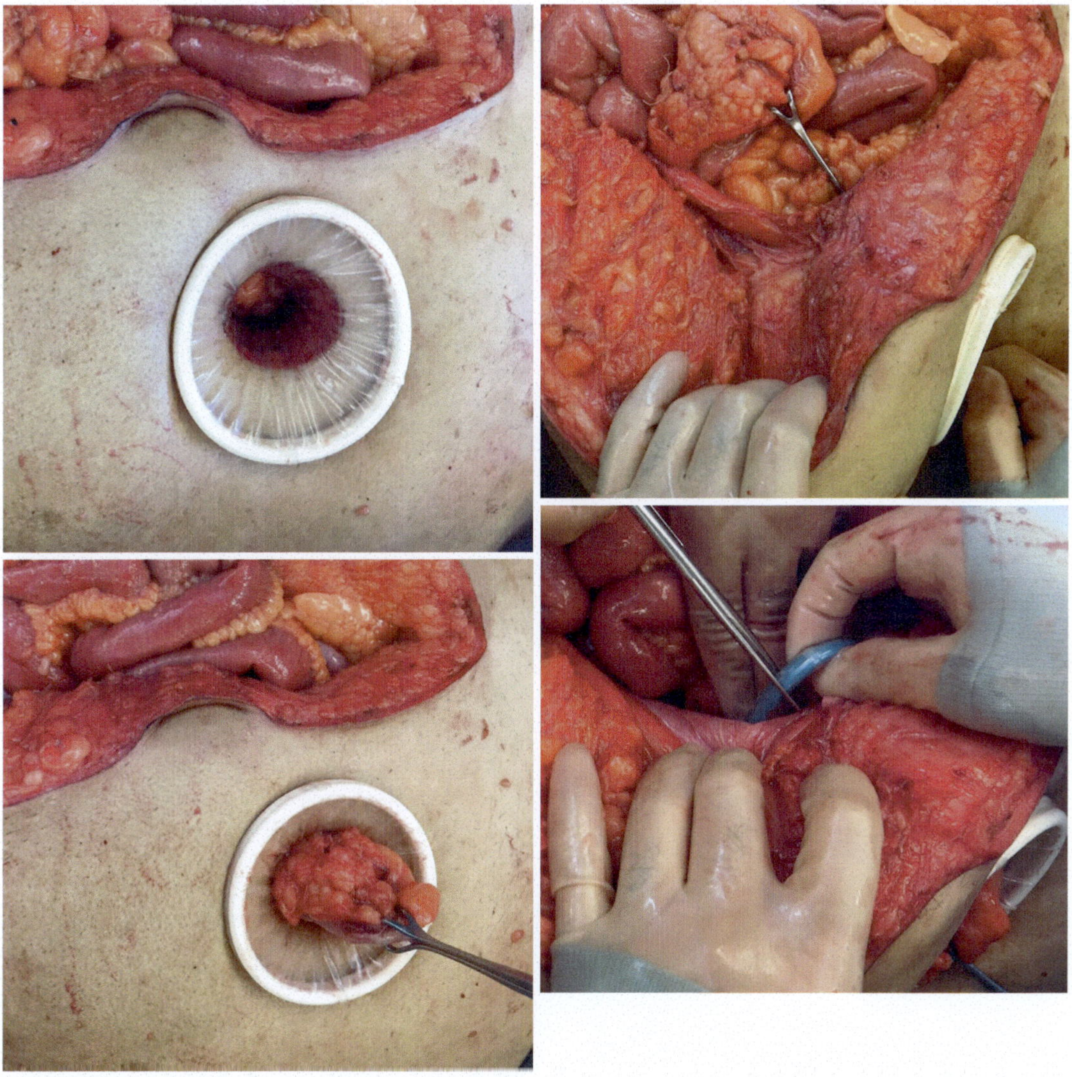

Fig. 48.4 Wound protector technique: a small Alexis wound retractor (**a**) is inserted through the aperture. Once the colon is passed (**b**, **c**), the inner ring is divided (**d**), and the plastic sheath is cut off and removed

of length. This often needs to be performed on both sides of the mesentery.

2. Push; don't pull! Aggressive traction on the cut end can tear the bowel and its mesentery as it moves through the abdominal wall. Gentle guidance of the bowel from within the abdomen is preferred.
3. Mature the stoma prior to closing the abdomen if any question remains about tension or viability.

Special Postoperative Care

1. A dedicated enterostomal therapy (EST) nurse helps tremendously with postoperative care, from patient education and emotional support to troubleshooting difficult stoma care situations. Continued follow-up with an EST can help patients learn to identify stoma care issues early on in their course.

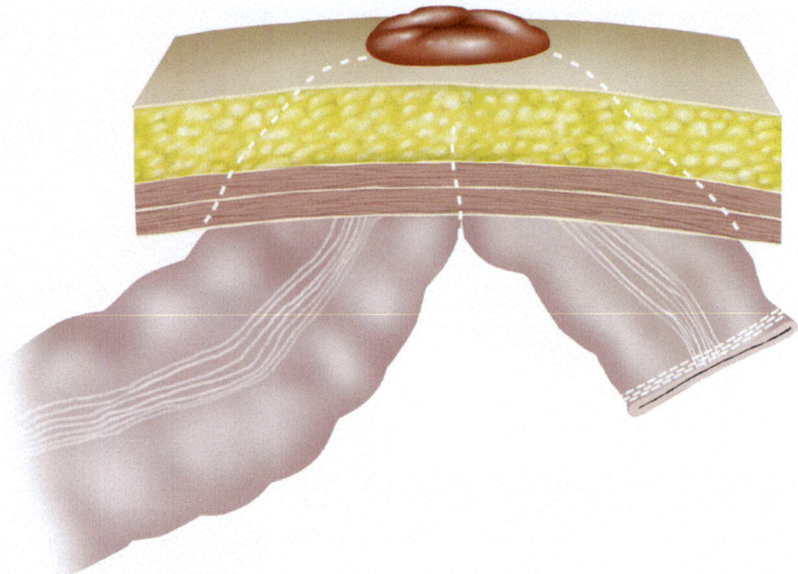

Fig. 48.5 Loop-end stoma technique: rather than unfurl the tip of the bowel and potentially risk compromising its blood supply, bring up a more proximal portion of the bowel using a Penrose underneath to help distribute the tension, and mature this in the same fashion as a loop ileostomy

Suggested Reading

1. Beck SJ. Stoma issues in the obese patient. Clin Colon Rectal Surg. 2011;24:259–62.
2. Chu DI, Dozoi EJ. Pearls for the small bowel and colon that will not reach. In: Pawlik TM, Maithel SK, Merchant NB, editors. Gastrointestinal surgery: management of complex perioperative complications. New York: Springer; 2015.
3. Mavroidis D, Kotun WA. Technique for atraumatic delivery of intestine through the abdominal wall during stoma formation. Dis Col Rect. 1996;39(4):461–2.
4. Meagher AP, Owen G, Gett R. An improved technique for end stoma creation in obese patients. Dis Colon Rectum. 2009;52:531–3.
5. Person B, Ifargan R, et al. The impact of preoperative stoma site marking on the incidence of complications, quality of life, and patient's independence. Dis Colon Rectum. 2012;55:783–7.
6. Whitehead A, Cataldo PA. Technical considerations in stoma creation. Clin Colon Rectal Surg. 2017;30(3):162–71.

Stoma Prolapse

49

Emily Steinhagen and Scott R. Steele

Clinical Scenario

A 70-year-old man who underwent abdomino-perineal resection 10 years ago for rectal cancer complains of a prolapsing stoma. The colon prolapses whenever he stands up, though it easily reduces when lying down. He has good stoma function; however, the exposed mucosa rubs against his appliance and is constantly irritated and bleeds a small amount.

Key Points

1. Stoma prolapse has an important impact on quality of life.
2. The majority of stoma prolapses are asymptomatic or minimally symptomatic. For these patients, working with enterostomal therapy nurse and changing to a different stoma appliance may be adequate.
3. The proposed mechanism for stoma prolapse is due to a mobile mesentery, increased intra-abdominal pressure, increasing size of the fascial defect, or a lack of fixation between the serosal surfaces of an everted stoma. Risk factors for stoma prolapse include increasing age, obesity, bowel obstruction at the time of stoma creation, and lack of preoperative site marking.
4. Loop stomas are more likely to prolapse compared to end stomas; typically and counterintuitively, the distal limb is involved (Fig. 49.1).
5. Preoperative stoma marking should be performed whenever possible.

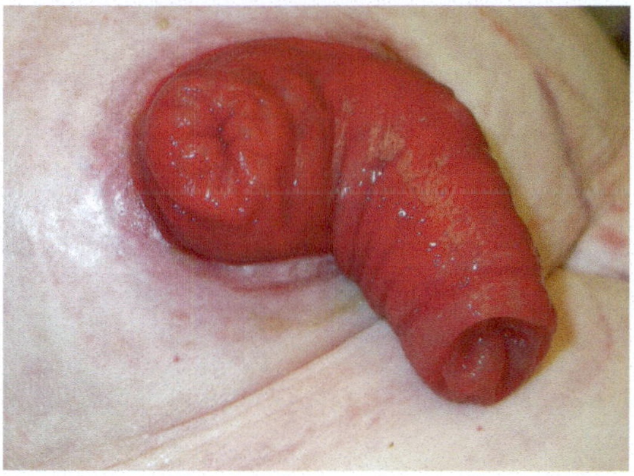

Fig. 49.1 Loop stomas are more likely to prolapse compared to end stomas; typically, the distal limb is involved

E. Steinhagen
University Hospitals Case Medical Center, Department of Surgery, Cleveland, OH, USA

S. R. Steele (✉)
Case Western Reserve University School of Medicine, Cleveland, OH, USA

Department of Colorectal Surgery, Cleveland Clinic, Cleveland, OH, USA

S. W. Lee et al. (eds.), *Colorectal Surgery Consultation*, https://doi.org/10.1007/978-3-030-11181-6_49

Operative Assessment

1. Stoma prolapse is categorized as fixed or sliding. A sliding prolapse can be easily reduced, and the patient will describe variation in the amount of prolapse. A fixed prolapse is unreducible.
2. How symptomatic is the prolapse? Mild symptoms can often be managed by reassuring the patient and changing the pouching system they use.
3. How much bowel is prolapsed? If the prolapse is excessive, particularly in the case of small bowel, a repair that requires resection may not be prudent.
4. Is the stoma a loop or an end stoma? This will often dictate surgical options.
5. Does the patient still require a stoma? The simplest approach is to reverse the stoma, when feasible.
6. Is there an associated parastomal hernia? This suggests that a local revision may not be the optimal approach.
7. Can the patient tolerate a laparotomy if necessary? Their fitness for surgery should affect operative planning as it is always prudent to have a backup plan in case of difficulty.

Operative Checklist

1. Ensure an understanding of the anatomy and the type of stoma, particularly if it was created by another surgeon.
2. Prepare the entire abdomen in case a local revision is unable to be performed.

Operative Approaches

1. End stoma
   (a) One technique for revising a prolapsing end colostomy is simple local revision. Detach the stoma at the mucocutaneous junction with electrocautery, and the redundant segment that is easily liberated is amputated, and the stoma is re-matured. Some practitioners perform seromyotomies to promote serosa-to-serosa fixation on the everted portion of the stoma to decrease the risk of recurrence (Fig. 49.2).

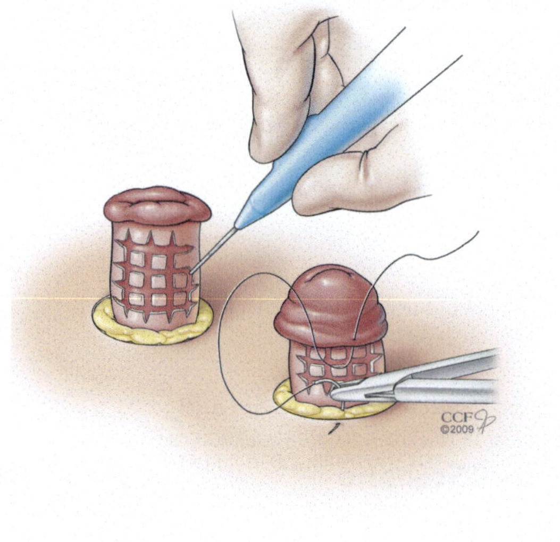

Fig. 49.2 Seromyotomies may promote serosa-to-serosa fixation on the everted portion of the stoma to decrease the risk of recurrence (Figure needs to be re-drawn). (With permission. © Cleveland Clinic)

   (b) In a long-standing stoma that has an easily reducible prolapse, incise a few centimeters proximal to the mucocutaneous junction [1]. The bowel is dissected and the redundant bowel is resected. The stoma is then re-matured by suturing it to the remaining mucocutaneous junction that had previously been matured. The mucocutaneous junction's blood supply comes from the surrounding skin (Fig. 49.3).
   (c) Intraperitoneal fixation may be an option in certain circumstances but requires either laparoscopy or laparotomy. With the prolapse reduced completely, the limb of bowel and/or mesentery leading up the prolapse is secured to the abdominal wall. When performed laparoscopically, two to three interrupted seromuscular stitches can be placed in the bowel wall, and a suture passer can be used to fix the bowel to the fascia. It is important to avoid full-thickness bites on the bowel, as this could predispose to fistula formation (Fig. 49.4).

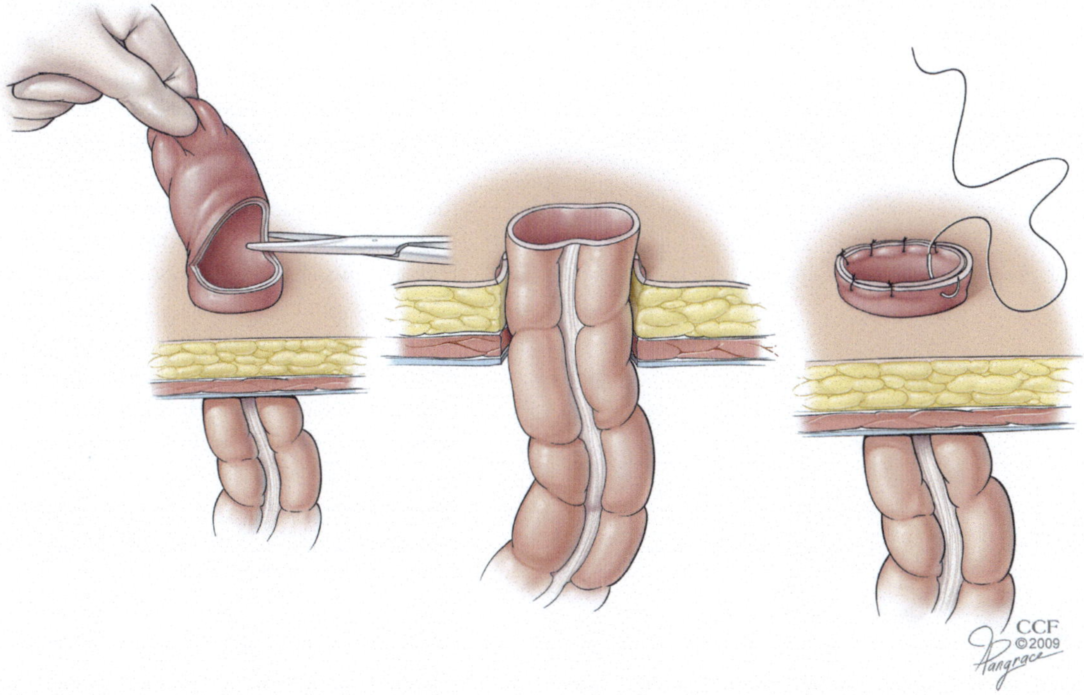

Fig. 49.3 Amputation repair. The prolapsed colon is transected and reanastomosed. (With permission. © Cleveland Clinic)

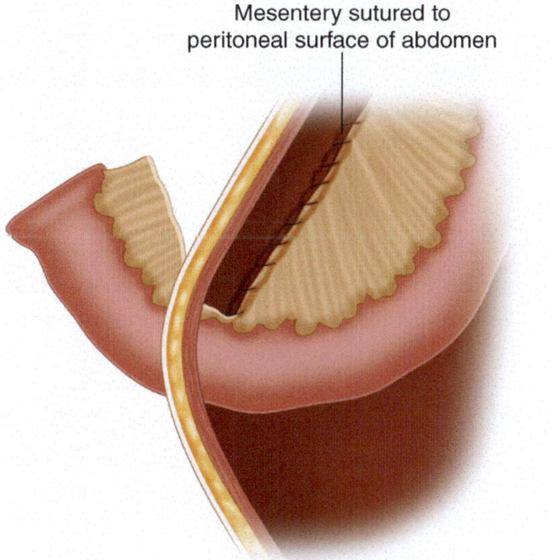

Fig. 49.4 Intraperitoneal fixation. The limb of bowel and/or mesentery leading up the prolapse can be secured to the abdominal wall

(d) Modified Delorme procedure: The mucosa is stripped from the prolapsed colon, and multiple interrupted plicating sutures are placed into the muscularis layer. The plicated colon is reduced, and mucosa-to-mucosa anastomosis is performed (Fig. 49.5).
(e) Strips of biologic mesh can be used to create seromuscular fixation to the fascia.
(f) A local revision with staplers may be possible [3]. With this technique, a GIA stapler is inserted into the lumen, and the prolapsed segment is divided. This is performed at two locations separated by 180 degrees on the prolapsing limb. This effectively bisects the prolapse. The mesentery is manually retracted to avoid ischemia. A third and fourth firing of the stapler then transects the prolapse 1 cm above the skin in a perpendicular fashion. This approach is simple and may be per-

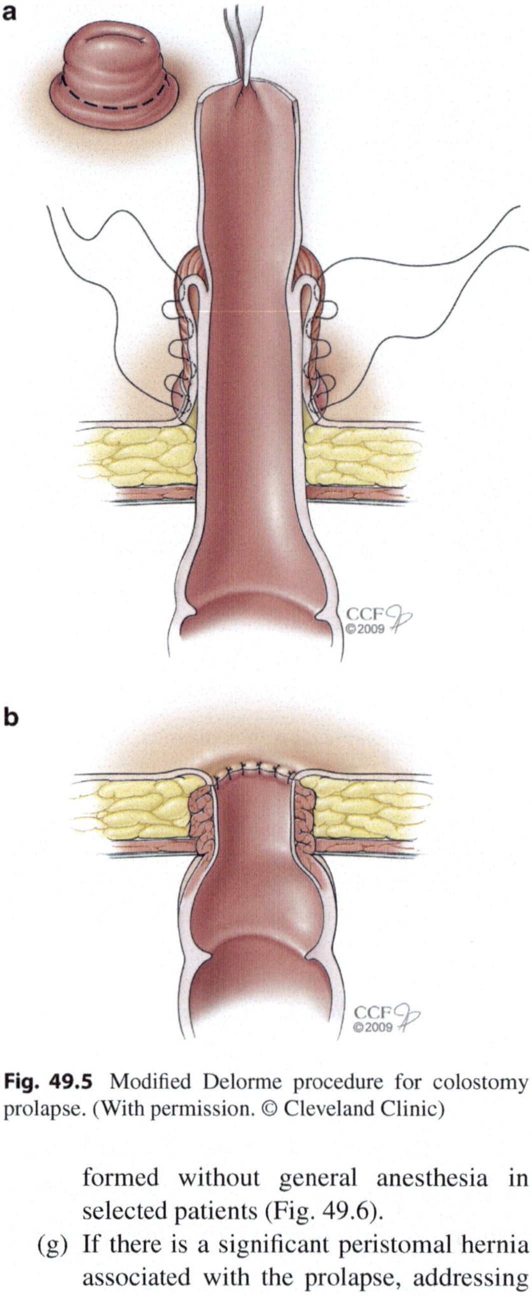

Fig. 49.5 Modified Delorme procedure for colostomy prolapse. (With permission. © Cleveland Clinic)

formed without general anesthesia in selected patients (Fig. 49.6).

(g) If there is a significant peristomal hernia associated with the prolapse, addressing the hernia takes precedence. The repair will often incorporate a solution for the stoma prolapse, but if it does not, an appropriate revision should also be performed.

2. Loop stoma
   (a) In a loop stoma that cannot be reversed, conversion to an end-loop (Prasad) stoma may address a prolapsed distal limb. The bowel can be divided and the distal end stapled. The stapled end is then placed below the fascia and back into the abdominal cavity or part of it opened at the level of the skin and matured as a mucus fistula. The proximal stoma is then re-secured to the skin. The size of the fascial opening may need to be reduced when this is performed (Fig. 49.7).
3. Incarcerated stoma
   (a) If the bowel is not necrotic, most presumably incarcerated stomas can be reduced with manual pressure. Holding the stoma with gauze to enable a firmer grip can be helpful, and the pressure should begin at the point most distal to the skin. The use of sugar to decrease edema has been successfully described, similar to the way rectal prolapse has been reduced. Anxiolytics and analgesics are also helpful in this situation.
   (b) If there is ischemia or gangrene, the stoma requires resection, and attempts at reduction should be avoided. In the presence of ischemic bowel, while it may be possible to perform a local revision, laparotomy may be required. Complete relocation may be appropriate depending on the circumstance.
4. Pseudoprolapse
   (a) Short-segment "pseudoprolapse" may occur during pregnancy. This is typically related to increased intra-abdominal pressure and changes in the position of abdominal organs due to the gravid uterus. It is a self-limited process, and the prolapse itself is usually relatively short in length. This process typically resolves after the pregnancy, and therefore surgical intervention should be avoided.

Technical Pearls (Tips and Tricks)

1. The size of the opening in the fascia and skin should allow the bowel to pass through without being unduly tight, but care should be taken to avoid making a very large opening.

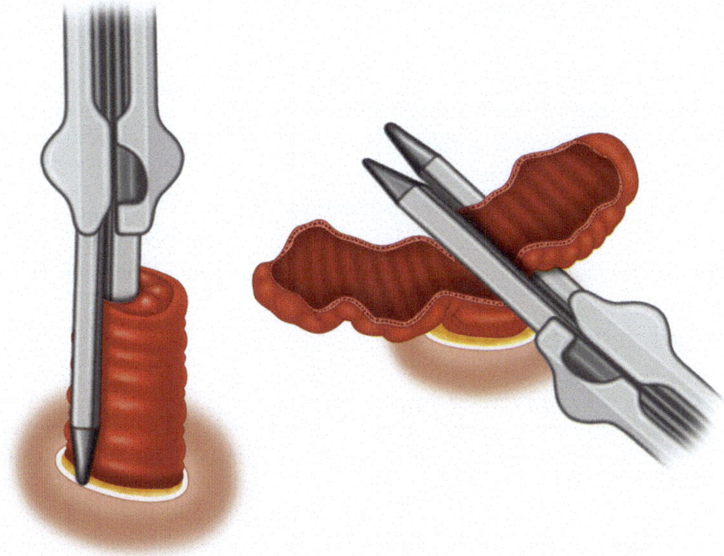

Fig. 49.6 GIA stapler technique. GIA stapler is inserted into the lumen and the prolapsed segment is divided. This is performed at two locations separated by 180 degrees on the prolapsing limb. This effectively bisects the prolapse. A third and fourth firing of the stapler then transects the prolapse 1 cm above the skin in a perpendicular fashion

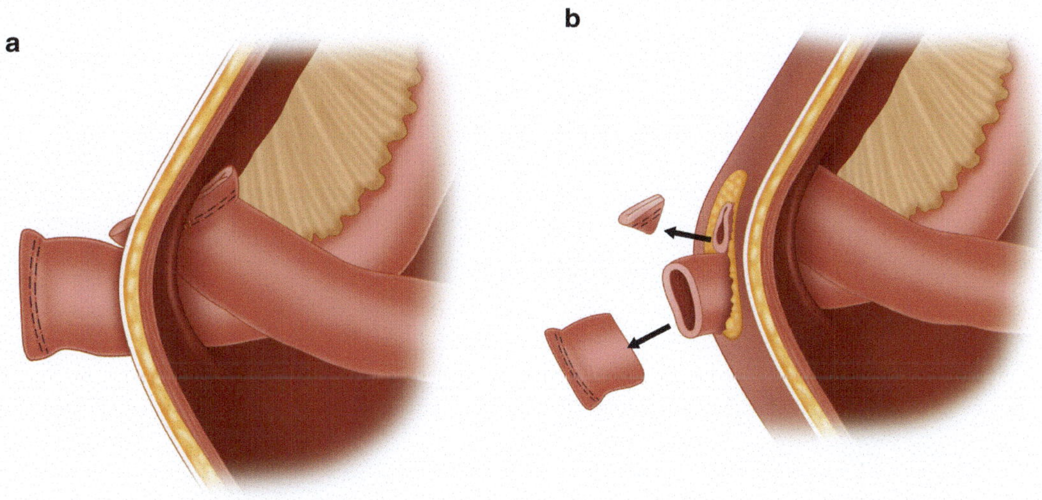

Fig. 49.7 Conversion to an end-loop (Prasad) stoma may address a prolapsed distal limb. The bowel can be divided and the distal end stapled. The proximal stoma is then re-secured to the skin. The size of the fascial opening may need to be reduced when this is performed

This may be more difficult when the bowel is distended.

2. Ideally, prolapse in a temporary stoma should be managed expectantly until the stoma can be closed.
3. In cases requiring operation, the type of revision should be tailored to the patient and the stoma.
4. In many cases, local revision can be performed.

Special Postoperative Care

1. Following revision, a diet may typically be resumed immediately (unless presenting with a bowel obstruction or ileus).
2. Perioperative antibiotics do not need to be extended before the perioperative dose.

Suggested Reading

1. Corman ML. Intestinal stomas. In: Corman ML, editor. Corman's colon and rectal surgery. 6th ed. Philadelphia: Lippincott, Williams, and Wilkins; 2013. p. 1396–451.
2. Fligelstone LJ, Wanendeya N, Palmer BV. Osmotic therapy for acute irreducible stoma prolapse. Br J Surg. 1997;84(3):390.
3. Hata F, Kitagawa S, Nishimori H, et al. A novel, easy, and safe technique to repair a stoma prolapse using a surgical stapling device. Dig Surg. 2005;22(5):306–9.
4. Leong AP, Londono-Schimmer EE, Phillips RK. Life-table analysis of stomal complications following ileostomy. Br J Surg. 1994;81(5):727–9.
5. Londono-Schimmer EE, Leong AP, Phillips RK. Life table analysis of stomal complications following colostomy. Dis Colon Rectum. 1994;37(9):916–20.
6. Park JJ, Del Pino A, Orsay CP, et al. Stoma complications: the Cook County Hospital experience. Dis Colon Rectum. 1999;42(12):1575–80.
7. Schiergens TS, Hoffmann V, Schobel TN, et al. Long-term quality of life of patients with permanent end ileostomy: results of a nationwide cross-sectional survey. Dis Colon Rectum. 2017;60(1):51–60.

Ileostomy Retracts Below the Skin

50

Titilayo Adegboyega and David E. Rivadeneira

Clinical Scenario

A 63-year-old female, body mass index (BMI) 55 kg/m^2, undergoes a sigmoidectomy, repair of colovaginal fistula, and drainage of pelvic abscess. A stapled colorectal anastomosis is created with positive leak test noted. The anastomosis is redone and with negative leak test. A diverting ileostomy is performed. Five days later, the ostomy nurse reports cellulitis around the ileostomy with mucocutaneous separation and retraction of the ileostomy.

Key Points

1. Ileostomies can retract in the early postoperative period.
   (a) Various steps can be taken to decrease potential ileostomy complications.
   (b) Preoperative ostomy marking, adequate mobilization of bowel intraoperatively to avoid tension, and appropriate postoperative ostomy care are important.
2. Local revision can usually be performed if healthy mucosa is seen above the fascia.
3. Abdominal approach for ostomy revision may be necessary to mobilize more bowel.

Operative Assessment

1. A good bedside exam with the entire appliance removed is usually sufficient to evaluate the ileostomy.
2. The degree of retraction should be determined and may vary from mucocutaneous separation to retraction of the stoma below the skin level to, in rare cases, retraction to or below the fascia.
3. Retraction of ileostomy is often an early complication, occurring within a month of creation, although later occurrences have been reported.
4. It is important to consider other complications associated with retraction such as soft tissue infection, intra-abdominal contamination, ischemia, or stenosis.
5. The mucosa of the retracted ileostomy should be evaluated to ensure healthy mucosa of the bowel within the subcutaneous tissue all the way to the level of the fascia. This was classically done using a test tube but now typically utilizes a blood collection tube.

T. Adegboyega
Huntington Hospital-Northwell Health, Department of Colorectal Surgery, Huntington, NY, USA

D. E. Rivadeneira (✉)
Surgical Strategic Initiatives, Northwell Health, New Hyde Park, NY, USA

Surgical Services and Colorectal Surgery, Huntington Hospital, Huntington, NY, USA

Hofstra University-Northwell School of Medicine, Hempstead, NY, USA
e-mail: DRivadeneira@northwell.edu

S. W. Lee et al. (eds.), *Colorectal Surgery Consultation*,
https://doi.org/10.1007/978-3-030-11181-6_50

Operative Checklist

1. Instruments and equipment
   (a) A basic abdominal tray is often sufficient for ostomy creation or revision.
   (b) In obese patients with thick abdominal wall, deep retractors should be available.
   (c) Adequate lighting is key and a headlight may be useful for revision.
2. Preoperative preparation
   (a) Stoma sites should be marked in cases where an ostomy is planned. This is particularly important in obese patients or those with multiple prior surgeries or scars on the abdominal wall.
   (b) In the case of ileostomy retraction and soft tissue infection, defining the degree on infection is essential. CT scan may be helpful to rule out intra-abdominal infection or abscess prior to proceeding with local revision.
   (c) Assess the viability of the retracted stoma either by bedside exam or endoscopy.

Operative Techniques

1. Initial ostomy creation.
   (a) Preventing retraction of any ostomy begins with adequate planning and application of basic surgical principles at the creation of the stoma. Preoperative teaching and marking are important components.
   (b) Although tension from a tethered mesentery is not a common problem for small bowel, in patients with inflammatory process such as Crohn's disease or peritonitis, the mesentery may be thickened and foreshortened, thereby restricting the mobility and reach of the small bowel.
   (c) The mesentery can be scored, releasing the peritoneum and lengthening the mesentery. Ideally, the most distal portion of the ileum should be used for the ileostomy.
   (d) When creating a loop ileostomy, a bridge or stoma bar can be used to support the stoma and prevent retraction.
   (e) The ileostomy should be created in a Brooke fashion, which elevates the bowel from skin level and reduces irritation of the skin.
2. If retraction of ileostomy occurs:
   (a) Most cases of retracted ileostomy are mild and can be managed effectively with stoma care utilizing approaches like convexity pouching, etc.
   (b) Prevent further complications by maximizing stoma care to prevent stool leaking into the subcutaneous tissue or onto the skin.
   (c) If revision is required, the major questions are whether it can be done locally through the stoma site or is laparotomy needed and can the stoma be reversed rather than revised at this time.
   (d) If the retraction is minimal and the ileostomy is without ischemia, local mobilization of the bowel and re-maturation in Brooke fashion can be done.
   (e) In the presence of significant retraction, local wound infection, ischemia, or significant tension, an abdominal approach is preferable.
   (f) Mobilization of the small bowel with lysis of adhesions may be needed to avoid tension at the recreated ileostomy. In addition, sacrificing some mesentery and relying on the arterial arcade to survive the stoma is usually required. Transilluminating the mesentery can be particularly helpful in this situation.
   (g) A more proximal segment of bowel may have better reach and can be used, if needed.
   (h) In situations where an end ileostomy is still under tension, a "loop-end" ileostomy can be created.
3. Obese patients are at risk for retracted stomas given the amount of subcutaneous tissue that needs to be traversed.
   (a) Coring out the subcutaneous tissue at the site of the ileostomy is helpful.
   (b) The abdominal wall tends to be thicker below the umbilicus. Siting the stoma more cephalad can permit better reach.
   (c) Creating a neoabdominal wall in morbidly obese patients has been described to decrease the thickness of the abdominal wall. This is done by excising a rectangular segment of fat at the ileostomy site and approximating the skin at the stoma site to the fascia, thereby compressing the depth of abdominal wall (Fig. 50.1a–e).

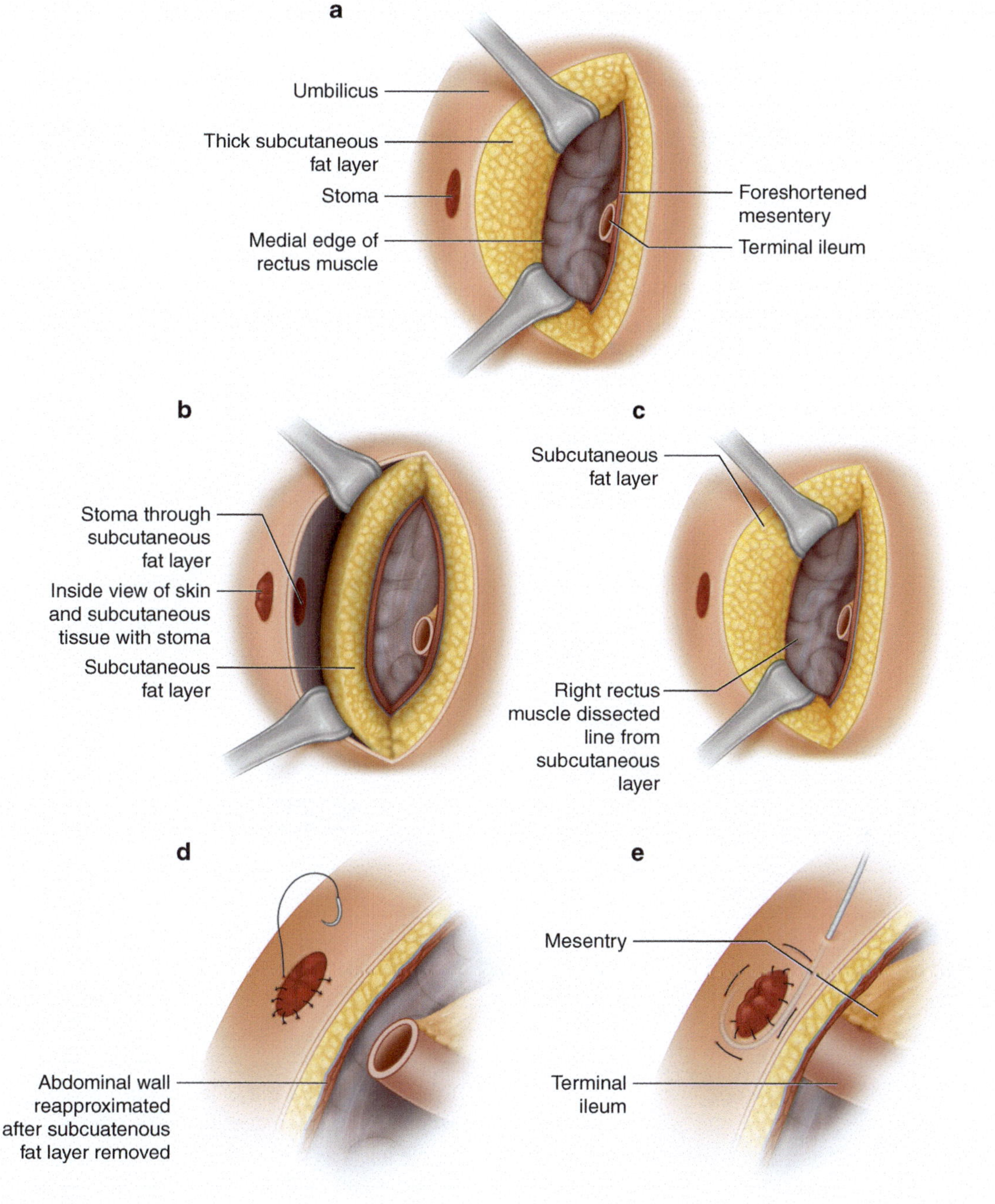

Fig. 50.1 (**a**–**e**) Creating a neoabdominal wall in morbidly obese patients. (**a**) Creation of a stoma below the level of the umbilicus. (**b**) The skin is retracted upward and the subcutaneous fat is fileted around the stoma. (**c**) The subcutaneous tissue is fileted above the fascia and a rectangular segment of fat is removed. (**d**) The skin is sutured to the fascial opening using an absorbable 2–0 chromic suture. (**e**) Four-O nylon sutures are placed to attach the skin to the underlying fascia. A closed sump drain helps to obliterate the dead space

Technical Pearls (Tips and Tricks)

1. Preoperative stoma marking is important.
2. Use the appropriate segment of bowel to ensure a tension-free ostomy is created.
3. The mesentery can be scored and dissected to increase reach, as needed.
4. A more cephalad ostomy location may be necessary to avoid retraction.
5. A loop-end ileostomy is an option when tension is still an issue.
6. Early recognition of ostomy complications and meticulous wound care are key to preventing further complications and skin breakdown. Most retracted stomas can be managed nonoperatively with stoma care.

Special Postoperative Care

1. Stoma care to address leaks and skin complications is important.
2. Antibiotics may be needed if there is soft tissue infection or intra-abdominal contamination.

Suggested Reading

1. Meguid MM, McIvor A, Xenos L. Creation of a neo-abdominal wall to facilitate emergency placement of a terminal ileostomy in a morbidly obese patient. Am J Surg. 1997;170:298–300.

Part VI

Technical Tips and Tricks for Difficult Anorectal Cases

Difficulties with the Stapled Hemorrhoidectomy Procedure

51

Sang W. Lee

Clinical Scenario

A 60-year-old male undergoing a stapled hemorrhoidectomy for symptomatic grade III internal hemorrhoids is found to have a recessed anus. Despite every attempt to fully engage the suture port, the dentate line and anoderm are visible through the fenestrated channel of the port.

Key Points

1. Inadequate protection of the anal canal with the retractor can lead to excision too close to the dentate line and significant morbidity.
2. Placement of the staple line too proximal to the hemorrhoidal apex can lead to inadequate resection and increased risk of recurrence.
3. Gaps between purse-string suture bites result in incomplete resection and greater risk of recurrence.
4. It is critical to ensure that the suture port is fully inserted and covers the dentate line and anoderm. Under no circumstances should the stapler be fired when the anoderm is not protected.

S. W. Lee (✉)
Department of Surgery – Colon and Rectal Surgery, Keck School of Medicine of University of Southern California, Los Angeles, CA, USA

Operative Assessment

1. It is critical to ensure that the suture port is fully inserted and covers the dentate line and anoderm. Under no circumstances should the stapler be fired when the anoderm is not protected.
2. It is important not to leave gaps between the bites when placing purse-string sutures. After the purse-string suture is cinched around the post of the anvil, the purse-string should be inspected to ensure that there is no gap.
3. Purse-string suture should be placed 1–2 cm above the hemorrhoid apex and 3–4 cm above the dentate line. Utilize the graduated markings on the anoscope to maintain a consistent level while suturing.
4. The final verification of the staple line distance from the anal verge can be accomplished by inspecting the marking on the outside of the stapler. The marking at the anal verge should read between 3 and 4 cm. If the marking is less than 2 cm, the level of the staple line is probably too close to the dentate line, and the purse-string suture may need to be replaced.
5. Vaginal examination, once the stapler is closed and prior to firing, is essential. Gently rocking the stapler should move independent of the vaginal tissues. Aiming the stapler posteriorly when closing the stapler mechanism can help avoid catching the vagina.

S. W. Lee et al. (eds.), *Colorectal Surgery Consultation*,
https://doi.org/10.1007/978-3-030-11181-6_51

Operative Checklist

1. The following should be included in the operative documentation:
   (a) Specific indication
   (b) Distance of purse-string suture placement with respect to the top of the hemorrhoid pedicles and dentate line
   (c) Mucosal and submucosal placement of the purse-string suture
   (d) Vaginal examination prior to firing of the stapler
   (e) Macroscopic appearance of resected specimen (was the excised tissue ring complete?)
   (f) Details of the staple line and its location relative to dentate line (was the staple line circumferential?)
   (g) Hemostasis

Operative Techniques

1. Detailed steps and techniques of staple hemorrhoidectomy are described elsewhere.

Technical Pearls (Tips and Tricks)

1. Dentate line and anoderm are visible through the channel of the port.
   (a) Milking out the anodermal skin by applying countertraction to ensure full insertion can be helpful. Withdraw the obturator. Confirm, with direct visualization, that the anal port completely covers and protects the dentate line and sphincters. The anoderm must not be visible through the channel of the anal port.
   (b) In patients with recessed anus, it may be difficult to fully place the anal port and to completely retract the anoderm out of the surgical field. In this case, four interrupted effacing sutures can be placed between the skin at the anal verge and anal margin several centimeters away from the anus. This will allow the anoderm to be everted out and away from the field (Fig. 51.1).
2. Purse-string placement.
   (a) Place the submucosal purse-string suture 1–2 cm above the hemorrhoid apex and 3–4 cm above the dentate line. Take care

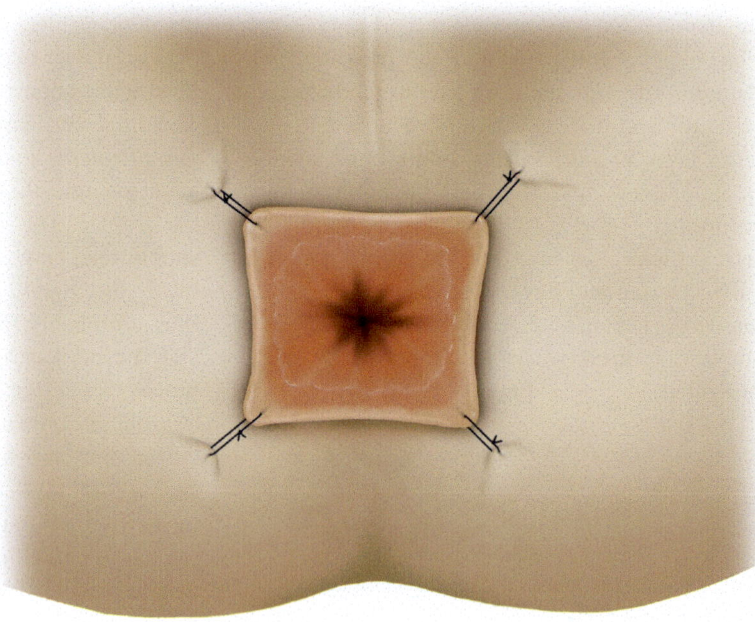

Fig. 51.1 In patients with a recessed anus, four interrupted effacing sutures can be placed between the skin at the anal verge and anal margin several centimeters away from the anus. This will allow the anoderm to be everted out and away from the field

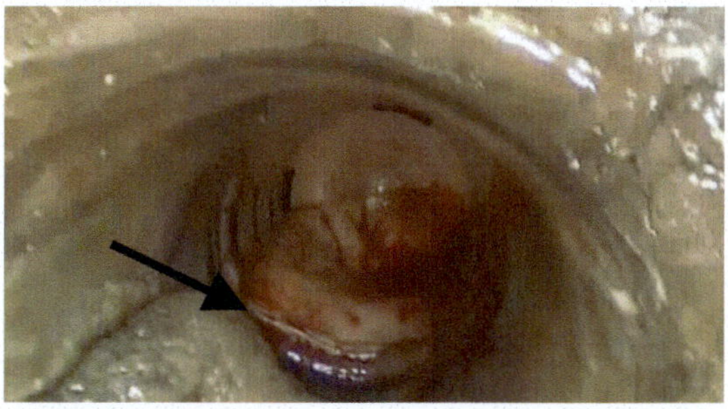

Fig. 51.2 Inspection of the staple line through the anoscope for hemostasis

to avoid incorporating deeper muscle layers. It is important not to leave gaps by starting each bite near the exit point of the previous bite.

3. Inspection for hemostasis.
   (a) Once the stapler is fired and removed, replace the anoscope without the surgical port and carefully inspect the staple for bleeding. Control staple line bleeding with 3-O absorbable sutures in a figure of eight fashion and avoid using electrocautery, when possible. The disposable anoscope has a large diameter that can tamponade bleeding; it is helpful to reexamine the anatomy with a small caliber anoscope to confirm hemostasis (Fig. 51.2).

Special Postoperative Care

1. Stapled hemorrhoidectomy is routinely performed as an outpatient surgery, though short stay hospitalization for observation as determined by the surgeon's discretion may be appropriate. The patient may resume their regular diet when recovered from anesthesia. Instruct the patient to maintain soft, bulked stools using fiber and stool softeners, as needed. Provide instructions for sitz baths several times a day, including after each bowel movement.

Suggested Reading

1. Nisar PJ, Acheson AG, Neal KR, Scholefield JH. Stapled hemorrhoidopexy compared with conventional hemorrhoidectomy, a systematic review of randomized controlled trials. Dis Colon Rectum. 2004;47:1837–45.
2. Pescatori M, Gagliardi G. Postoperative complications after procedure for prolapsed hemorrhoids (PPH) and stapled transanal rectal resection (STARR) procedures. Tech Coloproctol. 2008;12(1):7–19.
3. Rivadeneira DE, Steele SR, Ternent C, et al. Practice parameters for the management of hemorrhoids (revised 2010). Dis Colon Rectum. 2011;54:1059–64.
4. Tjandra JJ, Chan MK. Systematic review on the procedure for prolapse and hemorrhoids (stapled hemorrhoidopexy). Dis Colon Rectum. 2007;50:878–92.

Symptomatic Long Residual Rectal Cuff Status Post J-Pouch

52

Anuradha R. Bhama and Scott R. Steele

Clinical Scenario

A 32-year-old female underwent restorative proctocolectomy for ulcerative colitis 3 years ago and has developed severe diarrhea and urgency and bleeding from the rectum. Examination under anesthesia reveals a 5 cm strip of inflamed tissue between the dentate line and the stapled ileal pouch anal anastomosis (IPAA) (Fig. 52.1).

Key Points

1. In creating a J-pouch, the rectal cuff should ideally be <2 cm long (Fig. 52.2).
2. Medical management with topical steroids or 5-aminosalicylates is often effective for treatment of routine cuffitis.
3. Cuffitis may require mucosal stripping.
4. Patients with a long rectal cuff may experience severe diarrhea.
5. It is necessary to know several techniques to address a symptomatic, long rectal cuff.

A. R. Bhama
Department of Colorectal Surgery, Cleveland Clinic, Cleveland, OH, USA

S. R. Steele (✉)
Case Western Reserve University School of Medicine, Cleveland, OH, USA

Department of Colorectal Surgery, Cleveland Clinic, Cleveland, OH, USA

S. W. Lee et al. (eds.), *Colorectal Surgery Consultation*,
https://doi.org/10.1007/978-3-030-11181-6_52

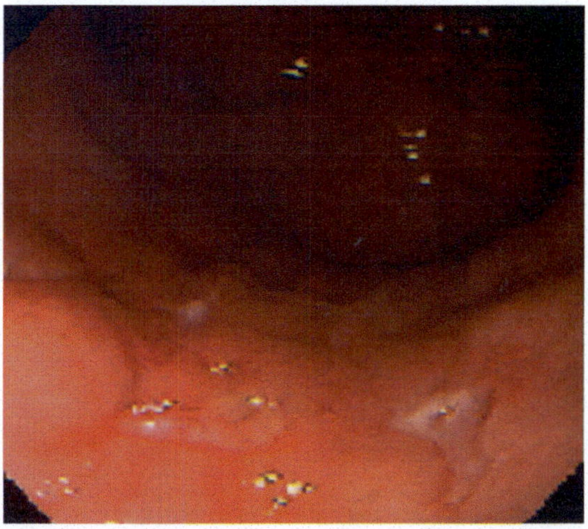

Fig. 52.1 Cuffitis

Operative Assessment

1. Has malignancy been ruled out?
   (a) Patient should undergo pouchoscopy with biopsies.
   (b) If neoplasia is identified, appropriate staging and oncologic resection are necessary.
2. Are there associated signs of Crohn's disease?
   (a) Perianal Crohn's – skin tags, fissures, fistulas.
   (b) Small bowel Crohn's.
   (c) Patients should be considered for pouch excision if extensive Crohn's disease is present.

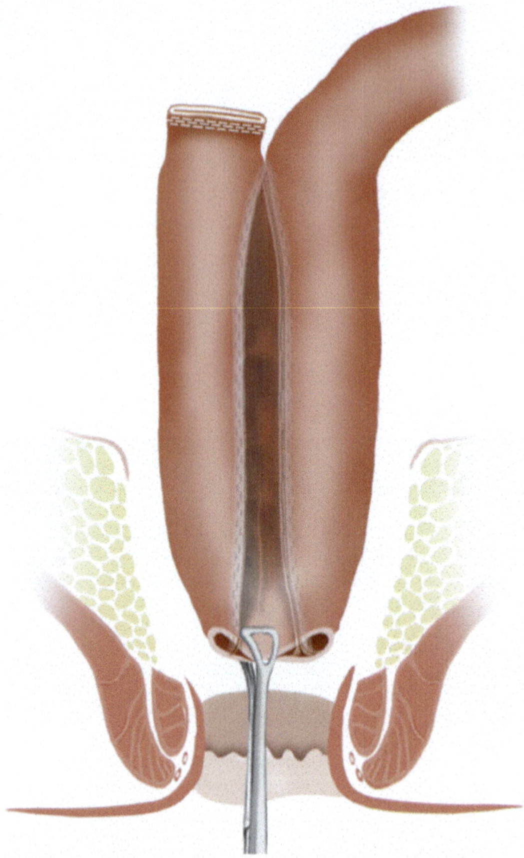

Fig. 52.2 Ideal anatomy of J-pouch rectal cuff

3. Does the patient require diversion?
4. Consider preoperative anal manometry to establish baseline sphincter function.

Operative Checklist

1. Additional helpful equipment
   (a) Surgical PPH (procedure for prolapse and hemorrhoids) stapler
      (i) Commercially available stapler kit
      (ii) 0 prolene suture
   (b) Mucosectomy/pouch advancement
      (i) Lonestar retractor
      (ii) Skin everting sutures
      (iii) Needle-tip bovie
      (iv) One percent lidocaine with epinephrine and spinal needle for submucosal injection
   (c) Redo pouch
      (i) Abdominal retractors
      (ii) Appropriate staplers to recreate J-pouch (100 mm blue load GIA)
2. Exposure
   (a) If performing PPH, mucosectomy, or pouch advancement from a perineal approach, it is necessary to have adequate visualization of the anal canal; use skin everting sutures (0 Vicryl sutures placed near the anal verge and anchored to the lateral skin of the buttocks), a Lonestar retractor, or lighted long right angle retractors or Hill-Ferguson retractors. A headlight may also help with visualization in the anal canal (see Chap. 51 for further details).
   (b) If performing transabdominal redo pouch, it is important to ensure visualization and lighting of the pelvis. A fixed retractor, lighted handheld retractors, or headlight can be helpful.
3. Positioning
   (a) For perineal procedures, lithotomy position.
   (b) For transabdominal procedures, the patient should be placed in modified lithotomy position with pressure points protected appropriately.

Operative Techniques

1. Mucosectomy using PPH stapler
   (a) The PPH stapler kit includes a 33 mm circular stapler, a circular anal dilator and obturator, and a clear purse-string suture anoscope. First perform a digital rectal exam with a lubricated finger and then introduce the anoscope and obturator to dilate the anal canal. Using the clear purse-string anoscope, a purse-string

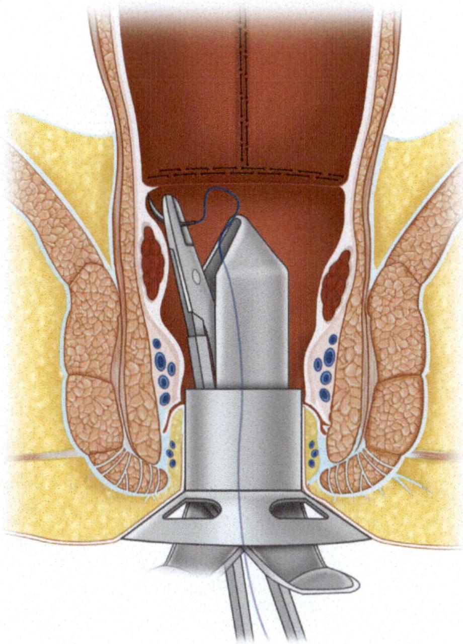

Fig. 52.3 PPH stapler

suture should be placed circumferentially at an appropriate height based on the specific anatomy. The anvil is inserted past the purse-string, which is then tied down around the anvil, and the stapler is closed and then fired. Per usual, confirm the vagina is free prior to firing the device (Fig. 52.3).

(i) The key here is removing the mucosa and submucosa only; therefore, the purse-string is the most important step. Only secure the mucosa and submucosa in order to avoid deeper resection for fear of having two staple lines next to each other and creating an area of ischemia.

2. Mucosal stripping
   (a) A Hill-Ferguson retractor can be utilized for optimal visualization. A submucosal injection of local anesthetic with epinephrine is used to promote hemostasis and to lift the mucosa off of the underlying bowel wall. The mucosa is excised using electrocautery, with care taken not to damage the underlying muscle. Dissection is carried cephalad up to the pouch, where the mucosa is transected. If necessary, the pouch may be advanced (see below) (Fig. 52.4).
3. Pouch advancement
   (a) Start by obtaining adequate visualization of the anal canal. Incise at the dentate line and extend dissection cephalad past the IPAA. Excise any remnant rectum and trim the distal edge of the pouch. Allis clamps can be placed on the distal pouch to assist in handling the pouch and ensuring that the anastomosis can be completed without tension. Advance the pouch distally and suture to the dentate line with 2-0 polyglycolic acid suture in four quadrants. The anastomosis is completed using 3-0 polyglycolic acid sutures (Fig. 52.3).
      (i) Understand that the pouch may not always be able to be advanced from below, and you should be prepared to mobilize from above and below.
4. Redo pouch
   (a) This should be approached transabdominally. Fully mobilize the pouch past the anastomosis down to the top of the anal canal. This mobilization should include the residual rectum down to the top of the anal canal. Transect distally leaving behind less than 2 cm of rectum.

Technical Pearls (Tips and Tricks)

1. For PPH – placement of the purse-string suture is the critical step of this procedure. Taking deep bites of tissue can cause rectal perforation posteriorly and rectovaginal fistula anteriorly. Ensure the suture contains only partial thickness rectal wall. Under these

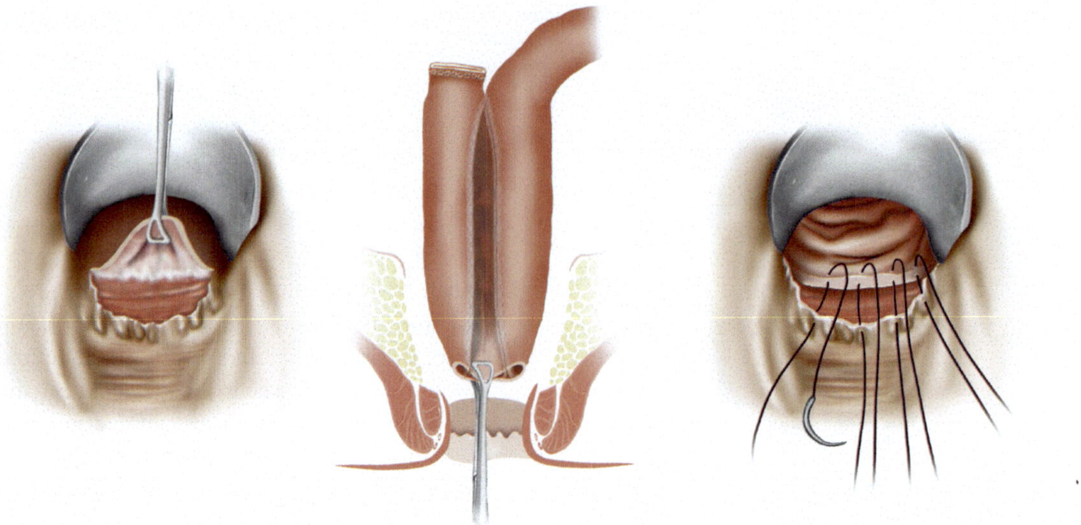

Fig. 52.4 Mucosectomy/pouch advancement. Incise at the dentate line and extend dissection cephalad past the ileal pouch anastomosis. Excise any remnant rectum and trim the distal edge of the pouch. Advance the pouch distally and suture to the dentate line with 2-0 polyglycolic acid suture in four quadrants. The anastomosis is completed using 3-0 polyglycolic acid suture

circumstances, the suture should be placed about 2 cm proximal to the dentate line.
2. For mucosectomy – epinephrine should be diluted at 1:100,000 concentration.
3. For pouch advancement – make incision at the dentate line and dissect cephalad using scissors; dissect out the ileal pouch using a combination of blunt and sharp dissection; resect the distal pouch for a fresh distal edge of the pouch; perform a hand-sewn ileoanal anastomosis at the dentate line. This operation frequently requires diverting loop ileostomy.
4. A redo pouch is a major undertaking and requires diverting loop ileostomy and consideration for ureteral stenting.

Special Postoperative Care

1. Pouch advancement/redo pouch – prior to loop ileostomy reversal, obtain gastrografin enema to ensure integrity of the pouch and patency of the anastomosis. Digital rectal exam should be performed prior to loop ileostomy reversal to ensure patency of the anastomosis. Consider anal manometry prior to loop ileostomy takedown to ensure sphincter function is adequate. After loop ileostomy takedown, follow up patients with pouchoscopy at recommended intervals.

Suggested Reading

1. Fazio VW, Tjandra JJ. Transanal Mucosectomy – ileal pouch advancement for anorectal dysplasia or inflammation after restorative proctocolectomy. Dis Colon Rectum. 1994;37(10):1008–11.
2. Litzendorf ME, et al. Completion mucosectomy for retained rectal mucosa following restorative proctocolectomy with double-stapled Ileal pouch-anal anastomosis. J Gastrointest Surg. 2010;14(3):562–9.
3. Ramirez RL, Fleshner P. Reoperative inflammatory bowel disease surgery. Clin Colon Rectal Surg. 2006;19(4):195–206.

Difficult Anterior Perineal Dissection During Abdominoperineal Resection

53

Sang W. Lee

Clinical Scenario

A 60-year-old male is undergoing an abdominoperineal resection (APR) for rectal cancer invading the anal sphincter complex. After completing the abdominal portion of the surgery, the perineal dissection was started. The posterior and lateral perineal dissection was completed, but the anterior dissection is very difficult because the plane is not well defined.

Key Points

1. Perform the anterior dissection last.
2. Palpate the Foley catheter to determine the location of the urethra and avoid injury.
3. In women, digitalization of the vaginal cavity can help define the dissection plane.
4. Apply posterior traction on the rectum to help dissect the anterior plane.
5. If possible, draw an imaginary line to the promontory of the sacrum and dissect along the line.
6. Review the rectal cancer protocol pelvic MRI to appreciate the location of the cancer in relation to the anterior plane and anticipate how you will address vaginal or urologic involvement.

S. W. Lee (✉)
Department of Surgery – Colon and Rectal Surgery, Keck School of Medicine of University of Southern California, Los Angeles, CA, USA

S. W. Lee et al. (eds.), *Colorectal Surgery Consultation*, https://doi.org/10.1007/978-3-030-11181-6_53

Operative Assessment

1. It is important to perform as much of the anterior dissection from the abdominal approach as possible before starting the perineal dissection. Ascertain if it is possible to perform more of the dissection from above.
2. Repeatedly palpating the Foley catheter can help determine the location of the urethra and define the correct plane.
3. Better define the rectovaginal plane by digital palpation through the vagina.
4. Keep in mind that the dissection plane is angled posteriorly. Draw an imaginary line to the sacral promontory and dissect along that direction.
5. Provide adequate posterior tension on the rectum.
6. By dividing the transverse perineal and rectourethralis muscles anteriorly, the posterior wall of the prostate may be better delineated.

Operative Checklist

1. Additional equipment
   (a) Pelvic tray including lighted pelvic retractors and self-retaining retractors for perineal dissection.
   (b) It is helpful to have an experienced assistant.

Operative Techniques

1. Detailed steps and techniques of abdomino-perineal resection are described elsewhere.

Technical Pearls (Tips and Tricks)

1. Anterior dissection technique.
   (a) Keep in mind that the dissection plane is angled posteriorly. Drawing an imaginary line to the sacral promontory and dissecting along that direction can be helpful. In men, palpating the Foley catheter can help determine the location of the urethra and define the anterior plane. In women, palpation of the posterior wall of the vagina will delineate the dissection plane. It is critical to provide adequate posterior tension on the rectum during anterior dissection. Given the space constraints in the low pelvis, using a long sponge stick to distract the rectum posteriorly can be helpful. Additional traction on the rectum can be provided by using the following two techniques.

2. Deliver the proximal rectal stump out of the pelvis.
   (a) Once the posterior and lateral perineal dissection is complete, the proximal rectum may be delivered out of the pelvis through the posterior perineal wound. The recto-urethralis muscle and the visceral fascia are divided under tension (Fig. 53.1).

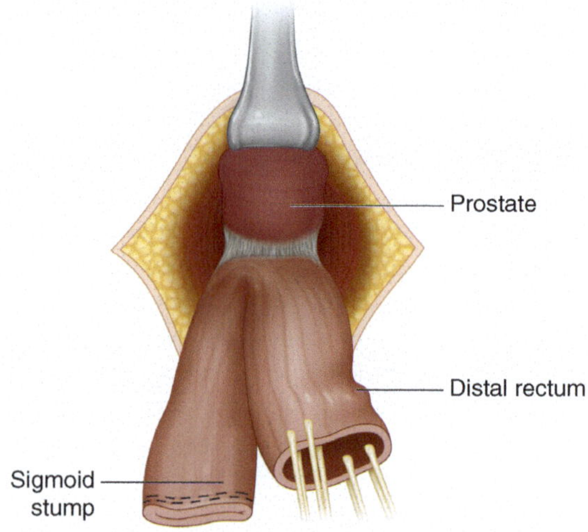

Fig. 53.1 Deliver the sigmoid stump out of the pelvis

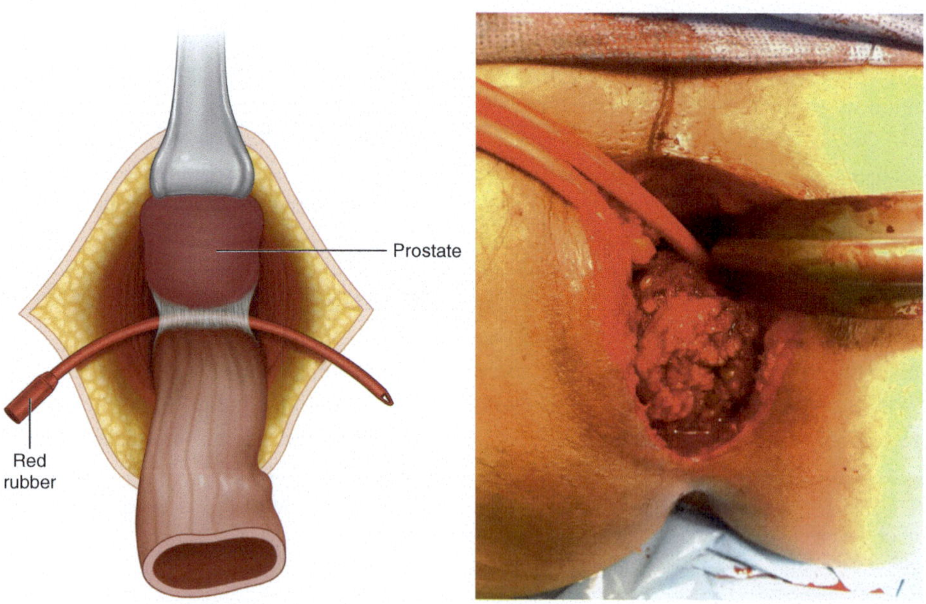

Fig. 53.2 (**a**, **b**) Red rubber catheter technique. By passing a red rubber catheter around the recto-prostatic plane, the proper anterior dissection plane can be defined. Application of electrocautery onto the red rubber catheter can complete the anterior dissection in difficult situations

3. Red rubber catheter technique.
   (a) Pass a red rubber catheter from the perineal wound into the pelvis, hook it around the rectum anteriorly, and pass the end back through the perineal wound. By pulling down on both ends of the red rubber catheter from the perineal side, tension will be applied across the anterior plane. Use the red rubber catheter as a guide to complete the anterior dissection (Fig. 53.2a, b). Alternatively an assistant placing their hand palm up in the deep pelvis can accentuate the correct plan of dissection.

Special Postoperative Care

1. Diet is advanced as tolerated, and ostomy teaching is provided.

Suggested Reading

1. Corman M, Nicholls J, Fazio VW, et al. Colon and rectal surgery. 4th ed. Philadelphia: Lippincott Williams & Wilkins; 1998.
2. Khatri VP. Advanced operative surgery. Philadelphia: Elsevier Saunders; 2013.

Anastomotic Sinus After Low Anterior Resection and Diverting Loop Ileostomy

54

Daniel L. Feingold and Garrett Friedman

Clinical Scenario

A patient with locally aggressive mid-rectal cancer undergoes neo-adjuvant chemoradiotherapy followed by a low anterior resection with a stapled colorectal anastomosis and a diverting loop ileostomy. Pre-reversal water-soluble contrast enema demonstrates a blind-ending sinus tract at the level of the anastomosis extending posteriorly.

Key Points

1. Before reversing a diverting loop ileostomy that has defunctionalized a low colorectal anastomosis, it is important to evaluate the anastomosis for patency and integrity. This evaluation is usually accomplished by performing a flexible sigmoidoscopy to evaluate patency as well as a water-soluble contrast enema study to identify any contrast extravasation (Figs. 54.1 and 54.2). Part of the justification for sigmoidoscopy is that a contrast enema study may not demonstrate a short anastomotic stricture due to the column of contrast above and below the stricture.
2. A blind-ending, non-healing sinus tract is actually a contained leak, and in the setting of festering inflammation in what is commonly an irradiated field, these tracts may be difficult to heal and may require multiple interventions.

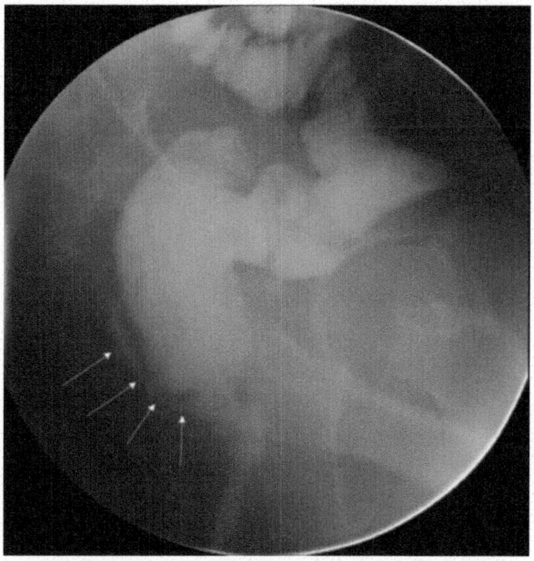

Fig. 54.1 Prestoma reversal gastrografin enema showing a posterior, blind-ending sinus originating from the low pelvic anastomosis

D. L. Feingold (✉)
Division of Colorectal Surgery, Department of Surgery, Columbia University, New York, NY, USA
e-mail: df347@cumc.columbia.edu

G. Friedman
Mike O'Callaghan Federal Medical Center, Department of Colon and Rectal Surgery, Las Vegas, NV, USA

S. W. Lee et al. (eds.), *Colorectal Surgery Consultation*,
https://doi.org/10.1007/978-3-030-11181-6_54

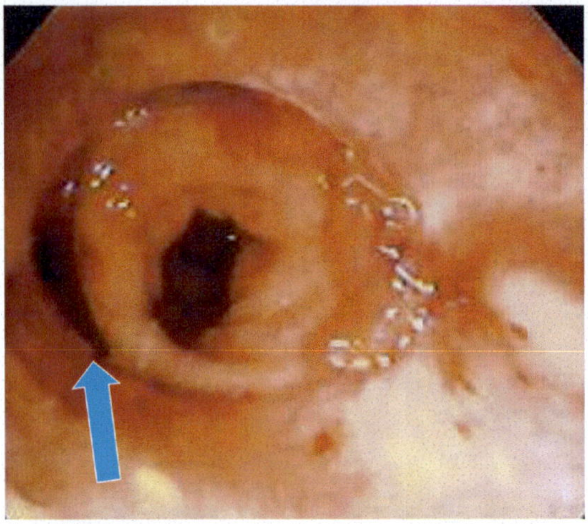

Fig. 54.2 Endoscopic view of a sinus

Technical Pearls (Tips and Tricks)

1. While the ideal time interval between low anterior resection and ileostomy reversal is not clear, the majority of diverted patients will complete their adjuvant chemotherapy prior to stoma reversal. If pre-reversal imaging demonstrates an otherwise asymptomatic sinus, waiting another 4–6 weeks and repeating the imaging may allow for healing. When repeating the enema study under these circumstances, it can be helpful to alert the radiologist to the results of the first study.
2. During a fluoroscopic examination evaluating a low pelvic anastomosis, it is important to use water-soluble contrast and to obtain views of the anastomosis in multiple planes to assess for possible contrast extravasation. With a low pelvic anastomosis, it is helpful to use a small Foley catheter without inflating the balloon rather than the large nozzle typically used for Barium enemas as the Foley is better tolerated by patients and the larger, stiffer radiology catheter may occlude the opening of a low sinus tract and give a false negative assessment. Post-evacuation images can sometimes demonstrate an elusive sinus. A pelvic CT scan with rectal contrast, as an alternative to fluoroscopy, may give additional information and should be considered in cases with persistent sinuses despite intervention.

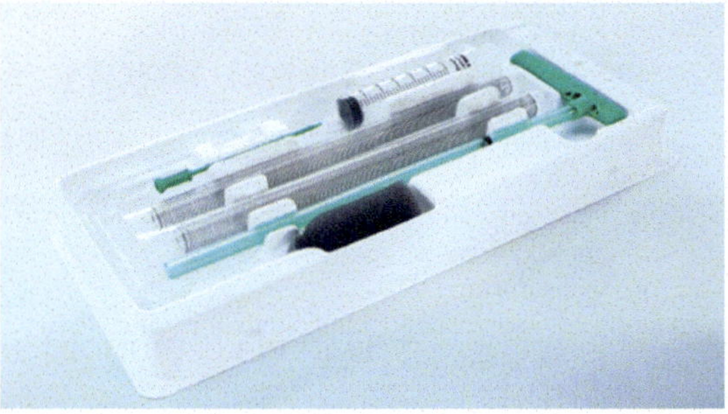

Fig. 54.3 Endo- SPONGE® (Braun)

3. Persistent sinuses accessible trans-anally may be amenable to exam under anesthesia with curettage and drainage typically with a mushroom-type catheter. This approach also addresses source control of the local sepsis, which may require antibiotic therapy, as well. As the sinus fills in and heals, repeat exam under anesthesia with downsizing of the drain can cause the sinus cavity to granulate in. Patients must realize that this approach requires time and multiple procedures.
4. Posteriorly located shorter sinuses may be amenable to marsupialization where the tract is laid open and sutured to prevent repeat sinus formation. Changing the morphology of the defect into a shallow ulceration can prevent ongoing festering in a narrow tract and can facilitate healing.
5. A growing experience supports the use of an endo-luminal vacuum platform (Endo-SPONGE) to heal anastomotic leaks (Fig. 54.3). While available case reports are enthusiastic regarding this technology, this approach may be impractical as it requires multiple, frequent returns to the operating room to change out the devices and patients find the trans-anal evacuation tubing difficult to tolerate.
6. Some sinuses will be amenable to advancing colon mucosa to cover the sinus opening as a flap or to primary suture repair. A variety of platforms can be used for this approach including trans-anal minimally invasive surgery (TAMIS), trans-anal endoscopic micro-

surgery (TEMS), and conventional trans-anal instrumentation. The chronic inflammation from the contained leak together with radiation changes can limit the ability of the anal canal to accommodate the exposure required for a colon advancement procedure. Endoscopic clipping may also be an option in some situations to obtain tissue coverage, but this requires pliability in the tissues in order to bridge the gap of the sinus opening and may not be feasible in most cases.

7. The local application of stem cells or harvested adipose cells may be options for future therapies and are currently under investigation. Similarly, the utility of endo-rectal stenting in a diverted but leaked anastomosis is not clear and may be another option. The performance of tissue sealing glues and fibrin products has not been reliable in this setting.
8. Patients with a persistent sinus often do not undergo stoma reversal due to concerns of the sinus tract becoming symptomatic or declaring a leak once the fecal stream is restored. Alternatives to leaving the patient with their stoma is to reverse the ileostomy and create a permanent end colostomy or to leave the patient protected by the existing ileostomy and repeat a low anterior resection and create a fresh anastomosis. Depending on the complexity of the anatomy, a Turnbull-Cutait procedure may be particularly useful in the latter case.
9. In rare cases, it may be reasonable to reverse the ileostomy in the presence of a persistent blind sinus tract though this requires a detailed discussion with the patient.

Suggested Reading

1. Habib K, Gupta A, White D, Mazari F, Wilson TR. Utility of contrast enema to assess anastomotic integrity and the natural history of radiological leaks after low rectal surgery: systematic review and meta-analysis. Int J Color Dis. 2015;30:1007–14.
2. Killeen S, Souroullas P, Tin HH, et al. Outcomes of asymptomatic anastomotic leaks found on routine post-operative water-soluble enema following anterior resection for cancer. World J Surg. 2013;37:2700–4.
3. Mussetto A, Arena R, Buzzi A, et al. Long-term efficacy of vacuum-assisted therapy (endo-sponge) in large anastomotic leakages following anterior rectal resection. Ann Gastroenterol. 2017;30:649–53.
4. Remzi FH, El Gazzaz G, Kiran RP, Kirat HT, Fazio VW. Outcomes following Turnbull-Cutait abdomino-perineal pull-through compared with coloanal anastomosis. Br J Surg. 2009;96:424–9.
5. Sirois-Giguère E, Boulanger-Gobeil C, Bouchard A, et al. Transanal drainage to treat anastomotic leaks after low anterior resection for rectal cancer: a valuable option. Dis Colon Rectum. 2013;56:586–92.

Part VII

Tips and Tricks for Difficult Colonoscopic Cases

Cannot Pass the Scope into the Cecum

55

David E. Rivadeneira

Clinical Scenario

A 58-year-old, thin [body mass index (BMI) 17 kg/m^2] female with prior history of hysterectomy and chronic constipation is scheduled for a surveillance colonoscopy. Another doctor performed her first colonoscopy 8 years ago, and she reports that a polyp was removed, and her doctor mentioned the procedure was done with significant difficulty. She remembers he mentioned she had a "twisted" colon. She woke up with severe bloating and abdominal pain.

Key Points

1. Understand that there are multiple reasons for not reaching the cecum during colonoscopy.
   (a) Experience. The ability to reach the cecum on colonoscopy (the cecal intubation rate) is proportionally related to the experience of the endoscopist. After around 300 colonoscopies, the cecal intubation rate should be greater than 90% (Fig. 55.1), and the time needed to reach cecal intubation is significantly less (Fig. 55.2).
   (b) Prep quality. Prep quality is an important factor that influences cecal intubation.
      i. Several prep solutions are available including polyethylene-glycol and sodium phosphate (Table 55.1).

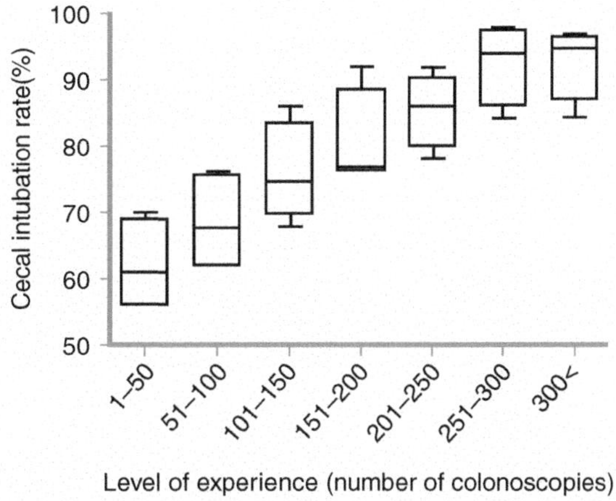

Fig. 55.1 Cecal intubation rate learning curves. The learning curve for average successful cecal intubation rates within 15 min based on the number of colonoscopies is shown ($p < 0.05$) with the Turkey test (error bars represent the 95% confidence interval). Cecal intubation rates reach the 92.5% at 250–300th procedures. (From Park HJ, Hong JH, Kim HS, Kim BR, Park SY, Jo KW, Woo Kim JW. Predictive factors affecting cecal intubation failure in colonoscopy trainees. *BMC Med Educ* 2013;13:5)

D. E. Rivadeneira (✉)
Surgical Strategic Initiatives, Northwell Health, New Hyde Park, NY, USA

Surgical Services and Colorectal Surgery, Huntington Hospital, Huntington, NY, USA

Hofstra University-Northwell School of Medicine, Hempstead, NY, USA
e-mail: DRivadeneira@northwell.edu

S. W. Lee et al. (eds.), *Colorectal Surgery Consultation*,
https://doi.org/10.1007/978-3-030-11181-6_55

ii. Split-dose preps have been associated with increased cecal intubation rates.

iii. Patients older than 65, males, diabetics, chronically constipated patients, and patients with a prior poor preparation have a higher incidence of inadequate preps and may benefit from a more individualized, more powerful prep (Table 55.2).

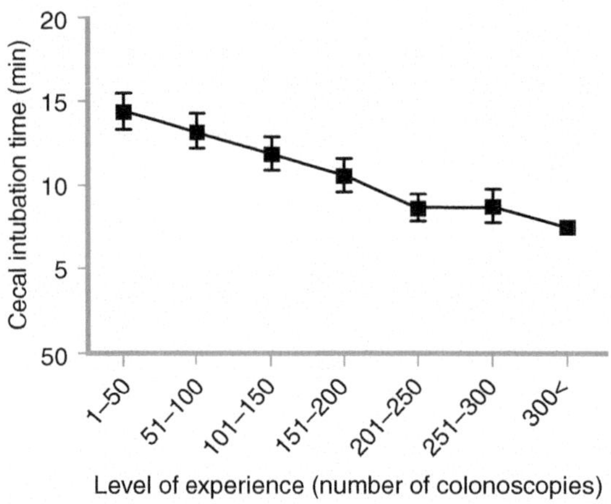

Fig. 55.2 Cecal intubation time learning curves. The learning curve for average cecal intubation times is shown. (Error bars represent the 95% confidence interval). A significant inverse correlation between cecal intubation times and level of experience is shown (From Park HJ, Hong JH, Kim HS, Kim BR, Park SY, Jo KW, Woo Kim JW. Predictive factors affecting cecal intubation failure in colonoscopy trainees. *BMC Med Educ* 2013;13:5)

(c) Loops/angulation/redundancy.

(a) Looping of the colonoscope usually occurs in the left colon.

(b) More common in women.

(c) Two-third of time spent during a colonoscopy is spent in the left colon.

(d) Most common loops are alpha and N loops (Fig. 55.3).

(e) Gentle transabdominal pressure can overcome excessive looping by fixing the colon in place allowing scope advancement.

(f) In long, redundant colons (where you "run out of scope"), repeatedly torqueing the scope in a clockwise rotation and pulling back can telescope the colon onto the scope and allow scope advancement.

(g) Suctioning out insufflation and utilizing less air can facilitate insertion; it is more difficult to advance through an overly distended colon.

(h) Certain patients will require changing their position from left lateral decubi-

Table 55.1 Summary of American Society for Gastrointestinal Endoscopy (SAGES), American Society of Colon and Rectal Surgeons (ASCRS), Society of American Gastrointestinal and Endoscopic Surgeons (ASGE) consensus recommendations on colon cleansing agents for bowel preparation during colonoscopy

Agent	Dosing	Recommendation	Level of evidence
Polyethylene glycol (PEG)	240 mL every 10 min until rectal output is clear or total of 4 L	Faster, more effective, better tolerated compared to dietary restriction with cathartics, gut lavage, or mannitol	Grade 1A
Sulfate-free PEG	240 mL every 10 min until rectal output is clear or total of 4 L	Better tasting, comparable to PEG in effectiveness and safety, acceptable alternative to PEG	Grade IIB
Low volume PEG/ PEG-3350 and bisacodyl	4 bisacodyl delayed-release tablets at noon, after bowel movement or 6 h, 240 mL every 10 min until 2 L is consumed	Equally effective to standard 4 L PEG, better tolerated, acceptable alternative to 4 L PEG	Grade 1A
Aqueous sodium phosphate	2 doses of 30–45 mL sodium phosphate with 8 oz of liquid 20–12 h apart	Equal alternative to PEG except for pediatric and elderly patients, bowel obstruction, renal failure, congestive heart and liver failure	Grade 1A
Sodium phosphate tablets	20 tablets on the evening before the procedure, 12–20 tablets 3–5 h before the procedure	Improved taste and palatability compared to aqueous sodium phosphate, but no improvement in patient tolerance	Grade 1A

tus to supine positioning to permit further insertion. Rarely, pronation or right lateral decubitus positioning may be helpful.
(i) Smaller diameter and more flexible scopes like pediatric or upper scopes may overcome angulated colons.
(j) Fluoroscopy may be used to help guide the scope.
(k) Biopsy forceps down the scope channel can help stiffen the scope to prevent a degree of looping.
(l) Variable stiffness scopes are widely available and are useful in certain situations.

Table 55.2 Predictive factors for quality of bowel preparation independent of colon cleansing agent

Patient-related factors	Procedure-related factors
Age >55 years	
Male gender	Adherence to bowel preparation instructions
Comorbidity	Timing of purgative administration
Diabetes	
Stroke disease	
In-patient status	
Low socioeconomic status	Appointment waiting times

Operative Assessment

1. Can this patient have a colonoscopy done safely?
2. What in the patient's history and physical exam indicate a possible difficult procedure?
3. What methods, techniques, and equipment may you need to increase the rate of cecal intubation safely in this patient?
4. If unsuccessful in performing the colonoscopy, what other modalities are available to survey this patient?

Operative Checklist

1. Prior history of a difficult colonoscopy may be an indicator of future difficult colonoscopy. It may be helpful to review prior procedure reports. This patient's presentation will almost assure you that her colonoscopy will be difficult, that her prior colonoscopy was reported as difficult, and that she was told she had a "twisted" colon and suffered significant abdominal distention and pain post procedure. Her thin body habitus and the prior hysterectomy may lead to sharp angulations in the sigmoid colon and looping.
2. Make sure the patient has prepped properly. In a patient with severe constipation, a clear liq-

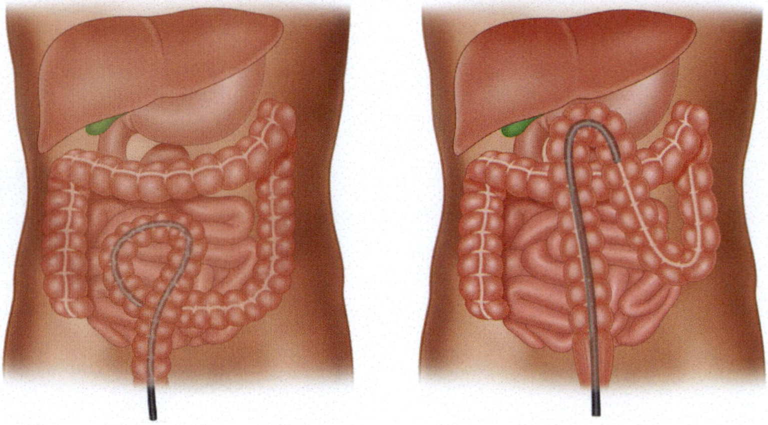

Fig. 55.3 Alpha and N loops

uid diet may be needed several days prior to the procedure. This patient may benefit from a split-dose approach.
3. May want to use CO_2 insufflation as opposed to ambient air. This will lead to rapid absorption and decreased post-procedure distention and pain.
4. Pediatric scope with a smaller diameter may be beneficial in a thin, female patient.
5. Fluoroscopy setup. Fluoroscopy to help navigate the colonoscope and reduce loops was used in the past but still may be a good option. If you plan on using this modality, make sure you have a fluoroscopy friendly table.
6. Variable stiffness colonoscopes: these scopes have the ability to adjust their stiffness through their tip and have been demonstrated to achieve a higher rate of cecal intubation (Fig. 55.4).
7. Magnetic endoscopic imaging (ScopeGuide): this technology uses built-in magnetic coils to provide a real-time, three-dimensional image of the configuration of the colonoscope during the procedure and help with loop reduction and scope advancement (Fig. 55.5).

Operative Technique

1. Two-third of time spent during a colonoscopy is in the left colon. One must master how to reduce a looping scope in order to efficiently and safely advance the scope. This is best done by repeated clockwise loop reductions that pull the colon onto the scope. This will then allow for 1:1 scope advancement.
2. Less air, more suction. Remember that more air will cause over-distention and more post-procedural pain.
3. Position changes: most will start the procedure in the left lateral decubitus position; however, if difficulty in advancing the scope is encountered, repositioning the patient in supine, right-lateral, and even prone position may aid in proper advancement.
4. External pressure applied to the abdominal wall will help fix the colon and is often useful in thinner patients.

Technical Pearls (Tips and Tricks)

1. Remember experience is key. The more you do the better you will become. Studies demonstrate a higher cecal intubation rate after greater than 300 procedures.
2. Ensure proper mechanical bowel preparation.
3. Certain patient characteristics are red flags for a difficult colonoscopy. Thin women, those with prior pelvic surgery such as hysterectomy, chronic constipation with elongated sigmoid colon segments, or large hernias, may all contribute to a difficult colonoscopy.

Fig. 55.4 Variable score stiffness

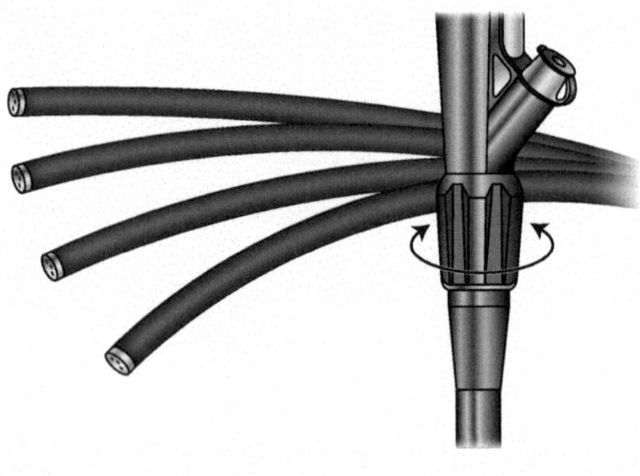

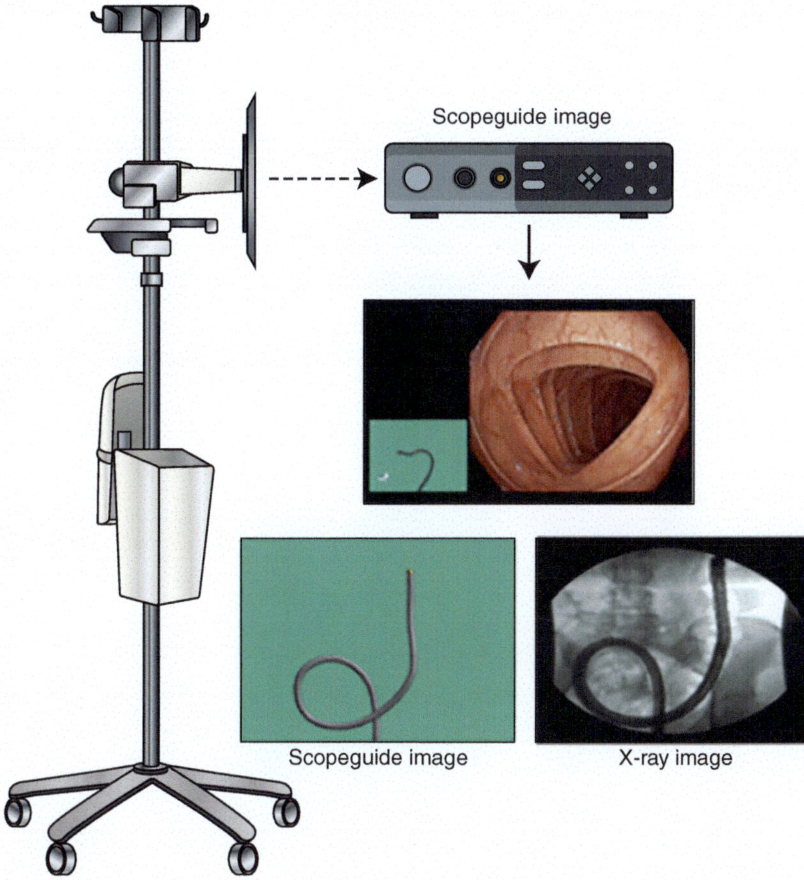

Fig. 55.5
Electromagnetic scope

4. Pediatric scopes, CO_2 insufflation, and variable stiffness scopes may improve cecal intubation rates.
5. Changing position, using external abdominal pressure, reducing loops with a clockwise reduction, and using less air and more suction are helpful maneuvers.
6. Use of fluoroscopy and/or magnetic endoscopic imaging (ScopeGuide) may visually aid in scope insertion.
7. Remember: do not force the procedure. If the colonoscopy is very difficult and despite reasonable attempts and the procedure is still unsuccessful, it is recommended to terminate the case. Alternatives in this situation may include a CT colonography (virtual colonoscopy) or a contrast enema study.

Special Postoperative Care

1. Allow patient to recover properly in the post-endoscopy unit. If the colonoscopy took a considerably long period of time to perform, then a longer period of recovery time should be expected.
2. Depending on the difficulty of the case and the clinical situation, serial abdominal exams looking for signs of possible perforation may be needed.

3. X-ray imaging to rule out a perforation, as clinically warranted.

Suggested Reading

1. Lee S, Ross H, Rivadeneira DE, Steele S, Feingold D, editors. Advanced colonoscopy and endoluminal surgery. Cham: Springer; 2017.
2. Park HJ, Hong JH, Kim HS, Kim B, Park SY, Jo KW, Kim JW. Predictive factors affecting cecal intubation failure in colonoscopy trainees. BMC Med Educ. 2013;13:5.
3. Romero R, Mahadeva S. Factors influencing quality of bowel preparation for colonoscopy. World J Gastrointest Endosc. 2013;5(2):39–46.
4. Ross H, Lee S, Mutch M, Rivadeneira D, Steele SR, editors. Minimally invasive approaches to colon and rectal disease: technique and best practices. New York: Springer Publishing; 2015.
5. Ross H, Lee S, Champagne B, Pigazzi A, Rivadeneira DE. Robotic colorectal surgery. New York: Springer Publishing; 2015.
6. Witte TN, Enns R. The difficult colonoscopy. Can J Gastroenterol. 2007;21(8):487–90.

56 Difficult to Remove Polyp

Daniel L. Feingold and Sang W. Lee

Clinical Scenario

During screening colonoscopy a medium-sized sessile polyp is found straddling a fold along the medial wall of the proximal ascending colon. The gastroenterologist feels that the polyp is not amenable to colonoscopic polypectomy and refers the patient for colon resection.

Key Points

1. Colorectal adenomas, depending on their size, location, and morphology, can be difficult to remove. A number of techniques are available to facilitate polyp removal in this situation.
2. Review the actual color colonoscopy photos to assess whether the polyp looks benign. Indistinct polyp borders, ulcerated and crater-like appearance, or disorganized vascular patterns suggest malignancy and will likely require an oncologic resection.

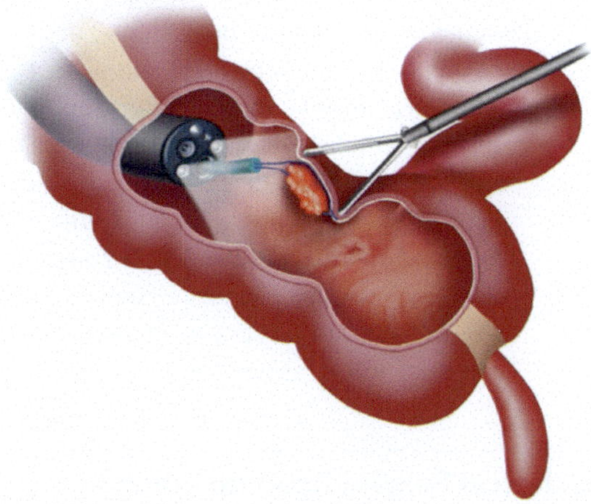

Fig. 56.1 Combined endolaparoscopic surgery (CELS) allows removal of difficult or large polyps while avoiding bowel resection

3. Consider obtaining pathology slides for in-house review. Polyps with high-grade dysplasia or intramucosal carcinoma are more likely to harbor foci of cancer and should be approached with caution when offering endoscopic treatment.
4. Possible surgical options such as intraoperative colonoscopic polypectomy, laparoscopic assisted polypectomy (Fig. 56.1), or partial colectomy need to be discussed with the patient.
5. Intraoperative colonoscopy will ultimately determine whether the lesion is likely to be benign or not. Although polyps partially

D. L. Feingold (✉)
Division of Colorectal Surgery, Department of Surgery, Columbia University, New York, NY, USA
e-mail: df347@cumc.columbia.edu

S. W. Lee
Department of Surgery – Colon and Rectal Surgery, Keck School of Medicine of University of Southern California, Los Angeles, CA, USA

S. W. Lee et al. (eds.), *Colorectal Surgery Consultation*,
https://doi.org/10.1007/978-3-030-11181-6_56

scarred from previously biopsies may not lift with submucosal injection, inability to lift with submucosal injection raises concerns for malignancy.

6. If the removed polyp feels firm, frozen section of the specimen can be performed to guide further therapy.

Operative Checklist

1. Additional resources and equipment
   (a) A colonoscope with CO_2 insufflation is required for intraoperative applications. Even with clamping of the terminal ileum, conventional ambient air colonoscopy causes significant colonic distension and prevents efficient abdominal manipulation of the colon. In addition, assorted ancillary equipment is needed like a choice of submucosal injection solution, injection needle, snares, and polyp retrieval trap and access to colonoscopic hemostatic clips, as needed.

Technical Pearls (Tips and Tricks)

1. Carefully torqueing the colonoscope and adjusting the view with the dials can orient the scope such that the target lays below and to the right. This orientation facilitates access for polypectomy. In certain cases it may be helpful to reposition the patient as well to get better orientation.
2. Submucosal saline injection can elevate the lesion bringing it into the lumen for better visualization of the target. Submucosally inject the polyp away from the scope lifting the polyp toward the scope for better access and visualization (Fig. 56.2). A mixture of saline with either Indigo carmine or dilute Methylene blue can facilitate visualization of the polyp and its borders. This injection also enables polypectomy by way of endoscopic mucosal resection (EMR). A variety of other lifting solutions is available each with a unique duration of lifting action, advantages and disadvantages. Failure of a lesion to lift ("non-lifting sign") may be due to fibrosis from prior attempts at removal and can signify presence of cancer.

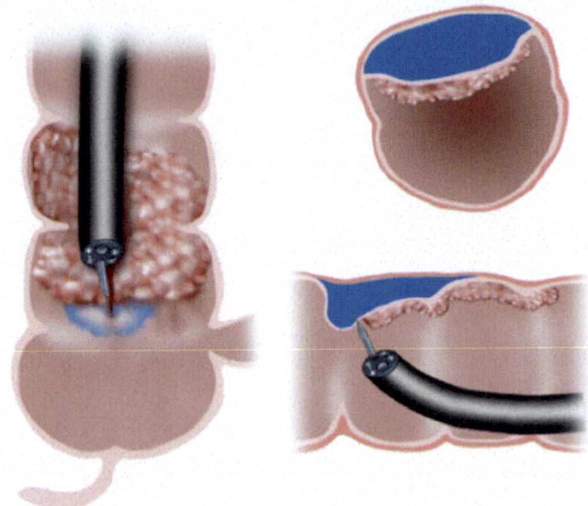

Fig. 56.2 Submucosal saline injection elevates the lesion bringing it into the lumen for better visualization of the target. Submucosally injecting the polyp away from the scope lifts the polyp toward the scope for better access and visualization

3. In certain situations, it may be helpful to retroflex the colonoscope and approach the target from its proximal side.
4. Cauterizing the edges of the polypectomy site can significantly decrease the chance of recurrence (Fig. 56.3).
5. Issues that limit conventional endoscopic polypectomy like unstable gas insufflation, accumulation of smoke and blood with poor suction capability, and one-handed tissue dissection can be overcome using more advanced platforms like transanal minimally invasive surgery (TAMIS) or transanal endoscopic microsurgery (TEMS). These setups are useful for removing distal sigmoid and rectal polyps.
6. Patients who do not have successful endoscopic polypectomy may be candidates for combined endoscopic and laparoscopic surgery (CELS) as an alternative to undergoing

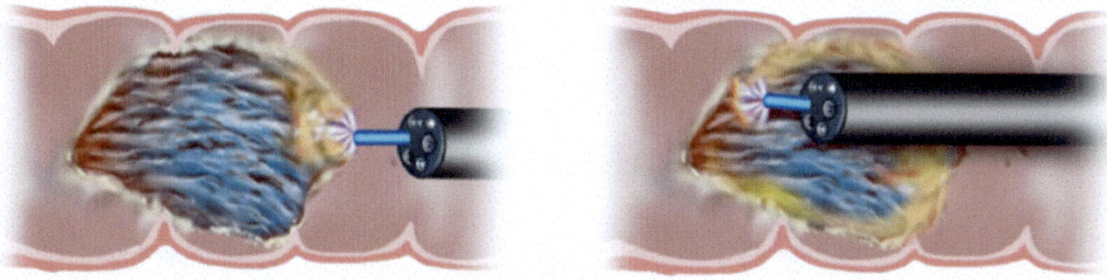

Fig. 56.3 Cauterizing the edges of the polypectomy site can significantly decrease the chance of recurrence

colectomy. The benefits of CELS include facilitating colonoscopic polypectomy by mobilizing the colon, direct assessment of the wall of the colon during polypectomy with the ability to repair a defect if one develops, performing colon wedge or sleeve resection excising the colon bearing the polyp lesion under colonoscopic guidance, and proceeding directly to laparoscopic colectomy, if needed.

7. Adenomas not amenable to colonoscopic or CELS removal should be addressed by colectomy. In this situation, an appropriate oncologic resection is recommended as a significant proportion of polyps treated by colectomy harbor occult cancer.

Special Postoperative Care

1. No special postoperative care is needed. Normal diet can be resumed as tolerated.

Suggested Reading

1. Jang JH, Balik E, Kirchoff D, et al. Oncologic colorectal resection, not advanced endoscopic polypectomy, is the best treatment for large dysplastic adenomas. J Gastrointest Surg. 2012;16:165–72.
2. Lee SW, Garrett KA, Shin JH, Trencheva K, Sonoda T, Milsom JW. Long-term outcomes of patients undergoing combined endolaparoscopic surgery for benign colon polyps. Dis Colon Rectum. 2013;56:869–73.

Bleeding After Colonoscopic Polypectomy

57

Howard M. Ross and Laura Greco

Clinical Scenario

Mr. Z. had piecemeal polypectomy of a 2 cm sessile adenomatous lesion located on a fold in the sigmoid colon. The patient was discharged promptly from the endoscopy unit but returned to the emergency department at midnight feeling light headed and weak. He began to pass significant bright red blood per rectum with clots. His hemoglobin dropped from 10 to 6 g/dl. Mr. Z was resuscitated with blood and taken emergently to the endoscopy unit. A pulsatile bleeding vessel was seen at the edge of the defect and was controlled with two clips.

Key Points

1. Incidence of bleeding after polypectomy can be as high as 1 in 200; however, clinically significant bleeding is extremely rare as biopsy forceps remove only superficial tissue without interrupting large blood vessels. In most cases of polypectomy, the site can be simply observed and hemostasis achieved without any specific intervention. A hemostatic therapy may be required if there is hemorrhage lasting more than 1–2 minutes, arterial bleeding, or heavy bleeding. Polypectomy in the right colon and removal of lesions greater than 20 mm are at increased risk of bleeding.
2. Early versus late hemorrhage after polypectomy.
   (a) Early hemorrhage is usually immediately apparent and is the result of insufficient hemostasis after polypectomy. This can, in most cases, be treated endoscopically. Bleeding occurring immediately after partial polypectomy of a larger polyp can usually be addressed by completing the polypectomy.
   (b) Late hemorrhage is often the result of dislodgement of a formed clot or delayed thermal injury to a blood vessel and can occur anytime up to about 21 days after polypectomy but most commonly occurs within the 1st week. This usually presents as blood per rectum or with the symptoms of acute blood loss anemia.
3. Familiarity with endoscopic techniques allows the surgeon to control post-colonoscopy bleeding.

H. M. Ross (✉)
Division of Colon and Rectal Surgery, Lewis Katz School of Medicine at Temple University and the Temple University Health System, Philadelphia, PA, USA
e-mail: Howard.Ross@tuhs.temple.edu

L. Greco
Department of Surgery, Temple University Hospital, Philadelphia, PA, USA

S. W. Lee et al. (eds.), *Colorectal Surgery Consultation*,
https://doi.org/10.1007/978-3-030-11181-6_57

Operative Assessment

1. The sites of polyp excision must be examined closely post-polypectomy.

Operative Checklist

1. The endoscopy suite must be equipped with tools to control post-polypectomy bleeding including clips, injectable saline with epinephrine, and cautery (Fig. 57.1).

Operative Techniques

1. Injection of epinephrine
   (a) Post-polypectomy bleeding can be addressed by injecting 1:10,000 epinephrine solution to vasoconstrict the vessels leading to hemostasis. Injection of epinephrine into the base of a polyp before endoscopic resection has been shown on meta-analysis to be an effective method of preventing post-polypectomy hemorrhage.
   (b) This method is used often in combination with clips or electrocautery for management of post-polypectomy bleeding. It can effectively slow hemorrhage to allow for better visualization of the bleeding vessel for more accurate clip or snare placement.
2. Clips
   (a) Clips are another method of achieving hemostasis. According to several studies, clips decrease the rate of rebleeding compared to cauterization or epinephrine injection but do not significantly decrease the risk of hemorrhage after polypectomy.
   (b) Clip Placement.
      (i) When clipping endoscopically, it is important to note the location of the working port on the colonoscope and to position the target area to be clipped in relation to that location. In order to achieve hemostasis, the vessel or area of bleeding must be clipped with an adequate amount of surrounding tissue captured in the clip to assure that it will remain in place. Angling the clip less than 90° from the desired area will allow for greater tissue capture within the clip. Multiple clips may be necessary to achieve hemostasis.
      (ii) Clips can also be placed in cases of failed hemostasis at the site of bleeding to localize the area radiographically.
3. Endoscopic band ligation
   (a) Several case reports have described the use of endoscopic band ligation for post-polypectomy bleeding. Endoscopic band ligation is most commonly used for management of esophageal varices and is also used for treatment of bleeding hemorrhoids. In these case reports, the band is introduced through the colonoscope and is deployed over a bleeding polypectomy stalk. This method has yet to be studied in

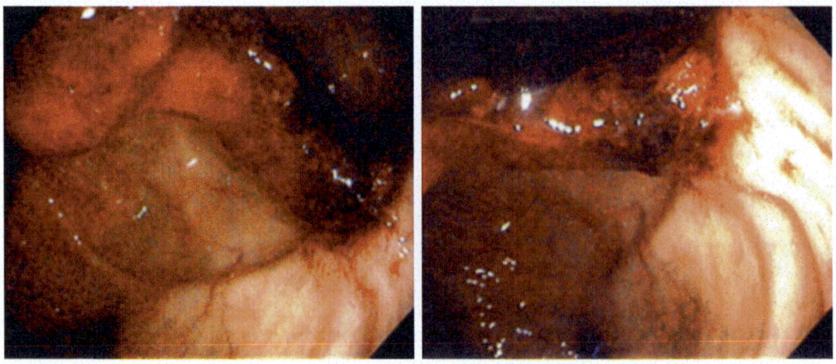

Fig. 57.1 Adherent clot via endoscopy on polypectomy site (left). Arterial bleeding once the clot is removed (right)

a larger trial, and, in the available case reports, banding is often used after multiple failed attempts with conventional interventions such as injection or application of clips or snares.

4. Bleeding not responsive to endoscopic intervention
   (a) Arterial embolization – Angiography can identify a source of arterial bleeding and selectively embolize the bleeding artery. Selective infusion of vasopressin can also be used angiographically to control post-polypectomy hemorrhage. Placement of endoscopic clips at the area of hemorrhage may provide assistance in radiographic visualization and identification of bleeding vessels.
   (b) Surgery – Operative intervention for post-polypectomy hemorrhage is rarely required given the efficacy of multiple endoscopic and angiographic methods to control bleeding. In cases where post-polypectomy hemorrhage results in hemodynamic instability or the bleeding is not responsive to endoscopic or angiographic intervention, surgery may be indicated. Surgical approaches include direct suture ligation of bleeding site or hemicolectomy.

Technical Pearls (Tips and Tricks)

1. Do not rush to leave a fresh polypectomy site. Patient observation may reveal bleeding.
2. Post-polypectomy bleeding is most commonly controlled with the above endoscopic interventions so maintain a low threshold to return to the endoscopy suite when bleeding is ongoing.
3. High volume irrigation and suction are extremely helpful in these cases.
4. In the rare case that surgery is required for a post-polypectomy bleed, endoscopically tattooing the polyp site upfront is helpful when trying to localize the site in the operating room. Alternatively, if the patient undergoes attempt at angiography, it is helpful to inject methylene blue through the super-selective angio-catheter to mark to area of bleeding that needs to be addressed in the operating room.

Special Postoperative Care

1. Ensure the bleeding did not result in any end organ damage that needs to be addressed.

Suggested Reading

1. Agha R, Miller M, George ML, Sabharwal T. Arterial embolisation to control haemorrhage following colonoscopic polypectomy. Int J Surg. 2008;6(5):420–1.
2. Amato A, Radaelli F, Dinelli M, Crosta C, Cengia G, Beretta P, Devani M, Lochis D, Manes G, Fini L, Paggi S, Passoni GR, Repici A. Early and delayed complications of polypectomy in a community setting: the SPoC prospective multicentre trial. Dig Liver Dis. 2016;48(1):43–8. https://doi.org/10.1016/j.dld.2015.09.007.
3. Gibbs DH, Opelka FG, Beck DE, et al. Postpolypectomy colonic hemorrhage. Dis Colon Rectum. 1996;39:806. https://doi.org/10.1007/BF02054448.
4. Kim JH, Lee HJ, Ahn JW, Cheung DY, Kim JI, Park SH, Kim JK. Risk factors for delayed post-polypectomy hemorrhage: a case-control study. J Gastroenterol Hepatol. 2013;28(4):645–9. https://doi.org/10.1111/jgh.12132.
5. Park Y, Jeon TJ, Park JY, Park SJ, Cheon JH, Kim TI, Kim WH, Hong SP. Comparison of clipping with and without epinephrine injection for the prevention of post-polypectomy bleeding in pedunculated colon polyps. J Gastroenterol Hepatol. 2015;30:1499–506. https://doi.org/10.1111/jgh.12994.
6. Parra-Blanco, et al. Hemoclipping for postpolypectomy and postbiopsy colonic bleeding. Gastrointest Endosc. 2000;51(1):37–41.
7. Rossetti A, Buchs NC, Breguet R, et al. Transarterial embolization in acute colonic bleeding: review of 11 years of experience and long-term results. Int J Color Dis. 2013;28:777. https://doi.org/10.1007/s00384-012-1621-5.
8. Slivka A, Parsons WG, Carr-Locke DL. Endoscopic band ligation for treatment of post-polypectomy hemorrhage. Gastrointest Endosc. 1994;40(2):230–2, ISSN 0016-5107. https://doi.org/10.1016/S0016-5107(94)70175-X.
9. Smith RE, Doull J. Treatment of colonic post-polypectomy bleeding site by endoscopic band

ligation. Gastrointest Endosc. 1994;40(4):499–500. ISSN 0016-5107. https://doi.org/10.1016/S0016-5107(94)70222-5.

10. Tolliver KA, Rex DK. Colonoscopic polypectomy. Gastroenterol Clin N Am. 2008;37(1):229–51. https://doi.org/10.1016/j.gtc.2007.12.009.
11. Tullavardhana T, Akranurakkul P, Ungkitphaiboon W, Songtish D. Efficacy of submucosal epinephrine injection for the prevention of postpolypectomy bleeding: a meta-analysis of randomized controlled studies. Ann Med Surg. 2017;19:65–73, ISSN 2049-0801. https://doi.org/10.1016/j.amsu.2017.05.035.
12. Waye JD, Rex DK, Williams CB, editors. Colonoscopy: principles and practice. 2nd ed. New York: Blackwell Publishing Ltd; 2009. ISBN: 978-1-405-17599-9. Ch. 25: Clips, loops, and bands-application in the colon.
13. Waye JD, Aisenberg J, Rubin PH. Practical colonoscopy. 1st ed. Chichester: Wiley; 2013. Ch. 14: Complications of colonoscopy.

58 The Thin Colon After Endoscopic Mucosal Resection

David E. Rivadeneira

Case Scenario

You are performing an endoscopic mucosal resection on a 3 cm villous adenoma in the ascending colon and you are concerned that the resection has been too aggressive and that the colon wall is very thin and risks perforation.

Key Points

1. Submucosal injection of either saline or viscous and hypertonic solutions (e.g., hydroxyethyl starch, sodium hyaluronate solution, 50% dextrose, and succinylated gelatin) underneath the lesion causing a lifting of the lesion will mitigate the risk of transmural thermal injury during the application of cautery.
2. It is imperative that the surgeon becomes comfortable placing clips. Available clips are now easier to place and can close larger defects.
3. The use of laparoscopy can aid in endoscopic resection and repair by means of combined endoscopic laparoscopic surgery (CELS), which can invaginate the colon wall laparoscopically and allow for better placement of clips and can suture the serosa side of an EMR site laparoscopically, if needed.
4. Endoscopic suturing of larger mucosal defects, typically performed after endoscopic submucosal dissection (ESD), has also been utilized.

Operative Assessment

1. Alert your staff and anesthesia personel that you will spend some additional time closing the defect.
2. Determine the extent of the defect that needs to be closed or reinforced.
3. Can this repair be done endoscopically with clips or does this need a CELS approach?
4. Intravenous broad-spectrum antibiotics, particularly if you suspect a perforation.

Operative Checklist

1. When performing EMR, it is beneficial to use CO_2 insufflation for the endoscopy as this leads to rapid absorption and less bowel distention, which will be important particularly if a CELS approach will be used.
2. Endoscopic clips. Preloaded devices are easier and faster to use.

D. E. Rivadeneira (✉)
Surgical Strategic Initiatives, Northwell Health, New Hyde Park, NY, USA

Surgical Services and Colorectal Surgery, Huntington Hospital, Huntington, NY, USA

Hofstra University-Northwell School of Medicine, Hempstead, NY, USA
e-mail: DRivadeneira@northwell.edu

S. W. Lee et al. (eds.), *Colorectal Surgery Consultation*,
https://doi.org/10.1007/978-3-030-11181-6_58

3. Laparoscopic equipment including bowel graspers and laparoscopic needle drivers for suturing.

Operative Technique

1. Endoclips are typically the first line option for repairing a thin colon wall after EMR. The QuickClip Pro (Olympus, Japan) two-pronged clips are available in different clip arm lengths, resulting in varied diameters of tissue (5–11 mm) that can be clipped. The clips can be rotated from the handle to align the clip with the targeted tissue. To deploy the mechanism, squeeze the trigger part way to advance the clip out of the sheath so that the clip partially opens. This step is critical and is referred to as "priming" the clip. One can still rotate the clip and adjust placement, as needed. When ready, squeeze the trigger the rest of the way to close the clip until a "click" is heard and felt. Several clips may be needed to close a defect.
2. Another available endoclip is the Resolution Clip (Boston Scientific Corporation, USA). Similarly, this is a two-pronged clipping device that has the additional benefit to open and close before finalizing deployment. It is preloaded and has a clip jaw span of 11 mm. Once delivered through the scope, the stopper is removed and the over-sheath grip is pulled back, exposing the clip. The trigger handle can then open and close the clip up to five times until the operator is satisfied with the grasp of the tissue.
3. Another device, the TriClip (Cook Medical Inc., USA) is the only three-pronged clip available and opens quite wide (12 mm diameter) but tends to have a lower radial grasping force than the other devices.
4. If performing a CELS approach, the patient needs to be in lithotomy position in order to have access for colonoscopy.
5. The use of CO_2 for the endoscopy is invaluable and minimizes bowel distention and allows for laparoscopic visualization and manipulation.
6. After a CELS technique we recommend an air leak test of the repair or of the reinforced serosal area.

Technical Pearls (Tips and Tricks)

1. Become familiar and comfortable with handling and placing endoclips. In terms of the learning curve, it is helpful to use these devices on easier cases and gain some experience so you are comfortable placing clips in more difficult situations.
2. Do not hesitate to use a CELS approach. Often the use of a combined laparoscopic and endoscopic technique will make a very difficult endoscopic repair much easier to approach.

Special Postoperative Care

1. Use intravenous antibiotics, if clinically indicated, such as with a full thickness defect.
2. If suspected of full-thickness injury to the colon, consider obtaining an upright chest x-ray post procedure to rule out free air.
3. Most clips used today are MRI compatible.

Suggested Reading

1. Choi KD, Jung HY, Lee GH, et al. Application of metal hemoclips for closure of endoscopic mucosal resection-induced ulcers of the stomach to prevent delayed bleeding. Surg Endosc. 2008;22:1882–6.
2. Garrett KA, Lee SW. Combined endoscopic and laparoscopic surgery. Clin Colon Rectal Surg. 2015;28(3):140–5.
3. Lee S, Ross H, Rivadeneira DE, Steele S, Feingold D, editors. Advanced colonoscopy and endoluminal surgery. Cham: Springer; 2017.
4. Romagnuolo J. Endoscopic clips: past, present and future. Can J Gastroenterol. 2009;23(3):158–60.
5. Ross H, Lee S, Mutch M, Rivadeneira D, Steele SR, editors. Minimally invasive approaches to colon and rectal disease: technique and best practices. New York: Springer Publishing; 2015.
6. Ross H, Lee S, Champagne B, Pigazzi A, Rivadeneira DE, editors. Robotic colorectal surgery. New York: Springer Publishing; 2015.

59 Cannot Remove the Snare During Colonoscopy

David E. Rivadeneira

Clinical Scenario

A 65-year-old male undergoing a routine colonoscopy is found to have a 3-cm pedunculated polyp in the sigmoid colon. The polyp is on a thick, broad-based stalk. You place a snare around what you believe is the base of the stalk and start to use cautery. About halfway through the stalk, you see just smoke coming from the cautery. You tell your assistant to increase the setting on the cautery and you notice that there is a "char" effect and you are unable to cut through the stalk completely. Now you are unable to open the snare and it is stuck.

Key Points

1. With the ever-increasing use of endoscopic procedures, surgeons and endoscopists must be prepared for potential complications associated with these procedures.
2. Polyps are often removed with snare and PolyLoop (Olympus, San Jose, CA) techniques.
3. Although more commonly encountered complications of bleeding and perforations can occur with these techniques, a snare or PolyLoop can at times become "stuck" and cannot be removed by usual methods.
4. These devices are more likely to become stuck when used on larger polyps.
5. Avoid or minimize electrocautery. There is increasing evidence that cold snare techniques are safer.
6. Changing to a "cutting" current mode may help finish getting through the tissue and allow device removal.
7. Use scissors or a wire cutter to cut the handle away from the snare or PolyLoop device. Then use an endoscopic sheer scissors to cut away the snare/loop and retrieve (Fig. 59.1).
8. If dealing with a PolyLoop, one can also cut away the handle and advance a snare through the scope, lasso the loop around the end of the catheter, advance utilizing a Seldinger approach to the loop, and finally cut the loop (Fig. 59.2).
9. If snare or PolyLoop is located in the rectum or sigmoid colon, then a trans-anal approach for removal can be done safely in the operating room. This can be done through plastic Hill-Ferguson retractors, a large working proctoscope, several commercially available

D. E. Rivadeneira (✉)
Surgical Strategic Initiatives, Northwell Health, New Hyde Park, NY, USA

Surgical Services and Colorectal Surgery, Huntington Hospital, Huntington, NY, USA

Hofstra University-Northwell School of Medicine, Hempstead, NY, USA
e-mail: DRivadeneira@northwell.edu

S. W. Lee et al. (eds.), *Colorectal Surgery Consultation*,
https://doi.org/10.1007/978-3-030-11181-6_59

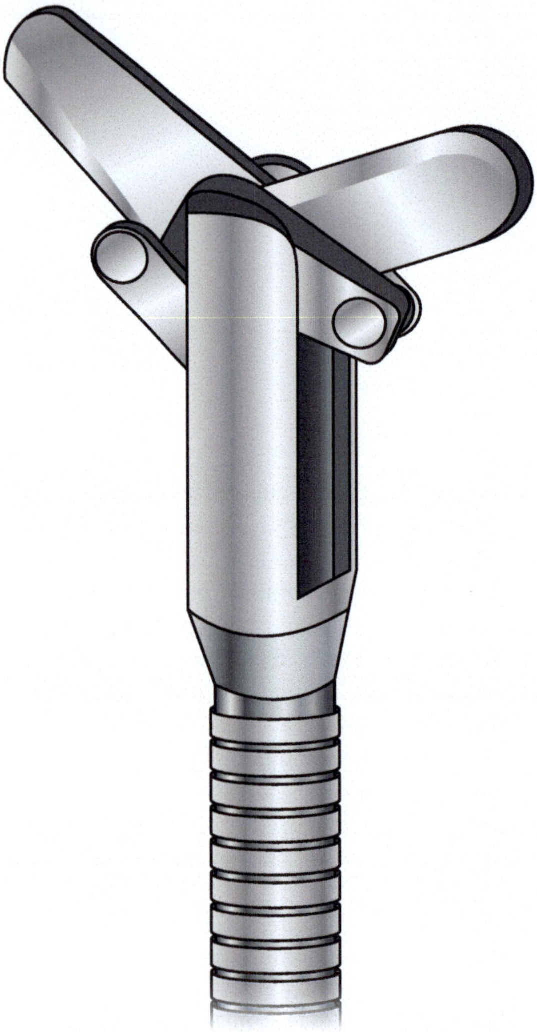

Fig. 59.1 Endoscopic sheer scissors

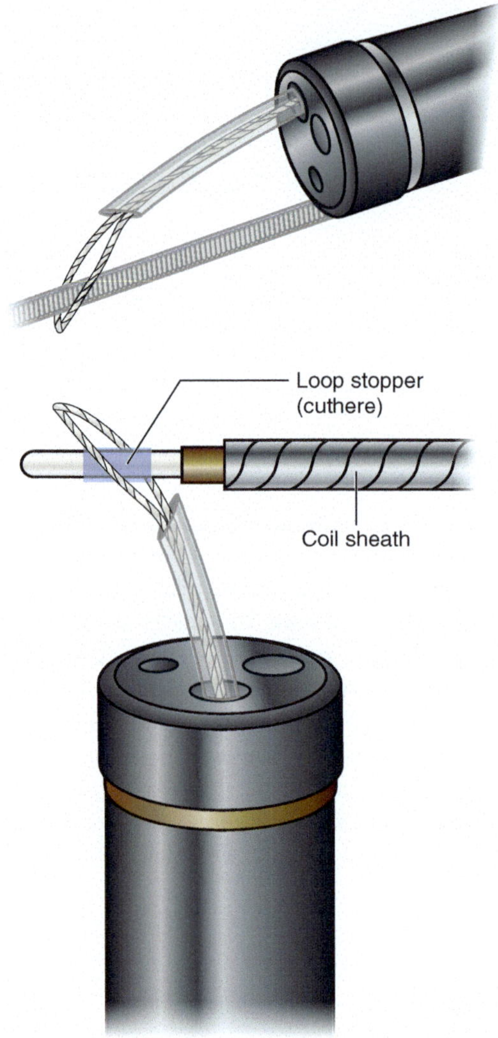

Fig. 59.2 Seldinger approach to the loop

trans-anal minimally invasive platforms (trans-anal minimally invasive surgery, TAMIS) (Fig. 59.3), and the use of laparoscopic scissors.

3. Is the patient stable? Do you need to approach this in the operating room or can you safely perform this in endoscopy suite?

Operative Assessment

1. Alert your staff and anesthesia personel that there is a problem. Communicate clearly that there is an issue with removing the snare or PolyLoop.
2. Additional anesthesia and time is needed.

Operative Checklist

1. Use heavy sheers or a wire cutter to remove handle away from catheter.
2. Use endoscopic scissors to cut snare or loop.
3. If snare or loop is in the rectum or sigmoid, then performing a removal in the operating

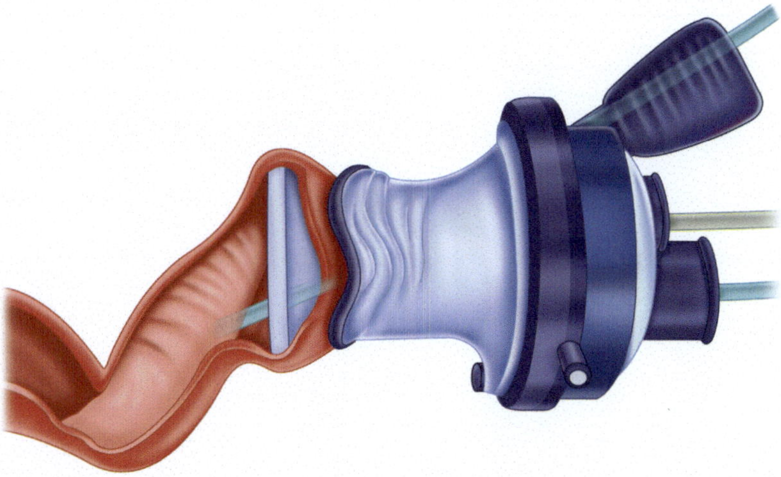

Fig. 59.3 Trans-anal minimally invasive platforms such as TAMIS or TEMS

room with plastic Ferguson retractor or large proctoscope and removal with laparoscopic scissors is possible.

4. Have trans-anal minimally invasive platforms such as TAMIS or trans-anal endoscopic microsurgery (TEM) available in the operating room.
4. If snare or loop is located in the sigmoid colon, then trans-anal platforms including TAMIS, TEMS, or large proctoscopes/plastic Ferguson retractors with the use of laparoscopic scissors for removal may be used.

Operative Techniques

1. "Cutting" current will help finish getting through the tissue and allow device removal.
2. Use endoscopic scissors to cut away snare or loop.
3. Use of trans-anal minimally invasive platforms such as TAMIS or TEMS may be used as well for snare or loops stuck in the rectum or sigmoid colon.

Technical Pearls (Tips and Tricks)

1. Avoid extensive cautery as this causes char effect of tissues and causes the snare to get sticky. Best to use cold snare techniques.
2. Alert your nursing and anesthesia team that more time will be needed.
3. Once handle has been cut off, then thread the catheter up the scope and use endoscopic scissors to cut snare or loop.

Special Postoperative Care

1. None needed; however, if the procedure is lengthy and complicated, obtain a KUB to rule out a perforation, if clinically warranted.

Suggested Reading

1. Lee S, Ross H, Rivadeneira DE, Steele S, Feingold D, editors. Advanced colonoscopy and endoluminal surgery. Cham: Springer; 2017.
2. Ross H, Lee S, Mutch M, Rivadeneira D, Steele SR, editors. Minimally invasive approaches to colon and rectal disease: technique and best practices. New York: Springer Publishing; 2015.
3. Ross H, Lee S, Champagne B, Pigazzi A, Rivadeneira DE, editors. Robotic colorectal surgery. New York: Springer Publishing; 2015.
4. Silva RA, et al. New technique for releasing a stuck loop. Endoscopy. 2006;38:437.
5. Tischer A, et al. Adhesion of snare and endoloop during polypectomy. Endoscopy. 2016;48:E117–8.

60 How to Address a Polyp Involving the Appendiceal Orifice

Howard M. Ross and Laura Greco

Clinical Scenario

An average risk patient undergoes his index screening colonoscopy at age 50. A 2-cm sessile lesion involving the appendiceal orifice is encountered (Fig. 60.1). Biopsy via cold forceps shows a tubulovillous adenoma.

Key Points

1. It is currently not possible to endoscopically completely remove a polyp involving the appendiceal orifice as current endoscopic equipment is larger than the appendix itself.
2. Laparoscopic partial cecectomy allows complete removal of an adenomatous lesion of the appendiceal orifice.
3. Laparoscopic cecectomy is readily performed completely laparoscopically and permits same-day discharge from the hospital.
4. Surgeons must be able to mobilize the cecum and right colon to resect the entire base of the cecum.
5. Simultaneous colonoscopic monitoring is important in achieving negative margins (Fig. 60.2).
6. Patents with polyps that are suspicious for cancer should undergo an oncologic resection.

Operative Assessment

1. Endoscopic resection of polyps at the appendiceal orifice was examined in 131 patients in a retrospective study from multiple tertiary care centers. Patients who had undergone endoscopic resection of polyps >2 cm in size or that took up >75% of the appendiceal orifice were significantly more likely to need additional procedures or surgery. Those with polyps >2 cm were more likely to have perforation secondary to procedure and those with polyps that occupied more than 75% of the diameter of the appendiceal orifice were significantly more likely to have polyp recurrence. For smaller lesions, the retrospective cohort study demonstrated that 94% of polyps could be resected endoscopically with overall low rates of bleeding and perforation.
2. Multiple studies have demonstrated that "radical appendectomy" or partial cecectomy is a

H. M. Ross (✉)
Division of Colon and Rectal Surgery, Lewis Katz School of Medicine at Temple University and the Temple University Health System, Philadelphia, PA, USA
e-mail: Howard.Ross@tuhs.temple.edu

L. Greco
Department of Surgery, Temple University Hospital, Philadelphia, PA, USA

S. W. Lee et al. (eds.), *Colorectal Surgery Consultation*,
https://doi.org/10.1007/978-3-030-11181-6_60

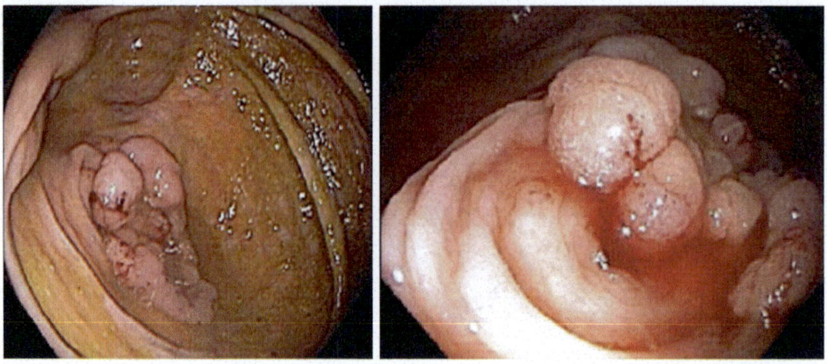

Fig. 60.1 Cecal polyp involving the appendiceal orifice

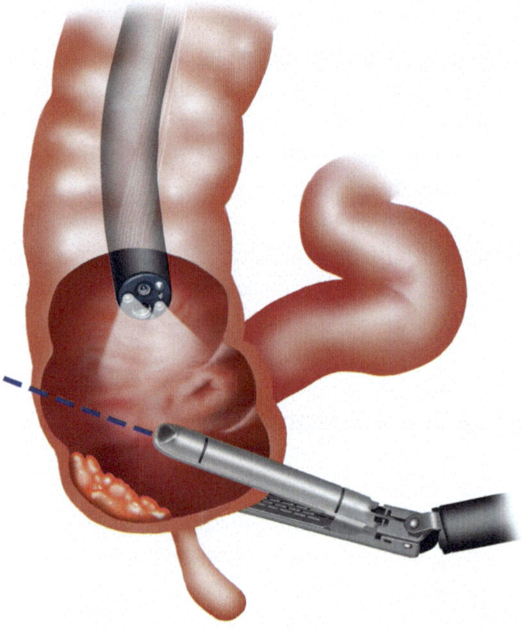

Fig. 60.2 Simultaneous colonoscopic monitoring is important in achieving negative margins

safe and feasible alternative to endoscopic resection, particularly in cases involving benign lesions that are too large to be safely excised endoscopically.

3. There have been several case reports describing the rare event of an intussuscepted or inverted appendix appearing as a polyp at the appendiceal orifice – these were more often seen in patients with comorbid conditions including Crohn's disease, endometriosis, or a mass of the appendix that was a lead point in adults. When evaluating what may appear to be a large polyp at the appendiceal base, an inverted appendix is a possible, though rare, finding and inadvertent endoscopic removal can lead to peritonitis and perforation.
4. An umbilical camera port and two left lower quadrant ports are placed and the ability to perform laparoscopic cecectomy is assessed by identifying the ileum and ileocecal valve and freeing the entire base of the cecum to permit cecectomy with a linear laparoscopic stapler.

Operative Checklist

1. Laparoscopic equipment including graspers to handle the small bowel and cecum, scissors to mobilize the cecum, laparoscopic linear stapler to transect the cecum, an instrument to divide the mesoappendix, and a specimen catch bag.
2. Patient positioning should include tucking the left arm.
3. For larger cecal polyps (>2 cm), a colonoscope with CO_2 insufflation should be available for intraoperative monitoring.

Operative Technique

1. The appendix can be grasped by its tip via a grasper. Attachments of the ileum to the pelvis should be freed and the cecum should be mobilized from lateral to medial.

2. The appendiceal artery should be divided with a stapler, clip, or vessel sealer.
3. Once the appendix and cecum are completely mobile, the appendix is grasped via an instrument held in the left hand and is retracted inferiorly and the surgical stapler is placed across the cecum taking care not to encroach on the ileocecal valve.
4. For large polyps, direct visualization with a colonoscope is essential in ensuring negative margins. It is imperative to verify that the ileocecal valve is not being incorporated into the staple line.
5. The specimen should be placed in a specimen bag and removed.
6. At a side table, the specimen should be opened to ensure grossly clear resection margins.

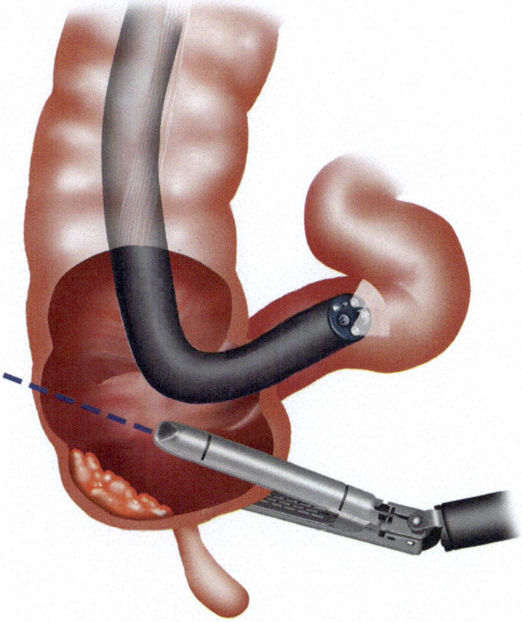

Fig. 60.3 For large cecal polyps that are extending out near the ileocecal valve, a colonoscope can be used to intubate the terminal ileum and protect the ileocecal valve from being incorporated into the staple line

Technical Pearls (Tips and Tricks)

1. Laparoscopic cecectomy is readily performed but requires mobilization of the cecum.
2. Evaluation of the appropriate lesion for laparoscopic cecectomy demands evaluation of the photograph from the initial endoscopy. Review must confirm the presence of the lesion at the appendiceal orifice.
3. For larger cecal polyps that extends near the ileocecal valve, a colonoscope can be used to intubate the terminal ileum and protect the ileocecal valve from being incorporated into the staple line (Fig. 60.3).

Special Postoperative Care

1. Recognize the potential for infection.
2. Patients may resume a diet on an enhanced recovery pathway, as indicated.
3. Prolonged antibiotics are not necessary.
4. Signs of obstruction should be evaluated to ensure the ileocecal valve was not involved in the resection if a partial cecectomy was performed.

Suggested Reading

1. Adrales, et al. Laparoscopic "Radical Appendectomy" is and effective alternative to endoscopic removal of cecal polyps. J Laparoendosc Adv Surg Tech. 2002;12(6):449–52.
2. Sakamoto, et al. Inramucosal adenocarcinoma of the appendix: how to find and treat. Endoscopy. 2003;35(9):785–7. https://doi.org/10.1055/s-2003-41577.
3. Song EM, Yang HJ, Lee HJ, et al. Endoscopic resection of cecal polyps involving the appendiceal orifice: a KASID multicenter study. Dig Dis Sci. 2017;62:3138. https://doi.org/10.1007/s10620-017-4760-2.

Part VIII

Medico-Legal Issues

Medico-Legal Issues in Minimally Invasive Colon and Rectal Surgery: A Primer

61

Daniel L. Feingold and Howard M. Ross

Clinical Scenario

A patient several days after sigmoid colectomy for diverticulitis develops an ileus and then starts having fevers and worsening abdominal pain. After appropriate evaluation, the patient is returned to the operating room where an anastomotic disruption is noted. An end colostomy is created. After waiting several months the patient undergoes an attempt at reversing the colostomy, but this is aborted due to severe pelvic fibrosis and scarring. A few months later, you are named in a lawsuit alleging malpractice that has resulted in the patient having a permanent colostomy.

Key Points

1. The threshold for acceptable clinical care from a legal perspective (i.e., the "standard of care") is generally defined as what a reasonable physician would do under similar circumstances. Whether a clinician met the standard of care in treating a patient is often a matter of opinion and, over the course of a lawsuit, the plaintiff's expert will opine that the defendant deviated from the standard of care and that the deviation caused harm to the plaintiff. A deviation from the standard that causes injury and damages roughly defines the terms medical "malpractice" or "negligence."
2. A critical concept in care is informed consent. A discussion between a fully trained, responsible surgeon and the patient must occur using terms the patient understands and should be documented. The discussion must include indications for the procedure, surgical and nonsurgical alternatives, and an explanation of reasonable expectations and risks. These discussions are usually based on the surgeon's education, training, experience, and practice and should include risks of particular importance to the specific patient undergoing surgery. For instance, particularly important risks may include things like stoma avoidance in a patient who was traumatized by a parent who "suffered" with a colostomy late in their life, preservation of function when dealing with anorectal disease, concerns for future fertility or sexual function, religious convictions that preclude accepting blood transfusions, specific concerns related to cosmesis, etc. It is also necessary to assess the degree of the patient's

D. L. Feingold (✉)
Division of Colorectal Surgery, Department of Surgery, Columbia University, New York, NY, USA
e-mail: df347@cumc.columbia.edu

H. M. Ross
Division of Colon and Rectal Surgery, Lewis Katz School of Medicine at Temple University and the Temple University Health System, Philadelphia, PA, USA

S. W. Lee et al. (eds.), *Colorectal Surgery Consultation*, https://doi.org/10.1007/978-3-030-11181-6_61

understanding and to give patients an opportunity to ask questions. A comprehensive discussion of the options, indications, risks, and benefits is crucial to avoid postoperative confusion and frustration. This is the opportunity to wean patients from the idea of certainty and to keep expectations realistic. In certain situations it may be appropriate to inquire about a family member or friend that the patient may rely on to help make medical decisions and invite the patient to return with that person or proxy at another visit.

3. Communicate, communicate, communicate! After surgery it is important to update the patient in terms of unique operative findings and their operative course. The concept of "full disclosure" does not provide clear guidance regarding what specifically needs to be discussed. For instance, is it important to tell a patient that an incidental serosal injury was made and repaired during the course of colectomy in a patient with adhesions from prior surgery? As a general rule of thumb, when in doubt disclose what you feel is relevant or significant information to the patient.
4. When to speak with a family member or proxy during the course of an operation depends on the circumstances of the operation. If a family member or another patient advocate is accessible, it may make sense to reach out when:
   (a) You discover significant unanticipated findings that influence the risk/benefit analysis for the surgery underway that may affect whether or not to proceed with the planned operation. Examples include:
      (i) Finding carcinomatosis during colectomy for what was thought to be non-metastatic colon cancer.
      (ii) Finding a second colon mass while exploring a patient for a known colon cancer.
      (iii) Finding unexpected inflamed bowel.
      (iv) When removing organs that were not included in the original operative plan, such as when the uterus needs to be removed in order to gain access to operate for rectal pathology.
      (v) In general, when another surgical service is consulted intraoperatively and joins the operation, it is reasonable to update the waiting family.
   (b) The patient deteriorates in the operating room. The main goal, of course, in this setting is to aggressively treat the patient and attempt to stabilize the situation. In the event the patient spirals to the point of imminent death, it may be helpful to personally update the waiting family so they understand the anesthesia and surgery teams taking care of their loved one are doing everything they can to try to save the patient but that you are concerned the patient may die. This usually brief interaction may help prepare the family for the news if the patient goes on to die despite your efforts.
5. The operative note transmits important information to future providers and is an opportunity for surgeons to explain their thought processes and intraoperative decision-making.
   (a) The operative note should typically be dictated by the attending surgeon as it is this surgeon who best understands the technical maneuvers that were performed in the operation.
   (b) The operative note should be dictated promptly after the operation.
   (c) Technical details should be specific. For instance, it is important to detail the identification of key structures like the left ureter in cases of sigmoid colon mobilization. Other relevant technical details should be included like the anatomic survey in an oncologic operation, the size of the circular stapler used in an anastomosis, that a leak test was performed for a pelvic anastomosis, the length of small bowel remaining after a

bowel resection in a patient with Crohn's disease, etc.

6. During the course of discovery as a lawsuit is progressing, plaintiff attorneys find a number of things helpful.
   (a) Missing or poor-quality documentation can make it difficult to support that the doctor met the standard of care. Many attorneys will expertly try to convince a jury that if an event or detail is not documented in the record, then it did not happen. The best way to protect yourself from this criticism is to adopt appropriate documentation habits as part of your daily practice. Clinicians often express frustration and dismay regarding the burden of documentation required in routine practice, but the reality is that quality documentation is important when defending yourself against a claim of malpractice. Good documentation may protect a surgeon from a lawsuit just as a seat belt does not improve a person's driving ability but protects the driver in the event of a crash. Similarly, long time intervals between the actual events and the date of the documentation can call into question the credibility of the record. It is in the clinician's best interest to complete operative notes and progress notes in a timely fashion and to "leave footprints."
   (b) Using poorly chosen words or phrases in the medical record. For instance, the term "missed enterotomy" can be construed as an admission of negligence due to closing a patient with an unaddressed enterotomy.
   (c) The medical chart is, in reality, a legal document; be smart. In general, it is important to avoid situations where clinicians criticize, contradict, or blame each other or the residents in the record. It is important to treat the record as a medico-legal document and not to use the patient chart as a medium to vent frustration or try to settle interpersonal conflicts between caregivers.
   (d) Diagnosis or treatment not reasonably supported by the medical records. For instance, performing a colectomy for alleged colonic inertia without first demonstrating an abnormal Sitz marker study.
   (e) Altering or supplementing medical records after the fact raises significant ethical and professional issues and is not condoned by jurors. The electronic footprint of modern-day electronic medical records provides plaintiffs with an easy way to analyze when the doctor entered specific information and gives the jury a roadmap as to how the record was altered. This conduct is discoverable and is generally not easily explained or justified.
   (f) Inconsistencies between the medical record and sworn testimony can lead to a believability issue. For instance, testifying that you got the phone call and came right in to the hospital to see the patient while the time stamp on the phone call was several hours before you actually came in.
   (g) Surgeons who do not take their deposition seriously or, worse, act inappropriately or unprofessionally during a videotaped deposition can hinder their defense as this testimony will certainly be shared with the jury at the trial.
7. During the course of discovery as a lawsuit is progressing, defense attorneys may find a number of things helpful.
   (a) Practice supported by the standard of care.
   (b) Honest, accurate, and timely documentation. Legal battles typically occur several years after the clinical events and appropriate documentation can facilitate an effective defense. It is better to have documented details of events or procedures rather than have to rely on what you testify as to your "usual and customary practice."
   (c) When defendant surgeons listen to and rely on their legal counsel. Often surgeon

defendants find themselves in the unfamiliar arena of a lawsuit with a sense of anger, embarrassment, loss of control, and anxiety from the uncertainty of the process. Relying on the experienced defense attorney representing you can help you navigate through the process and prepare you for your deposition testimony and, ultimately, your trial appearance.

8. Transparency, communication, and honesty are required. Many claims are filed after a poorly understood bad outcome, out of a sense of injustice or due to a "fundamental lapse in risk management." Speaking frequently, patiently, plainly, and humbly with patients and their families and listening to patients' concerns go a long way toward strengthening the physician-patient relationship and preventing suits. Talking with the family on a regular basis while their loved one is hospitalized helps prevent miscommunication and misunderstandings and keeps everyone on the same page.
9. In the event of an interaction with a dissatisfied patient or family member that you feel may possibly lead to litigation, contact your risk management team early on. These professionals are typically expert in all medicolegal facets and can provide invaluable advice.
10. Memories fade. Consider having a written document that details the events as you remember them in conjunction with your attorney in the event you are notified of pending litigation or have an untoward patient event.

Suggested Reading

1. Christiansen SM, Oetting TA. Delivering bad news and discussing surgical complications: real world advice for physicians everywhere. EyeRounds.org. Posted December 15, 2016. Available from: http://EyeRounds.org/tutorials/delivering-bad-news.htm.
2. Jena AB, Seabury S, Lakdawalla D, Chandra A. Malpractice risk according to physician specialty. N Engl J Med. 2011;365:629–36.
3. Raper SE, Rose D, Nepps ME, Drebin JA. Taking the initiative: risk-reduction strategies and decreased malpractice costs. J Am Coll Surg. 2017;225:612–21.

Index

S. W. Lee et al. (eds.), *Colorectal Surgery Consultation*,
https://doi.org/10.1007/978-3-030-11181-6

The manufacturer's authorised representative in the EU is Springer Nature Customer Service Centre GmbH, Europaplatz 3, 69115 Heidelberg, Germany. If you have any concerns regarding our products, please contact ProductSafety@springernature.com

Printed and bound by CPI Group (UK) Ltd, Croydon, CR0 4YY
30/09/2026
02225233-0019